D1614791

Needles, Herbs,
Gods, and Ghosts

LINDA L. BARNES

Needles, Herbs,
Gods, and Ghosts

*China, Healing,
and the West to 1848*

HARVARD UNIVERSITY PRESS

Cambridge, Massachusetts

London, England

2005

Library of Congress Cataloging-in-Publication Data

Barnes, Linda L.
Needles, herbs, gods, and ghosts : China, healing, and the West to 1848 / Linda L. Barnes.
p.   cm.
Includes bibliographical references and index.
ISBN 0-674-01872-9 (alk. paper)
1. Medicine, Chinese—Popular works.   I. Title: China, healing, and the West to 1848.
II. Title.

R601.B37 2005
610′.951—dc22   2005050278

To Devon

Acknowledgments

I thank my editor, Ann Downer-Hazell, whose steadfast faith and advocacy have accompanied this book's many phases. I also thank Sara Davis and Camille Smith, who carried it through production; Wendy Nelson, whose painstaking copyediting made everything better; and my anonymous reviewers for their invaluable comments and corrections. I am deeply grateful to Dr. S. T. Lee and the Lee Foundation of Singapore for their generous publication subsidy, without which I could not have illustrated the book so richly.

Extraordinary scholars have taught me, first among them Arthur Kleinman—a key mentor and one of my closest readers. John Carman remains the staunchest supporter of the integrative study of religion and healing. Ted Kaptchuk's historical eye provided valuable insights. Tu Wei-ming taught me about Chinese religions. TJ Hinrichs provided much of what I know about the history of Chinese medicine.

I thank an earlier writing group that included TJ Hinrichs, Bridie Andrews, Eric Jacobson, and Cathy Kerr. I also thank my project manager, Justine de Marrais, for all her backup support.

Jack Eckert of the Boston Medical Library in the Francis A. Countway Library and Susan Halpert and Elizabeth Falsey of Houghton Library have patiently borne with my endless requests for sources. Joanne Bloom Toplyn at Harvard's Fine Arts Library located images for which I often had only concepts or partial names. I thank them all.

Kimberley Patton, my oldest and dearest friend, weathered with me the years and life circumstances that surrounded this work. Maribeth Kaptchuk, Joan Martin, Emilie Townes, Susan Sered, Jayne Guberman, Jack Maypole, Greg Plotnikoff, and Ellen Highfield provided staunch friendship and deepened the scope of my critical thinking. Howard Bauchner, Ben Siegel, and Kathi Kemper have been worthy colleagues, friends, and mentors.

I thank my father, Louis B. (By) Barnes; my mother, Florence Maddix; my stepfather, Forrest Maddix (who kindly proofed the text for me); and my brother, Ted Barnes. Each nurtured the self who could write this book. Finally, I thank my husband, Devon Thibeault. He met me as I was completing my dissertation, hung in when I decided to dismantle it and start over to write this book, and married me in the midst of everything. He has endured my working on it over most weekends and vacations for years. He has been my heart's companion.

Contents

Illustrations

Needles, Herbs,
Gods, and Ghosts

Introduction

The history of Western knowledge about the Chinese and their healing practices, and in some cases the adoption of such practices, dates
back to the thirteenth century. It involves the initial investigations of
China by European countries, subsequent colonialism and diaspora,
and eventually the United States. This book addresses Western representations that contributed to how the Chinese and their healing traditions were imagined across these different periods and settings. I use
the term *imagined* deliberately. In 1714 Scottish doctor John Bell observed: "In the cliffs of the rocks you see little scattered cottages, with
spots of cultivated ground, much resembling those romantick figures
of landskips which are painted on the China-ware and other manufactures of this country. These are accounted fanciful by most Europeans,
but are really natural" (Bell [1763]1965, 1:334). Years later, historian
Hugh Honour (1961) drew similar connections between material culture and the formation of impressions: "The willow-pattern plates off
which we ate each day afforded a vivid glimpse of the Chinese landscape . . . Chinese costumes were likewise familiar to me for I, like
other children, occasionally went to fancy-dress parties dressed as a
mandarin—complete with embroidered silk suit, straw slippers, a pig-
tail hanging from the back of my head and drooping moustaches
gummed to my upper lip . . . And even when, years later, I discovered
that they had all been made in Europe, the original impression remained at the back of my mind" (1–2). Memory, history, and imagination converged in representations of the Chinese and their healing

practices. Such perceptions have served as lenses through which later viewers approach related subjects.

One can simultaneously view a phenomenon in multiple ways, just like one can see the drawing of a goblet as two faces staring at each other. I have, accordingly, composed this study to be read from different perspectives. The first perspective focuses on the *racializing* of the Chinese in the context of emerging Western categories of what I am calling humankinds. The second focuses on how those grounded in Christian traditions engaged in a process we might awkwardly call the *religionizing* of the Chinese. The third addresses the interaction between traditions of healing, with attention to how Western observers viewed and reported on Chinese traditions. This perspective includes the *medicalizing* of the Chinese.

This book is not a history of Chinese medicine (for overviews of that history, see Hinrichs 1998; Sivin 1998, 1988; and Hart 1999). It is instead a history of cross-cultural interactions, involving Western translations and interpretations, in the mode of historian Jonathan Spence (1998). The writers from whom I draw were themselves involved in racializing, religionizing, and medicalizing the Chinese. Their reports regularly contained aspects of all three. Through a focus on Chinese healing traditions, broadly defined, I hope to illuminate how these three dynamics converged, and what they produced.

Racializing Chineseness

Changing Western understandings of what it meant to be Chinese informed how Westerners perceived, described, and received Chinese healing practices. Meanings assigned to "Chineseness" converged with unfolding formulations of race and racial identities, with race configured as a Manichaean opposition between black and white poles of a spectrum, along which "Others"—including the Chinese—were positioned. As constructions of blackness and whiteness solidified, perniciously normative understandings of racial identity, and of whiteness in particular, permeated meanings of "European" and "American." To understand how this happened requires detecting points along the way when key typologies coalesced, providing subtexts to some responses to Chinese healing.

Western perceptions of the Chinese were not uniform. John James

Clarke (1997) suggests that Orientalism consisted of "a wider range of attitudes, both dark and light . . . [in which] the West has endeavored to integrate Eastern thought into its own intellectual concerns in a manner which, on the face of it, cannot be fully understood in terms of 'power' and 'domination'" (8–9). Although the larger history is set squarely within Western imperialist expansion, observers were not unaffected or unmoved by what they witnessed and experienced. I illustrate some of the complexities of these responses with examples of how the West appropriated certain cultural forms, remaking them in its own image, while being changed in the process.

Religionizing the Chinese

The second perspective involves the part played by Western and Chinese religions. On the Western side, there were the tributaries of the Christian river, the dam-ups between them—particularly conflicts between Roman Catholics and Protestants—and spillovers into representations of Chinese practices. Christian theology and Christianity as a religious system, and the influence of both on methods of studying religion, generated attempts to identify distinct religious and doctrinal systems in China. Chinese religion was frequently represented as consisting of three traditions, or teachings—Confucianism, Daoism, and Buddhism. This formulation omitted much: "Such common rituals as offering incense to the ancestors, conducting funerals, exorcising ghosts, and consulting fortunetellers; belief in the patterned interaction between light and dark forces or in the ruler's influence on the natural world; the tendency to construe gods as government officials; the preference for balancing tranquility and movement—all belong as much to none of the three traditions as they do to one or three" (Teiser 1996, 21). Lawrence Thompson (1975) suggests that the confluence of these religious worldviews and practices represents a manifestation of Chinese culture. There was no separate Chinese term for "religion" until outsiders from the West insisted on one. In China, family dynamics, social networks, and political structures were all permeated by religious ways of seeing, and being in, the world—what C. K. Yang (1961) refers to as "diffused religion" (295). With these fluid attempts at definition in mind, I have included practices that might not seem relevant to readers familiar with Western concepts of "religion."

My task is to address the connection of these practices within this broader conceptualization.

The degree to which matters of healing permeate the religious, and vice versa, is an often-overlooked dimension in religious studies. In China, healing practices grew from the same roots and paradigms as other versions of Chinese religiosity. Even acupuncture and herbal medicine—ostensibly secular—were grounded in concepts of the body as a microcosm, a miniature version of a cosmos, composed of the same vital psychophysical stuff called *qi* (pronounced "chee"). The world, indeed the cosmos, constituted a sacred network, wherein the "ten thousand things"—all of reality—comprised the triad of Heaven, Earth, and Human Being, all engaged in an ongoing dynamic relationship of co-creation. Thus, the term *secular* calls for considerable caution.

I refer to "Chinese healing practices," rather than "medicine," to encompass the range of strategies developed by the Chinese in the pursuit of healing. Given the nature of Chinese religion, this notion of "healing practices" draws in not only acupuncture and herbs, but also therapeutic measures—such as burning paper houses and furniture to send them via their smoke to the *yin* world of the dead, and aligning graves according to the tenets of geomancy. It includes affliction caused by angry ancestors and their ghosts, and imbalances in a person's *qi*. It encompasses diagnostic measures like divination, pulse reading, and a spirit medium's trance. It spans longevity practices, pilgrimages, meritorious deeds to offset bad karma, and petitions to local gods.

Medicalizing the Chinese

I have avoided using the term *medicine* in connection with this broad range of Chinese practices. There is a corresponding term (*yi*), but my intent is to explore the wider history of different understandings of healing, within which particular elite traditions were referred to as "medicine." Historian Nancy Siraisi (1990) suggests, "Attitudes, beliefs, and doctrines embedded in medicine may illuminate fundamental cultural assumptions about the human body, illness and wellness, the characteristics and relations of the sexes, and the stages of human life from infancy to old age" (ix–x). Similar claims can be made about

Western understandings of "medicine" as these informed perceptions of the Chinese and their practices. Embedded cultural codes, operative on both sides, structured encounters between these cultural worlds. Such codes governed European attempts to translate and interpret Chinese typologies.

Much confusion grew out of differences in the two cultures' concepts of "person." Did a person consist of body, mind, and soul, or *jing, qi,* and *shen?* Over the course of the narrative, I will discuss meanings assigned to these terms. Suffice it to say here that such differences intruded when Western observers struggled to understand Chinese readings of the body, represented in diagrams that looked nothing like Western anatomical drawings.

Responses to Chinese healing were repeatedly shaped by Western anatomical models and by a dynamic tradition of vitalism. Western observers routinely misunderstood the practices they witnessed, even when reporting them with considerable accuracy. Their translations introduced distortions and false equations. They selectively appropriated pieces of Chinese practice, and then rewrote them. It is useful to ask: Why these particular misunderstandings?

Just as the Chinese were racialized, they were also gradually *medicalized,* particularly as Western physicians increasingly reported on their encounters with Chinese bodies. One aspect of this process involved the insertion of the Chinese into constructions of the monstrous and the pathological. The Chinese also had a history of "recording the strange," in both dynastic histories and medical cases (see Grant 1998, 45). In Western practice, however, what Larissa Heinrich (1999) has called "the Sick Man of Asia" emerged, in a convergence of race and pathology, represented as needing a cure from the West.

The Order of Things

To weave these threads together, I have divided the book into five time periods. This division is admittedly Eurocentric, precisely because this is a study of Western perceptions and responses, but I do not take Western time frames as normative. Chapter 1 begins with the period corresponding to the dispatching of Christian emissaries to investigate potential consequences for Europe from thirteenth-century Mongol expansion. These religious delegates, along with several other reporters, produced some of the earliest narratives with details about Chinese healing. Chapter 2 begins in 1492, with European expeditions to Asia and the Americas, and continues until 1659. Foreign observers sent detailed reports to Europe, including comments about Chinese approaches to healing.

The same dynamic continued during the period addressed in Chapter 3 (1660–1736), with two major differences. First, this period saw a new phenomenon—the production by Western authors of detailed studies of Chinese pulse theory, acupuncture, and moxibustion. Second, growing numbers of writers in Europe who had never gone to China wrote about Chinese practices, based on sources sent by firsthand observers. Chapter 3 ends with one of the great compendia of China reports, Fr. Jean-Baptiste Du Halde's *Déscription géographique, historique, chronologique, politique, et physique de l'empire de la Chine et de la Tartarie chinoise* (1735), translated as *The General History of China* (1736). It included discussions of many dimensions of Chinese healing.

Chapter 4 addresses the period 1737 through 1804, closing with the publication of John Barrow's *Travels in China*—one of the last major sources resulting from the embassy of Britain's Lord Macartney. The broader context of an intensified European chinoiserie—a fascination with things Chinese—served as a setting for new discussions of Chinese practices. The United States was no longer required to trade with the Far East through the British East India Company, and officially entered the China trade, producing some of the first reports by American observers. Chapter 5 examines representations of Chinese healing generated in Europe and the United States between 1805 and 1848—the year before the beginning of major Chinese immigration to the United States and other parts of the world.

Closing—and Opening—Thoughts

Earlier histories have provided frames of reference for this book. Works like those by Joseph Needham and Lu Gwei-Djen (*Celestial Lancets*, Lu and Needham 1980, comes to mind) provide little sense that Western countries were actively engaged in making sense of the Chinese as a people, or that descriptions of healing practices were only one thread in a larger fabric. Although I deeply admire the contributions of Needham and his colleagues, in this book I attempt to address that lack.

I do not conceptualize religions, medicines, or forms of healing as single, coherent systems, whether in China, Europe, or the United States. Nor were the Chinese, European, or American contexts static frames within which these systems emerged. The model I use involves interacting forms of pluralism, influencing each other to varying degrees, changing over time, and responding to new, mutually influenced constellations of ideas and practices. Moreover, I have given these Western observations of Chinese healing practices a far more systematic presentation than was available at their time. Beyond their explicit citations of earlier works, we cannot always be certain what knowledge specific individuals had of the particular sources I have used, although sometimes one can speculate with reasonable certainty. In short, Western representations of Chinese healing practices were a matter, not of an unbroken dialogue, but of intermittent contacts, flurries of representation, periods of indifference, and multiple forms of incomprehension.

Nevertheless, tropes recurred in response to specific Chinese practices. Writers sometimes knowingly referred back to earlier reports and entered China with these tropes in mind. In such cases, I have tried to identify and understand cultural factors that shaped the different responses, and to track not only similarities but also critical differences. This book is an inquiry into a series of changing configurations, whose unfolding has captivated my own imagination for these past twenty-five years.

First Impressions:
Until 1491

Early European impressions of the Chinese, and of healing in China, involved not only the Chinese but also the Mongols, founders of the Yuan dynasty (1279–1368). These impressions merged in Western imaginations. As late as the nineteenth century, those opposed to Chinese immigration to the United States fanned fears of the "Mongol hordes." It was the height of irony that a people whom the Chinese once despised proved the source of images with which they themselves would be imagined.

Cultural exchange between China and the West began at least as early as the second century BCE, as Roman traders traveled the Silk Road into northern China. In 115 BCE, Chinese emperor Han Wudi (r. 147–87 BCE) sent an envoy west. Much later the Tang dynasty (618–907) favored open trade, leading to commerce with Italy and the entry of Nestorian Christianity and Islam.[1] Still, by the twelfth century, European knowledge of China had faded to near oblivion.

In 1211, led by Temüjin (1163?–1227)—styled "Chinggis Khan" (Universal Khan)—the Mongols invaded northern China, then headed west, attacking the eastern Seljuq empire and Russian and Turkish armies in the Crimea. Chinggis was reported to be pitiless toward those who resisted. When his son-in-law was killed at Nishapur, the town was laid waste "in such a manner that . . . not even cats and dogs should be left alive" (Boyle 1969–1970, 9). Chinggis's death in 1227 resulted in his empire's division into four parts. His third son, Ögedai (d. 1241), conquered northern China by 1234 and, two years later, much of Sichuan.

Subsequent conquests encompassed western Persia, Asia Minor,

Russian principalities, Poland, and Hungary. Chronicler Matthew Paris (1200–1259) recorded that in 1240, "a detestable nation of Satan . . . broke loose from its mountain-environed home, and . . . poured forth like devils from the Tartarus, so that they are rightly called 'Tartars' or 'Tartarians'" (Boyle 1969–1970, 11). "Cathay," as China was known in Europe, derived from "Khitan," a tribe conquered by the Mongols. Distinctions between Mongols, Khitans or Cathayans, and Chinese were rarely clear to Europeans. Cathay was thus long associated with the Khan and the Mongols, and both of these, with the Chinese.

Observers and Pseudo-Observers

In 1245 Pope Innocent IV dispatched Franciscan Giovanni de Plano Carpini (1182?–1252) to carry two bulls to Chinggis's grandson Güyük Khan (r. 1246–1248). Giovanni, sixty-five, was so corpulent that he required a donkey to travel any distance. His arrival coincided with the installation of Güyük as Khan. Observing that the Mongols were planning another Western campaign, Giovanni refused to take envoys back with him, to avoid revealing Europe's weaknesses. He reached Avignon in 1247, later writing *The Journey of Friar Giovanni of Plano de Carpini to the Court of Güyük Khan*. Widely read, its popularity grew after Vincent de Beauvais (d. 1264) incorporated it into his encyclopedic *Speculum historiale*, whose 3,793 chapters covered world history through 1250.[2]

Güyük Khan was followed by his cousin Möngke (r. 1251–1259). Shortly after Giovanni's return, a messenger informed French king Louis IX that the mother of Möngke Khan was Christian, making Möngke friendly to the faith. Louis concocted the idea of allying with the Mongols to attack the Saracens, and in 1253 he dispatched Franciscan friar William of Rubruck—Willem van Ruysbroeck—also known as Rubriquis (ca. 1215–ca. 1270), with the offer. William and two companions reached Karakorum, the seat of Möngke's power, where he encountered travelers from throughout the world known to Europe. Returning to his convent at Acre in 1255, William's *Journal of Friar William of Rubruck, 1253–1255* remained largely unknown. However, Franciscan Roger Bacon (1214–1294)—physician and alchemist—incorporated details into the geographical section of his own *Opus majus* (ca. 1262). Through Bacon, English readers like explorer Richard Hakluyt and Protestant minister Samuel Purchas later encountered the friar's account, which they republished and popularized.

Ögedai's son Qubilai (r. 1260–1294) founded the Yuan dynasty in 1279. When Qubilai moved his capital to Beijing—known to Europeans as Cambaluc (Turkish *Khan-balik,* "city of the Khan")—so many missionaries, merchants, diplomats, and other travelers journeyed East that Francesco Balducci Pegolotti's *La pratica della mercatura* ([1340]1936) detailed the route. In Yangzhou lies the tombstone of Katerina Ilioni (d. 1342), daughter of Domenico Ilioni, from a Venetian merchant family.

In 1265 Qubilai welcomed merchants Niccolò and Matteo Polo—a scene represented by Western artists as a European monarch welcoming missionaries. Niccolò later sent his son Marco to China, where he arrived in 1275 (see Figure 1). Marco Polo (1254–1323) claimed to have spent seventeen years in China, learning Mongolian and Chinese. *Les récits de Marco Polo* (The Travels of Marco Polo) was supposedly dictated in 1298, while Polo was a prisoner of war in Genoa, to fellow

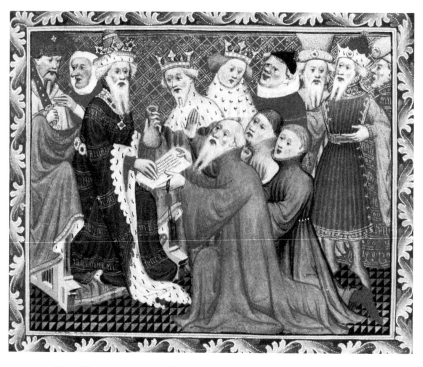

Figure 1. The Khan presents golden tablets to Marco, Niccolò, and Matteo Polo. *Les livres du Graunt Caam,* ca. 1400. (MS Bodl.264 fol.220.) Courtesy of the Bodleian Library, Oxford University.

prisoner and romance author Rusticello of Pisa.[3] Filled with Arthurian romance-genre material, entire passages may derive from Rusticello's other work, making it unclear where Polo's own narrative began and left off—or whether he went to China at all (Spence 1998). Nevertheless, the book achieved international renown.

Latin Christian missionaries went to China, among them Italian Franciscan Odoric of Pordenone (1286?–1331). Odoric reached Beijing in 1325 accompanied by James of Hibernia, the only Irishman known to have gone to China during this period. Returning to Europe in 1330, Odoric later described attending court banquets: "For we Minor Friars have a place of abode appointed out for us in the emperor's court, and are enjoined to go and bestow our blessing on him" (Komroff 1928, 239). Odoric traveled throughout China, producing a report reveling in superlatives—more ships in Canton's harbor than in "all Italy"; Hangzhou, the "greatest city in the whole world"; the Khan's golden chariot drawn by four elephants *and* four horses (Steiner 1979, 39).

As popular as Polo's and Odoric's books were, *The Voiage and Travayle of Sir John Maundeville Knight* (ca. 1371; Maundeville 1887) surpassed them both and had been translated into at least nine languages by the end of the century. "Maundeville," represented as a knight and a physician, never existed; the real author might have been a French romance writer. Plundering Giovanni, Odoric, and others, "Maundeville" thrilled readers with giants, men whose heads grew beneath their shoulders, and supposedly authentic details about China. Nor was there occasion to challenge his account as, shortly after its publication, China became increasingly closed to outsiders.

Locating the East in Space, Time, and Humankinds

Europeans did not encounter new peoples in an intellectual vacuum. Existing classifications relating space, time, and humankinds influenced what they saw. Christian geography had long interpreted the East as the site of paradise. Medieval maps located divine power in the East, at the top of the map where God sat enthroned. Jerusalem, sacred center of the world, lay in the middle. The "T-O map" assigned the upper half of the globe to Asia, dividing the bottom half with the Mediterranean, represented as a vertical line between Europe and Africa. The divisions corresponded to the sons of Noah—Shem, Ham, and Japheth—from whom "the whole world branched out" (Genesis

9:19). Geographers assigned Asia to Shem, seen as the eldest. They gave Africa to Ham and Europe to Japheth, producing the "Noachide" map that inserted Eastern peoples into Christian constructions of sacred space and history.

The East had also long been associated with marvels and monsters. Spatial distance from Jerusalem equaled distance from holiness. Christian mapmakers positioned Jews and Muslims nearer to the margins of maps, and the "monstrous" races even farther out. The Chinese thus existed ambiguously in the East, home of God *and* monsters. Defining the Mongols as Shem's descendants made them human, even as their brutal campaigns linked them with Christian villains.

Different authors modified the Noachide myth accordingly. Some claimed that the Khan descended from Ham. One version of the Maundeville manuscript said: "I will tell you why he is called the great Khan . . . Ham for his cruelty took the best part, which is called Asia . . . and from Ham's lineage came the Saracens and the various men who dwell on the islands around India" (Friedman 1981, 103). Conflating "Ham" with "Khan" linked Mongols with Saracens, viewed as enemies of Christendom. Other writers traced the Mongols to Ishmael, rejected son of Abraham. The logic of such identifications rested on metaphors for groups construed as having rejected, and been rejected by, God.

Paris had identified the Mongols as "Tartars," a corruption of *Tatar*. The word became associated with Tartarus, or Hell, locating Mongols among Satan's ranks. The phrase *Mongol hordes* entered western languages, suggesting countless demonic warriors. Although *horde* derived from *ordu* (Turkish for "camp"), this distortion lodged itself in European collective memory. It then took little to identify the Khan with the Antichrist, who was expected to conquer the world, march to Jerusalem, and lay his crown on Golgotha. One could also look to the monstrous biblical tribes Gog and Magog, whom Alexander the Great was said to have confined behind a great brass gate in mountains to the East. (*Magog* and *Mongol* sounded enough alike for some to equate the two.) Their escape would herald the end of the world.

Of Humankinds

Like Aristotle, medieval mapmakers assumed that environments influenced human appearance and character, while not always agreeing

on the specifics. Ethiopians, or "Aithiopes"—"burnt faces"—and Indians were routinely confused with one another. *Ham,* sometimes
spelled *Cham,* conflated *Cain* with *Ham* (as well as with *Khan*), based
on shared negative associations and similar sounds. Yet Ham's descendant Nimrod—like Ham—was also said to have fathered African
peoples, condemned to serve the descendants of the other two brothers due to Ham's having witnessed Noah drunk and unclothed. This
stigma appeared in both Christian and Muslim sources, providing a
rationale for enslaving Africans. The shared stigma did not prevent
Christians from depicting Muslims as black and, in some cases, with
dogs' heads. Abraham's son Ishmael was identified with Saracens and
Muslims, and also depicted as black. Color polarities merged with
moral and religious polarities, particularly regarding "enemies" of Christendom whose "blackness" could only be made pure (white) through
baptism.

Some authors portrayed Mongols as cannibals. Paris wrote, "They
are inhuman and beastly, rather monsters than men, thirsting for and
drinking blood, tearing and devouring the flesh of dogs and men"
(Komroff 1928, xiii; see Figure 2). Giovanni commented, "For they eat
dogs, wolves, foxes and horses and, when driven by necessity, they feed

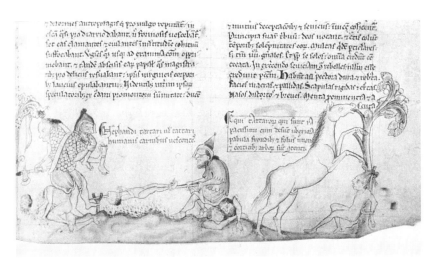

Figure 2. Mongol cannibalism. Matthew Paris, *Chronica Major,* 13th century.
(CCC MS 16, ff 166r.) Courtesy of the Masters and Fellows of Corpus
Christi College, University of Cambridge.

on human flesh" (Guzman 1991, 34). Such narratives borrowed from older texts representing northern barbarians as eating "things polluted and base, dogs, mice, serpents, the flesh of corpses, yea unborn embryos as well as their own dead" (45). Imputed cannibalism symbolized extremes in difference, or nonhumanness.

Actual encounters with Mongols focused on physical differences. Giovanni wrote: "In appearance the Tartars are quite different from all other men . . . their eyes are little and their eyelids raised up to the eyebrows . . . Hardly any of them grow beards, although some have a little hair on the upper lip and chin and this they do not trim. On the top of the head they have a tonsure like clerics . . . the rest of their hair they allow to grow like a woman, and they make it into two braids which they bind, one behind each ear. They also have small feet" (Dawson 1955, 6–7). The eyes and beards of Mongol and Chinese men became common tropes. William of Rubruck wrote, "As is general with all those eastern people, their eyes are very narrow" (Yule 1914, 1:59). The *Maundeville* author added, "They have small eyen as little birdes" (Maundeville 1887, 175). The description contained gender ambiguities. The Mongols were nearly beardless, had tonsured hair like clerics (celibate men), and wore the rest long, like women. They had small feet. The particulars converged in a feminized figure, whose differences could not be construed as truly masculine. Mongol warriors might or might not be real men, given their "feminine" traits, geographic marginality, and "monstrous" brutality.

Giovanni praised Mongol women's chastity and honesty. Likewise, he admired the obedience and honesty of the Mongols toward their superiors, while finding their eating and drinking habits dirty. He reserved his strongest criticism for interactions with outsiders: "At first indeed they are smooth-tongued, but in the end they sting like a scorpion . . . Any evil they intend to do to others they conceal in a wonderful way so that the latter can take no precautions nor devise anything to offset their cunning" (Dawson 1955, 16). The *Maundeville* author reiterated the assessment: "They are commonly false for they holde not their promise" (Maundeville 1887, 175). The discrepancy between honesty toward one's own and dishonesty toward others may have been exaggerated; it may also have indicated a situational ethos among the Mongols.

A Crueler Traffic

By the fourteenth century, European slave trafficking flourished. Christians fell prey to Muslim raids, enslavement, and ransom bargaining, while Genoese merchants purchased Muslim slaves in North Africa (Verlinden 1995). Not only were enslaved Africans transported to Italy and in some cases to China (Irwin 1977); Russians, Circassians, Scyths, Hungarians, Bulgarians, and Greeks were sold in Spanish and Italian markets. Venetian merchants provided the Mongols with banking services and collaborated with them in the slave trade.

Tartars were brought from Middle Eastern markets and sold in Spain and Italy. Of 357 persons sold in Florence between 1366 and 1397, 274 were "Tatars" (Phillips 1985). One child was recorded as being of Chinese descent, although her name was Tartar. Ledgers from 1360 include a fifteen-year-old Tartar girl, "Catais"—a name regularly given captives along the road from Cathay. In 1441, Father Benedetto delle Croci of Venice paid Matteo di Settimo of Treviso with a fifteen-year-old Tartar boy. Alessandra Strozzi advised her son Filippo to choose a Tartar slave, who would be "sturdy and suited to hard work" (Origo 1955, 361). Marco Polo's will released "Peter the Tartar" from bondage. Tartar girls and women were forced into concubinage, reconfiguring Tuscan ancestries (Phillips 1994). It is not clear how many of these Tartars were Chinese or even Mongol. Many slaves in Venice were called "Tartars" (Spence 1998). Still, local paintings showed figures with Asian features, like some of the spectators depicted in the fourteenth-century *Martirio di frati francescani a Thanah* (The Martyrdom of the Franciscan Brothers at Thanah) in the Basilica of San Francesco at Siena, suggesting some encounter (see Figure 3).

Multiple tropes pertaining to nature and appearance were initially applied to Mongols but—with boundaries between Mongol and Chinese blurred by distance and ignorance—often spilled over onto the Chinese. Observers compared European practices with those of different Asian peoples. When European and Asian practices looked the same, observers assumed they *were* the same, regardless of underlying differences. The absence of a European practice in Mongol or Chinese culture was often construed as a deficit. European observers regarded as normative not only their version of humankind but also their religion and medicine. Core differences between these world-

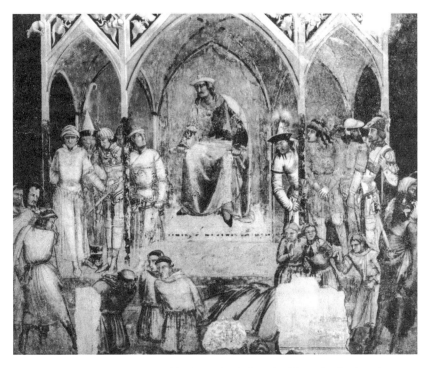

Figure 3. Franciscans martyred before the Sultan in Thanah. Ambrosio Lorenzetti, Basilica of San Francesco, Siena, 14th century. Courtesy of Historic Photographs, Fine Arts Library, Harvard College Library.

views and those of the Mongols and Chinese would lay the foundations for centuries of misunderstanding.

Their Physicians Know a Great Deal

European travelers encountered Mongol and Chinese healing traditions in light of their own concepts of medicine, as in the list of master physicians given by Geoffrey Chaucer (d. 1400) in *Canterbury Tales* (1387–1400):

> With us ther was a Doctour of Phisyk
> In al this world ne was ther noon him lyk
> To speke of phisik and of surgerye . . .
> Wel knew he the olde Esculapius,
> And Deyscorides, and eek Rufus,

Olde Ypocras, Haly, and Galyen,
Serapioun, Razis, and Avycen
Averrois, Damascien, and Constantyn,
Bernard, and Gatisden, and Gilbertyn (Prol., lines 413–415, 431–436)[4]

One can reasonably speculate that William of Rubruck held analogous preconceptions about medicine when he wrote: "Their physicians know a great deal about the power of herbs and diagnose very cleverly from the pulse; on the other hand, they do not use urinals nor know anything about urine; I saw this myself, for there were many of them in Karakorum" (Dawson 1955, 144). But what might his frame of reference been?

In Europe, Claudius Galen (ca. 129–ca. 216) continued to influence the Greek intellectual world of Alexandria, Constantinople, and Syria. Through Arabic translations, Al-Kindi (d. 873?), Isaac Israeli (832?–932?), Rhazes (al-Razi, 865?–925?), Avicenna (Ibn Sina, 980–1037), Averroes (Ibn Rushd, 1126–1198), and Moses Maimonides (1135–1204) drew on Aristotle for their philosophy and Hippocrates and Galen for their medicine, producing texts that became foundational for later generations. For example, Hunayn ibn Ishaq, or Johannitius (d. 873), an Iraqi Christian, composed the treatise later given the Latin title *Isagoge*. Arabic pharmacology filtered through Dioscorides, author of a first-century *materia medica*. Stationed with Roman legionaries in the Near East, Dioscorides encountered previously unknown herbs, some entering through international trade. Other Arabic works included medicinals from Southeast Asia, India, Africa, and China (Conrad 1995). Constantinus the African (ca. 1020–1087), a Tunisian Christian monk in southern Italy, translated Galen, the *Isagoge,* and Arabic medical treatises into Latin. At the monastery in Salerno, medical teaching grounded in such texts began around 1100. Consequently, Arabic medicine reconfigured European medicine, even during the Crusades, indirectly providing limited Chinese medical knowledge.

Of Fire, Air, Earth, and Water

Two key influences informed Western encounters with Chinese approaches to healing. The first was Galen's humoral theory, the second, anatomical dissection. Both would structure Western understandings of Chinese healing from the thirteenth throughout the mid-nineteenth century. Although the specifics will become fully clear only over the course of the larger narrative, some particulars function as recurring motifs.

The theory of humors presumed that all things consisted of core principles, called *elements*—fire, air, earth, and water. Elements themselves were not matter. Rather, they joined with matter to constitute four *qualities*—heat, cold, dryness, and moisture. Everything one consumed consisted of these elements. When digested, they became *fluids* called "humors"—blood, phlegm, yellow bile, or black bile, corresponding to fire, air, earth, and water. The veins contained a combination of humors but, because the humor "blood" predominated, its name was given to the mix as a whole.

Each of the main organs had a humoral *complexion,* as did a person's general system. Each complexion corresponded to a *temperament*—blood to "sanguine," phlegm to "phlegmatic," yellow bile to "choleric," and black bile to "melancholic." One's complexion and temperament simultaneously described a physiological type and a psychological profile. Health involved the equilibrium of the humors appropriate to a given person's complexion; disease lay in their imbalance, or improper mixture. Thirteenth-century English physician Gilbertus Anglicus therefore argued in his *Compendium medicinae* (ca. 1240) that one could classify all diseases as hot, cold, moist, or dry, as diagnosed by touch and observation (Getz 1991). To restore balance appropriate to a particular system, physicians attended to all the body's fluids, including excreta. They determined the nature of an excess, and then purged or offset it. Excessive heat—excess blood—required bloodletting, for example; a hot headache needed cooling therapies, the avoidance of "too much thinking, staying awake, bathing, and sexual excitement" (Getz 1991, xx). Medicines, dietary recommendations, and behavioral modifications corresponded to this strategy of opposites.

Like Aristotle, Galen had sought to understand the force that generated and sustained life—the "vital" or life (*vita*)-giving virtue. This "virtue" manifested through the beating of the heart, rhythms of the pulses, and breathing. Galen called it *pneuma* (Latin, *spiritus*). *Pneuma / spiritus* was inborn, its essence an innate heat. Although inborn, *pneuma/spiritus* required nurturing, deriving sustenance from "digesting" air, first in the lungs, and then in the heart and arteries, and being nourished by a combination of respiration and blood. The thoracic cavity and arteries carried a mixture of blood and *pneuma* to the rest of the body, with the heart as the central agent. The organs involved, because they conveyed *pneuma/spiritus,* were sometimes referred to as "spiritual members" (Temkin 1973). As *pneuma/spiritus* moved through the body, it transmuted into *animal spirits.* "Animal" referred not to the body's fleshly aspects, but to *anima,* or soul (making the later term *animal soul* technically redundant). Each animal spirit played a part in different aspects of cognition, motion, and sensation. Thus, the eye contained certain animal spirits, enabling it to see (Siraisi 1990). The animal soul also had a nutritive or "vegetative" aspect, facilitating nutrition, growth, and reproduction.

Christian authorities sometimes suspected Galen of denying the soul's immortality, an issue they resolved by differentiating between the immortal soul bestowed by God and the animal soul. The latter was intrinsic to *pneuma/spiritus,* the innate principle of life. Both animated the body with vital heat and life force. This humoral model, with its version of vitalism and theories of balance and imbalance, would repeatedly shape and distort how Western observers encountered Chinese theories of vitalism, especially concepts like *qi, yang,* and *yin.*

Of Criminals and Cadavers

A second Western construction of the body would also repeatedly obstruct an understanding of Chinese theory. The body, in Greek-descended medicine, was a structure animated and nourished by *pneuma/spiritus.* Knowing the body required knowing its structure and the workings of its parts. When the parts' ability to function suffered, the knowledge of structures enabled one to discern which part was affected, and how and why (Kuriyama 1999). If the deepest understanding of such relationships was divine, studying the body approximated divine knowledge. One studied the body through dissection.

Animal dissection entered Salerno's curriculum around 1120. By 1250 forensic autopsy was relatively common in Italy, France, and Germany. Later in the century, such autopsies entered medical education. The word *anatomy* came to mean cadaver dissection. Local authorities provided the corpses of executed criminals, whose dismemberment resembled executions. Public dissections occurred in churches and halls, usually in winter to delay decomposition. Anatomy texts instructed viewers about the order of operation, beginning with parts likely to rot quickly and describing what viewers should expect to see.

Cadaver dissection became part of medical education only after the death of William of Rubruck (ca. 1270) and a few years before Friar Odoric set out on his missionary journey. But within William's lifetime, Galenic medicine—particularly humoral theory and animal dissection—was well established. This combination may have provided William's frame of reference when observing Karakorum's physicians. Yet even had he known more about dissection, he would have encountered little corresponding practice among the Mongols. Although Chinese physicians enjoyed favor in Karakorum, where multiple medical traditions coexisted, the last recorded dissection had occurred during the Song dynasty (960–1127). The absence of a tradition of dissection and related understandings of anatomy would become a persisting bone of contention in the assessment of Chinese practices.

Their Physicians Know a Great Deal about the Power of Herbs

William does not tell us whether the physicians he saw were Mongol or Chinese, but Chinese physicians were active in both Karakorum and Beijing. Qubilai appointed as medical overseer of the empire a West Asian physician, Isaac (Aixie), who had served Güyük as astrologer and physician at Karakorum (Olschki 1960). Such doctors introduced Chinese medical theory into Mongol settings. By the early 1300s there existed a Chinese-style Office of the Chief Physician, responsible for preparing medicines for the emperor, along with other medical duties (Buell and Anderson 2000).[5]

The *Huangdi neijing* (Inner Classic of the Yellow Emperor) and the *Nanjing* (Classic of Difficult [Topics]) were two key sources for Chinese physicians. The *Neijing* consisted of two parts—the *Suwen* (Basic Questions), which was primarily theoretical, and the *Lingshu* (Divine Pivot), primarily therapeutic with a focus on acupuncture. Edited during the first century BCE (or possibly during the previous century), its contents date from as much as six hundred years earlier and were revised over the centuries (see Unschuld 2003; Harper 1998; Yamada

1979). The *Nanjing* was also compiled during the first and second centuries BCE, gathering "all aspects of theoretical and practical health care perceivable within the confines of the yinyang and Five Phases doctrines, as defined by the original medicine of systematic correspondences" (Unschuld 1986b, 4).

The *Neijing* and *Nanjing* texts were grounded in the same cosmology that informed Chinese religious worldviews. Chinese thought had, from early on, reflected a fascination with the nature of change, expressed through concepts like *qi, yin* and *yang,* and the theory of *wuxing,* or the Five Phases. *Qi* constituted the psycho-spiritual-material stuff of which everything consisted; its written character represented steam rising from hot rice, associated with vapor, air, or breath. *Qi* could assume degrees of density, whether as a rock, a person, an ancestor, a ghost, or a god. A person consisted of different aspects of *qi,* including *yuanqi*—"original" or "primordial" *qi.* Mengzi (Mencius, 372?–289? BCE), a lineage descendant of Confucius (551–479 BCE), argued that self-cultivation engenders awareness of the identity of one's own heart and the heart of Heaven, because *qi* is the substance of both. Thus, there was no clear divide between matter and spirit as in European thought. Body, *spiritus,* animal soul, and immortal soul would all have been viewed as variations on *qi.*

Qi's dynamism expressed itself through the ceaseless transformations of *yang* and *yin,* concepts drawing their meanings from images of light and shadow on a mountainside. *Yang* reflected brightness, heat, light, the masculine, and penetration; *yin* was shadows, coolness, darkness, the feminine, and receptiveness. Each continuously transformed into the other, the transformation encompassing every kind of change, including the human body. Where *qi* circulated, life flourished; where it stagnated, sickness arose. There developed a theory of *jingluo*—vessels or channels of *qi* in the body (often translated as "meridians").[6] These channels could be palpated at different points, facilitating assessment of the flow of *qi* in the larger system.

Another conceptual system, associated with physician Zou Yan (ca. 350–270 BCE), entailed five processes, sometimes mistakenly translated as "elements"—wood, fire, earth, metal, and water. Each referred to a type, or *phase,* of change. Wood represented an active, growing change; fire, a change at its peak, on the verge of decline. Metal represented decline moving toward deep rest; water was the deepest rest,

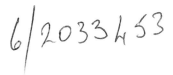

about to return to activity. Earth, a neutral state, buffered the others. Like *yin* and *yang*, the Five Phases constantly transformed into one another. By the time of the Song dynasty, Five Phase theory was regularly used to explain the causes and stages of illness.

Confucian scholar Dong Zhongshu (ca. 179–104 BCE) had posited that every facet of reality existed within networks of connections, or "systematic correspondences." During the Song-Jin-Yuan periods, Chinese medical thinkers reworked this theory in relation to herbal medicine. They joined the *Huangdi neijing* tradition, the *bencao (materia medica)* literature on the properties of individual drugs, and the work of Zhang Ji (150–219), author of the *Shanghan zabinglun* (Treatise on Cold Damage and Miscellaneous Disorders).[7] Drawing on Zhang's efforts to integrate the medicine of systematic correspondences with the use of different drugs, their interest in cold as an illness-causing factor inspired new approaches to categorizing herbs and their properties, including flavor, characteristics of a drug's *qi,* and related aspects of the dynamic between *yin* and *yang.* These categories enabled one to classify an herb and explain how and why it worked. One could challenge the assignment of particular herbs to certain categories, but the process represented a theoretical pharmacology. (Many treatises from the period also include sections labeled simply "Treatment of Symptoms"; Unschuld 1985.) Herbal practice based on these developments could have been what William witnessed in Karakorum.

Galenic medicine likened the body to a stove that cooked—"decocted"—food and air, circulating and distributing the "cooked products." If each plant and animal matter had a humoral complexion, then one could ingest that humoral dimension in an herbal formula or food. European physicians classified foods according to humoral properties. Anglicus, for example, judged how things looked, felt, or tasted. One would not serve fish—white, wet, and cold—to someone with a phlegmy disorder (Getz 1991). Dietetics, therefore, functioned as a key humoral therapy, along with related lifestyle adjustments (sleep was considered cooling; thought, heating).

Chinese medicine had an analogous tradition of "iatro-dietetics," wherein "all material things were considered part of an organismic cosmos in which all the parts belonged, interacted, and responded to the same dynamism" (Mote 1977, 226). One consumed food according to its therapeutic properties, to promote and sustain the cor-

rect balance of *yin* and *yang*. During the Yuan dynasty, Hu Sihui's
Yinshan zhengyao (Proper and Essential Things for the Emperor's Food
and Drink, 1330) argued, "Many diseases can be cured by diet alone"
(Mote 1977, 226). Hu, coming possibly from a mixed Chinese and
Turkic family, served as the imperial dietitian under several of
Qubilai's descendants in the early 1300s. His book merged Chinese
medical theory and folk beliefs with Mongol and West Asian approaches to nutrition and food preparation. Guests at court feasts
could expect dishes from Mongolia, China, India, and Iran. For that
matter, medicinal substances were available from the farthest reaches
of the empire (see Buell and Anderson 2000).[8]

William made no mention of specific medicines. Polo (1579),
however, described several, as when Yunnan hunters killed crocodiles
("serpents") for their gall, to use against rabid dog bites, for difficult
labor, and to cure tumors. He saw camphor trees in Fujian and referred, in passing, to the district of Succiu (Suzhou), which exported
rhubarb. Rhubarb may well have reached Europe even earlier, by the
eighth or ninth century, carried by Arab traders. Tenth-century Persian and Arab pharmacologists wrote about it extensively, singling out
the Chinese sort (Foust 1992). Dioscorides may have encountered
varieties of rhubarb imported to Greece and Rome from the Black
Sea and northern Caspian. Anglicus prescribed it as a purgative to
expel "evil humors," along with bloodletting and diet, using it for feeble sight, "corrupte wyndes in a mannes body," hiccups, "casting and
spewing" (vomiting), and distemper of the liver, generally with other
herbs (Getz 1991, 167–168, 217–218). The reference in Polo only fueled mercantile interest. Pegolotti (1936 [1340]) listed "riubarbero,"
as "China rhubarb," native to northwest China and eastern Tibet. Of
the almost three hundred herbs in his compendium, camphor and
galangal also came from China.

Some herbs were used medicinally in both China and Europe, al-
though in quite different ways. For example, the Chinese practiced
"moxibustion," burning the down from the leaves of mugwort, or
Artemesia vulgaris, at strategic points along the meridians. In contrast,
Anglicus used "mug-wede," "mug-worte," or "mugwort," as medieval
European herbals called it, for earache—one stamped it with oil of rue
and a little wine, roasted it in a cabbage leaf, and laid it to one's ear.
For hemorrhoids, one steeped mugwort and other herbs in wine, and

consumed only this tonic for nine days (Getz 1991). Mugwort was sometimes classified with plants that could take on magical properties and corresponding therapeutic attributes, and was worn as an amulet (Siraisi 1990). Herman of Sancto Portu suggested carrying it as protection from venomous beasts (Stannard 1999).

William did mention hearing about a province where, regardless of one's age upon entering, one aged no further once within (Komroff 1928). He may have been referring to the Chinese alchemical tradition, particularly longevity practices involving elixirs thought to confer immortality. In Europe, the earliest Latin translations of Arabic alchemy works appeared by the mid-twelfth century. Trade routes between China and the Arabic world yielded a cross-fertilization of alchemical theory and practice as early as the Tang dynasty. Some Arabic writers speculated that alchemy originated in China (Needham, Ho, and Lu 1980). Chinese ideas therefore filtered into Europe through Arabic works long before the observers' accounts.

They Diagnose Very Cleverly from the Pulse but Do Not Use Urinals

Diagnosis, in Galenic medicine, included assessing the pulse, which was less associated with the heart and blood than with innate heat—an aspect of blood as a humor. Pulse changed over one's lifetime, playing out in musical rhythms and slowing with age. Humans therefore possessed an intrinsic musical aspect, corresponding to the world's own music *(musica mundana)*. What William witnessed in Karakorum was different—a diagnostic tradition involving palpation of the meridians and related flows of *qi* that was also conceptualized as pulse taking. By the early Song, the pivotal source on this approach, the *Mojing* (Classic of the Pulse) of Wang Shuhe (210–285), had inspired more than seventy other works. William's reference to pulse taking suggests that he remained unaware of important differences in how European and Chinese doctors conceptualized the body. Had he grasped these differences, he might have devised an alternative term to refer to the Chinese practice.

Urine was another case of difference. Like excrement, it allowed the Western physician to assess the patient's humoral state. Medieval manuscripts show physicians inspecting flasks of urine. Chinese physicians tended to rely instead on other signs and inquiries for diagnostic purposes, but in some cases they did use urine *as* medicine. It came under the smaller subheading of the use of what the Chinese called "human drugs," which also included semen, saliva, milk, blood, hair, nails, bone, and teeth (Cooper and Sivin 1973)—practices with some parallels in the West.

The Method of the Nine Needles

One may be surprised to find no mention of acupuncture, the therapeutic insertion of needles at selected points. Surely, had William observed it, he would have said something. Acupuncture is the primary therapy of the *Lingshu* section of the *Neijing*. Between the Han and Song dynasties, some ninety acupuncture treatises were written. In 1023, Song emperor Renzong ordered the designing of a bronze training figurine, marked with meridians and point locations. Following the Song, however, acupuncture specialists were relegated to a lower status in the hierarchy of practitioners, alongside practices considered technical or manual, in contrast with the more "scholarly" study of *materia medica*.

Acupuncture was sometimes negatively associated with alchemy or amulet healing, and with a category of women healers linked to moxibustion, shamanism, and midwifery. Family medicine book author Yuan Cai (ca. 1140–1190) argued that "women who claim to be dealing in acupuncture needles and moxa must not be allowed into the household" (Leung 2003, 396). Yuan acupuncturist Hua Shou criticized his contemporaries, writing, "In a later age, [healing] by prescriptions and drugs became extremely prevalent, and the way of acupuncture was thus halted and ignored, moxibustion barely got transmitted." Song Lian, who authored the preface for Hua's book, added, "Those who transmit the method of the nine needles are rare" (Leung 2003, 383).

Why nine needles? Early techniques for cautery (the therapeutic application of heat), together with early understandings of the meridians, provided a foundation for what would emerge as acupuncture. Medical manuscripts discovered at Mawangdui, dating from the second century BCE, "[explain illness as] pathogenic conditions of vapor [*qi*] in the vessels, associate the occurrence of certain ailments with particular vessels, and recommend cauterizing the vessels to cure ailments" (Harper 1998, 5).[9] Donald Harper reminds us that the *Neijing*'s authors were informed by meridian theory, and suggests that this therapeutic paradigm paved the way for acupuncture, understood as pricking the meridians to address vapor (*qi*)-related conditions. Some of the earliest associations with *mai*—another term for channels, or meridians—included blood and *qi*, with conceptual links "between the body and earth, and between blood vessels and streams" (83). Networks of channels conducted blood and *qi*, in some way analogous to how water flowed through the earth, but differences between the two fluids were not specified.

Harper (1998) and He and Lo (1996) also provide persuasive evidence that self-cultivation practices significantly influenced the early stages of conceptualization of the *mai*. By the time of the *Lingshu,* meridian theory posited a circuit of twelve interconnected channels.[10] Cauterization involved burning mugwort leaves (a precursor to using just the down) and other substances at points along the meridians—a practice with explicit analogies to divination strategies. In particular, the word *jiu* (cauterize) also referred to the brand pressed against a tortoise shell to produce divinatory cracks, and had exorcistic overtones. Cautery practice contributed to knowledge of the meridians and eventually to the identification of points where needles could be inserted (Harper 1998). Although metal needles originally were used primarily for draining infection, Keiji Yamada suggests that by the late third to early second century BCE, such needles had largely replaced the application of heat; by the time of the *Neijing,* acupuncture had become the dominant meridian-related therapy. Needles also continued to be used for lancing abscesses, linking these different treatments, particularly in relation to the expulsion of harmful *qi*.

At the same time, the term *needles* requires elaboration. The *Lingshu* refers to nine needles, versions of which persisted down to Hua Shou's day. A few were heavier variations on the needles with which we are familiar. The others looked like hooks, scalpels, and slender knives; these were used for treating cataracts, lancing boils, and minor bloodletting—the latter arising alongside acupuncture. The *Suwen* section of the *Neijing* specified bloodletting points, like the "foot major-*yang* vessel," which one "needled" to release blood. Given the connection between blood and *qi*, bloodletting expelled excesses in both, freeing the system from a pathogen.[11]

Had William seen the nine needles, he might have been reminded of European surgery, which included "shaving, bleeding, leeching, cupping, scarifying, and treatment by surgical operation and manipulation" (Getz 1991, xxxvii). Bloodletting was critical to European practice, because blood contained all four humors. Cupping provided a variation. It involved heating the air inside a small globe to create a warm vacuum, as a warming therapy. Often, small cuts were made in the skin under the cup, the suction enhancing bleeding. Scarifying, an extreme application of heat, entailed touching the skin with a hot iron rod or putting burning matter on it. Both approaches generated open sores, which were then kept open. Infection was induced, the resulting pus evidence that the body was purifying itself. Bleeding, leeching, scarifying, and cauterizing were all cleansing operations. There were sufficient apparent similarities that an early observer might have been excused for imagining that the Chinese and European practices grew from the same conceptual framework.

Divinations, Auguries, Soothsayings, Sorceries, and Incantations

Given *qi's* fluid nature in its many forms, a neglected ancestor could become an angry ghost. A civil servant embodying Confucian ideals could, after death, become a city god. Given the theory of correspondences, one could examine the cracks in burnt tortoise shells or bovine scapulae and discern therein answers to questions. Analogous practices flourished among the Mongols. Giovanni commented, "They pay great attention to divinations, auguries, soothsayings, sorceries and incantations" (Dawson 1955, 12).[12] Entering Möngke's dwelling one day, William noticed someone exiting with a charred sheep's scapula:

> When the Chan wishes to do anything he has three of these bones brought to him before they have been burned, and holding them he thinks of that matter about which he wishes to find out whether he is to do it or not; then he hands the bones to a slave to be burned . . . When the bones, therefore, have been burned until they are black they are brought to the Chan and he therefore examines them to see if with the heat of the fire they have split lengthwise in a straight line. If they have, the way is clear for him to act; if, however, the bones have cracked horizontally or round bits have shot out, then he does not do it. (164)

So important was divination that troops could not go to war without favorable augury. William speculated that the Mongols would have returned to attack Hungary, but the diviners had not yet received favorable readings. He explained, "Khan . . . means also a diviner or soothsayer. All diviners are called Khan amongst them. Whereupon their princes are called Khan, because the government of the people depends on divination" (92–93). Other Mongol "soothsayers" oversaw carts with figures of the gods, served as astrologers, conducted rituals, and presided over sacrifices. They also supervised ritual purification: everything and everyone entering the court had to pass between two fires, as did everything belonging to someone who had died. From these proceedings, the soothsayers received a share.

Anyone in the camp who sickened was quarantined. The soothsayers "do not allow anyone to cross these bounds, for they are afraid an evil spirit or wind may come in with those entering" (106). One of William's tales involved a convoluted mix of sorcery, sickness, death, and revenge. A Nestorian Christian woman received a gift of furs, which passed through the purifying fires. The soothsayers took more than their share, which the woman's servant pointed out. The mistress reprimanded the soothsayers, shortly after which she fell ill. The soothsayers had the maid lay her hand on the painful places of the mistress's body and extract what she found—a piece of felt that when laid on the ground crawled like an animal and when placed in water became a leech. They accused *her* of sorcery and of taking the furs, and tortured her for seven days seeking a confession, during which time the mistress died. Faced with the servant's refusal to confess, Möngke allowed her to live. Still requiring a culprit for the mistress's death, the soothsayers blamed the nurse responsible for the mistress's daughter. The nurse was also a Nestorian Christian, and her husband was a Nestorian priest; she confessed to using oracles and charms to endear herself to her mistress. The Khan had her executed and sent her husband "to his bishop in Cathay for sentence, although he had not been found guilty" (199).

The Khan's chief wife then bore a son who, the soothsayers divined, would have good fortune and long life. The child died shortly thereafter. His mother accused the soothsayers of false prophecy. *They* blamed the dead nurse, claiming to see her ghost carrying the dead child.

Learning that the deceased nurse had had two children, the Khan's wife had them killed. Möngke dreamed about them and asked for them the next morning. When he discovered what his wife had done, he imprisoned her without food for seven days and had the children's executioners killed. Had the Khan's wife not borne his children, she too would have died. As it was, the Khan left the *orda* (tent camp) for a month (Dawson 1955).

The tale pits the soothsayers, all men, against women who accuse them and women affiliated with the accusers. Women are blamed for sorcery and charms. Illness and death required explanation, sometimes extracted by torture. At the same time, the narrative foregrounds the soothsayers' own guilt—their theft, failed prophecy, efforts to allocate fault—and the resulting deaths of others. The story also points to religious differences: the soothsayers are called in when a Nestorian Christian woman falls sick; her Christian nurse turns to oracles and charms. Both instances corroborate Giovanni's description of the attention paid to soothsaying, regardless of other allegiances. Here one finds a gap between the Nestorian Christianity of China and the Latin Christianity of the Franciscans, who believed that soothsayers trafficked in the demonic.

Giovanni pointed to the Mongols' engagement with local gods: "When they receive an answer from the demons they believe that a god is speaking to them" (Dawson 1955, 12). Devotees made offerings and enacted directives from the gods. William told a similar tale: "Some of the soothsayers also invoke demons and they assemble in their dwelling by night those who wish to consult the demon and they place cooked meat in the middle. The *Kam* who is performing the invocation begins to chant his incantations, and, holding a tympanum, strikes it heavily on the ground. At length he begins to rage and has himself bound. Then the devil comes in the darkness and gives him meat to eat and he utters oracles" (Dawson 1955, 200–201). An English translation of Polo's travels described trance possession and ritual healing in "the Province named Cingui" (in Yunnan):

In thys Province, and in the other two afore specifyed, there be no Phisitions, but when they doe fall sicke, they cause to come unto their houses certayne Ministers, which use inchantmentes by the power of the Divell, and declare the sickness that the diseased hathe, and these Ministers sound their instrumentes in honor of theyr Idols, in so muche that the Devill entereth into one of those Ministers, Inchanters, or Idols, and falleth downe as though he were dead, and those Ministers, or Maysters of the Idols, demaunde of hym that lyeth inchanted, or in a trance, wherefore that man fell sicke, and hee aunswereth, for that he hathe angered such or such an Idoll, and then those Maysters or Ministers of the Idols saye unto him that is inchanted, we request thee to pray unto that Idoll that is angrie wyth the sicke bodye, to pardon hym, and will make hym Sacrifice with hys owne bloud. (Polo 1579, 83)

This place had "no Phisitians"; the practice of diagnostic trance possession also lay beyond familiar frameworks of sacred healing, leaving only the construct of ceremonies involving the devil. Polo interpolated Christian assumptions concerning witchcraft: The process became "inchantment," the officiants "Ministers," "Inchanters," and "Maysters of the Idol."

And if hee that is in thys trance, doe beleeve that the disease is mortall, hee aunswereth, thys sicke man hathe so displeased the Idoll, that I knowe not whether he will pardon hym or not, for that hee hathe determined that hee shoulde dye, and if he thynketh that hee shall escape hee sayeth, if hee wyll lyve, it behoveth hym to gyve unto the Idoll so manye Sheepe that have blacke neckes, and to dress so many sortes of meates dressed with spices, sufficient to make the sacrifices unto the Idoll that is angry with him, and for the ministers that serve him, and for the women that serve in his temple, whiche is all fraude and guile of the inchanters for to gette victuls, by this meanes all are damned unto Hell. To this banket there is convited the maisters and ministers of the Idols, the inchanters and women that serve in ye temple of that Idoll. And before they sitte downe to the Table, they doe sprincle the broath aboute the house, singing and dauncing in the honor of that Idoll. And they doe aske the Idoll if he have forgiven the sicke man. And sometimes the Feende aunswereth, that there lacketh such or suche a thing, whiche immediately they do provide: and when he answereth that he is pardoned, then they do sitte downe to eate and to drinke that sacrifice which is drest with spices, and this done, they go unto his house with great joy. If the paciente heale, it is good for him,

but if he dye, it is an everlasting payne for him, and if he recover, they
do beleeve that the divelishe Idol hath healed him, and if he die, they
say that the cause of his deathe was for the great offence that he had
done unto him, and so they be lost as brute beasts in all that Countrey.
(Polo 1579, 83–84)

The account was rooted in the Christian understanding of idols, which
by definition represented false religion. Sacrifice was suspect. The mo-
tivating source could only be "the Devill" or "Feende," the practices
"all fraude and guile," and those involved "damned to Hell." Insofar
as the demonic was irretrievably associated with the offspring of
fallen angels and women, there was no room for the potentially benevolent demons of Chinese legends who might intervene to help the
living.

To illustrate: A minor demon pilfered Tang emperor Xuanzong's
jade flute and his concubine's embroidered perfume bag. A larger
demon, Zhong Kui, caught the smaller one and ate him. Zhong Kui in
life had been a virtuous scholar who had committed suicide after failing the imperial examinations. The grateful emperor, his property restored, bestowed posthumous honors upon Zhong, who in turn swore
to pursue harmful demons (Ebrey 1996). His posthumous recognition
influenced not only his living relatives but also Zhong, who, still capable of human sentiments, acted nobly in death. The pervasiveness of qi
made such things possible. Polo's account, however, contributed to
the impression that the East stood in grave need of Christian conversion.

The effect was compounded by Polo's story of "the kingdom of
Dagoian," recast by Odoric as the island called Dondin ("unclean").
"They who dwell in that island," wrote Odoric, ". . . have also among
them an abominable custom; for the father will eat the son, the son
the father, the wife will eat the husband, or the husband the wife."
When a father fell ill, his son had a priest consult "an idol" through
whom "a demon" would reply. Should the prognosis be mortal, the
priest was said to suffocate the sick man, after which the family cooked
him and invited friends to feast, preferring to consume their dead and
spare them from corruption by worms (Yule 1914, 2:101–103). The
fabricated story proved such tabloid fare that the *Maundeville* author
plagiarized it almost verbatim.

"Credo in unum Deum"

Europe at the time was rife with its own religious therapies. Saints exorcised the possessed and, after death, continued to heal through their relics. Surgeon Henri Mondeville noted with frustration that the common people divided afflictions into "those caused by spells, in which a surgeon was useless; those due to misfortune; and those coming from glorious and almighty God, that it was he who sent it, and that thus surgeons can do no good, because they cannot oppose God" (Pouchelle 1990, 55). When asked if they sought healing, many replied, "Not by human hands, that is not possible and would not please God, since if he wished it, I should be healed at once" (43). Even so, Mondeville's book opened with a dedication to Jesus, the Virgin, and twin physician saints Cosmas and Damian. He incorporated prayers, incantations, and a Trinitarian structure into treatments. Medicine also applied a penitential conception of the patient's role: The surgeon expected the afflicted to submit, like a sinner obeying God in trust.

In China, the Mongols asked both William and Odoric to expel demons. As William and his party traveled through steep and jagged rocks, his guide requested "a prayer which could chase away the demons because in this place the devils were known to carry away men without their knowing what was happening to them." William did not interrogate the guide's fears, or suggest that the real culprits might be bandits. Demons were expected in the wilderness. "Then we sang loudly *'Credo in unum Deum'* [I Believe in One God] and by the grace of God we passed through safe and sound." The guide and his men, impressed, requested that William write out charms for them to wear on their heads, as one might ask of a soothsayer (Komroff 1928, 122–123). Instead, William offered to teach them the *Credo* and Lord's Prayer. When his interpreter could not translate either one, William wrote them out—confirming the guide's notion of what religious authorities should do.

The friars, Odoric commented, found their reputation as exorcists spreading. People journeyed for many days to bring their sick to them. The friars ordered the demons to leave the bodies of the possessed in Jesus' name. The exorcised submitted to baptism, after which the friars cast felt figures of "their idols" into a fire. In a dramatic scene of

Heaven-to-hell combat, some demons leaped to rescue the idols. "And so the friars take holy water and sprinkle it upon the fire, and that straightway drives away the demon from the fire; and so the friars again casting the idols in the fire, they are consumed. And then the devil in the air raises a shout, saying:—'See then, see then, how I am expelled from my dwelling-place'" (156). Idols figured in other narratives of healing as well. Foreign monks and priests sometimes cared for sick members of the Khan's family, as in the case of Cota, Möngke's second wife, "an idol worshipper." She was treated by an Armenian monk, Sergius (who, it later emerged, was only an unordained cloth-weaver, and thus a religious fraud). Accompanied by William, Sergius had Cota prostrate herself before the cross, and taught her to make its sign. When she worsened, Möngke again summoned Sergius, who promised to cure her or suffer beheading. William wrote:

> Now he [Sergius] had a certain root which goes by the name of rhu-barb, and he used to cut it up almost to a powder and put it into water with a little cross he had from which the figure of our Savior had been removed. He declared that he was able to tell by means of this whether a sick man was going to get well again or going to die; for if he was go-ing to get well it would stick to his chest as if glued to it, otherwise it would not stick. At that time I still believed that the rhubarb was some sacred thing he had brought from the Holy Land of Jerusalem. He used to give some of that water to all ailing people to drink with the in-evitable result that their bowels were all disturbed by so bitter a potion. This change in their bodies they put down to a miracle . . . I mentioned to him the holy water which is made in the Roman Church, for it is most efficacious in driving out demons and I understood that she was troubled with a devil. At his request we made some holy water for him, and he mixed some rhubarb with it and plunged in the cross to soak all night in the water. (Dawson 1955, 167–168)

Diagnosis depended on the herb and cross, steeped together, lending prophetic properties to the cross, expressed through adherence. Wil-liam assumed the rhubarb must have come from Jerusalem, enhanc-ing its miraculous dimensions. Nor was he surprised that a demon had afflicted a non-Christian woman. Exorcism through holy water, infused with sacred words, made sense. The ensuing mix—rhubarb,

cross, holy water, and priestly authority—illustrates how herbal and religious categories of healing converged.

William observed protective objects of "sorcery" around Cota's bed:
"a silver chalice such as we use, which had perhaps been taken from a
church in Hungary, and it was hung up on the wall full of ashes and on
top of the ashes was a black stone." He complained that the Nestorian
priests not only did not criticize such objects, but also promoted them.
Even Sergius consulted with a soothsayer and his wife, inviting them to
"sift dust and divine for him." The Lady Cota recovered sufficiently for
William and two Nestorians to visit. Venerating the cross, she drank
more of the holy-water-rhubarb medicine, placing some on her chest.
William read the Gospel of John over her, applying the therapeutic
power of the word. Möngke, hearing of his wife's improvement, summoned the priests. They found him inspecting a sheep's blackened
scapulae. "He took the cross in his hand," wrote William, "but I did not
see him kiss it or adore it; instead he looked at it wondering I know not
what" (Dawson 1955, 165–169). When William later fell ill, Sergius
gave him the rhubarb tonic, which made William worse—particularly
because he drank two bowls, thinking it holy water. "I thereupon . . .
said to him [Sergius]: 'Either go about like the Apostle truly working
miracles by the power of prayer and the Holy Ghost, or act as a physician in accordance with the science of medicine. You give men, who
are not prepared for it, a strong dose of medicine to drink as if it were
something holy; if this came to the knowledge of the public you would
incur the worst possible scandal'" (181). Here we find the emerging
separation of religious and medical authority in Europe, and between
their respective domains of curing. The struggle lay between religion
and medicine, on the one hand, and divergent religious therapies—
those of the Mongols, and two calling themselves Christian.

It is easy to sustain the impression that medieval Europe possessed little direct information about Asia. This impression is exacerbated when
discussions of authors like Polo remain unrelated to the social contexts in which their journeys to China transpired. The store of knowledge based on real encounters was more extensive than we may
realize. Yet knowledge was often piecemeal, available primarily to the
literate. Travelers and authors had not necessarily heard about one an-

other or about each other's narratives. Some works—like those of Giovanni, Polo, Odoric, and Maundeville—reached relatively wide audiences; others, like William's, were barely read until a later period.

The Mongol empire fell to indigenous rebels whose leader captured Nanjing in 1356 and founded the Ming dynasty (1368–1644) as Zhu Yuanzhang. The Ming's founders inherited a China that eighty-nine years of Yuan rule had reconfigured, not least in its expanded boundaries. For a time, China reached outward, sending seven diplomatic missions between 1405 and 1433, led by Grand Eunuch Zheng He (1371–1433), a Muslim, to enroll other nations as tributary states as far as the east coast of Africa. Confucian scholar officials, jealous of Zheng's power and opposed to foreign trade and contact, brought the voyages to an end. As Jacques Gernet (1972) observes, "Anticommercialism and xenophobia won out, and China retired from the world scene" (139). Ming rulers increasingly closed China to foreigners and prohibited Chinese citizens from going overseas. As Christian missions largely collapsed during the upheaval of the Mongols' fall, their version of Western influence ceased to operate.

The visitors described in this section encountered China obliquely, under the rule of the Mongols. Nevertheless, they brought back fleeting observations that contributed to the racializing of the Chinese, along with comparative impressions related to practices of healing. Key pieces were put in place, albeit in abbreviated form—Chinese diagnostics and herbalism, encounters with food informed by a therapeutic worldview, hearsay of longevity practices, and accounts of divination, gods, mediumship, and exorcism. For close to two hundred years, however, there would be no new European reports.

CHAPTER 2

A New Wave of Europeans:
1492–1659

This period opens with European explorations in 1492 and the establishing of Jesuit, Dominican, and Franciscan China missions. It encompasses uprisings of the Tungus, who, unified as the Manchu, invaded China in the 1620s and founded the Qing dynasty in 1644. Earlier China narratives fueled European imaginations. Cristobal Colón read Polo and Maundeville, inspiring his westward search. In 1493 a papal bull bisected an unsuspecting world, assigning to Portugal routes around Africa to East Asia, and to Spain the Western Hemisphere. The Portuguese settled in Malacca in 1511, and in 1530 they established a base on Macao, gaining access to Canton and China's southeast coast.

After Fernando Magellan (ca. 1480–1521) entered the Philippines in 1521, Spain traded Chinese silks and porcelains in its American colonies, bringing back to China peanuts, Indian corn, sweet potatoes, and two million pesos per year in silver (Chinn 1969). Chinese sailors joined Spanish galleon crews, and the Spaniards were also accompanied by Chinese servants or slaves—known as "chinos" (Israel 1980; Lai 1999). By the turn of the sixteenth century, Chinese shipbuilders, servants, textile workers, farmers, and barbers were in California and Mexico (Dubs and Smith 1942).

British pirates challenged the Portuguese and Spanish, capturing the *Madre de Dios* in 1592. The cargo—"benjamin, frankincense, galingale, mirobalans, aloes, zocotrina, camphire"—included medicinal drugs (Honour 1961, 42). In 1600, English merchants formed the British

East India Company, with twelve "factories" (establishments for overseas agents, or "factors"). The agents and other traders were restricted to Amoy and Macao. In 1637, Charles I dispatched Captain John Weddell to expand China trade, without great success. Still, the 1651 Navigation Act required British merchants in North America to purchase goods through the Company, in London, instead of trading directly with China. Dutch merchants, having organized the Dutch East India Company in 1602, settled on Java in the city of Batavia (Jakarta). In 1624 they opened trade with Chinese and Japanese merchants on Formosa (now Taiwan).

The Reporters

Traders and missionaries continued to produce China narratives. Cornishman Peter Mundy (ca. 1597–1667), who sailed with Weddell, wrote about his years in Macao and Canton (Mundy [1634–1637]1919). Occasionally Westerners got caught in the Chinese government's efforts to regulate foreign trade. Galeote Pereira, from a Portuguese noble family, was captured by coastal patrollers in 1548 and held until 1553, when he bribed his way to freedom. His account was translated into Italian in 1565, and into English in 1577 as *History of Travale in the West and East Indies.* Protestant minister Samuel Purchas (1577–1626) included it in his multivolume anthology *Purchas His Pilgrimes* (1625), which offered "a theologicall and geographicall historie of Asia, Africa, and America." Another group of authors included physicians, although none during this period actually entered China.

China missions and missionary narratives were set against the backdrop of the Protestant Reformation and Catholic Counter-Reformation. The Thirty Years' War started in 1618, engulfing Europe and intensifying the imperative to spread partisan religious perspectives. Anti-Catholic sentiment was equally extreme in some British colonies. In 1647, Massachusetts Bay passed laws excluding Jesuits. Ignatius of Loyola (1491–1556) had founded the Jesuits in 1534 to fight heresies (including Protestantism) and convert "heathens."

As explorers, missionaries, and teachers, the Jesuits compiled detailed observations of other cultures. In China they employed a three-part strategy: proselytizing among Chinese scholar-officials to gain influence at court; accommodating as much as possible to Chinese religious and ritual traditions; and incorporating European science and technology into missionizing, to demonstrate Christianity's affinity for advanced civilization (Zürcher 1990). By calling Chinese sages "philosophers," Jesuits avoided defining Chinese teachings as being religious and therefore in conflict with Christianity. Kong Qiu, or Kong Fuzi (551–479 BCE), whose name Jesuit Matteo Ricci (1552–1610) romanized as Confucius, was "the equal of the pagan philosophers and superior to most of them" (Ricci [1615]1942, 30). The Jesuits also rationalized the religious dimensions of ancestor veneration, to avoid confronting potential converts about a core expression of Chinese religious life. Still, the missionaries never entirely overcame literati uneasiness toward "foreign" teachings, particularly from celibate priests who failed the Confucian obligation to perpetuate their family lines.

Some reports from the eight hundred missionaries in China between 1552 and 1795 were read only within their orders; others reached wider audiences. Portuguese Dominican Gaspar da Cruz (d. 1570) visited Canton in 1556, publishing *Tractado em qu se cōtam muito por estēço as cousas da China* (Treatise in Which Matters of China Are Extensively Related, 1570; Boxer 1953). Spanish author Bernardino de Escalante ([1577]1992) later paraphrased da Cruz, without acknowledging his source. John Frampton's English translation of Escalante (Frampton 1579) was abridged by Purchas (1625), bringing da Cruz to wider audiences in a roundabout way.

Missionary scrutiny encompassed everything, to the point of espionage. Augustinian Martín de Rada (1533–1578) went to China in 1575, instructed to "learn the quality of the people of the land, and understand their manners and customs, and what trade and commerce they have; and if they keep their word and speak the truth in what they promise, and what merchandise can be taken from here and brought from there, so that the trade may be profitable to both parties, together with all the other matters and secrets of the country which can be found and learnt" (Dawson 1967, 28–29). De Rada wrote about his three months in Fujian (Boxer 1953).

New narratives frequently reiterated content from earlier ones, mixing a dense recycling of information with new observations. Augustinian Juan Gonzalez de Mendoza (1545–1618) wrote the church-sponsored *Historia de las cosas más notables, ritos y costumbres del gran reyno de la China* (History of the Most Notable Things, Rites and Customs of the

Great Kingdom of China, 1585), drawing on Pereira, da Cruz, and de Rada. Three years later Richard Hakluyt—geographer, collector, and editor of travel narratives—"englished" (translated) Mendoza (1588). By the end of the seventeenth century, Mendoza's work had entered forty-six editions and seven languages.

Spanish Jesuit Diego de Pantoja (1571–1618) went to Macao in 1597 and Beijing in 1601. A long letter he wrote was published as *Relación de la entrada de algunos padres de la Compañía de Iesus en la China* (Relating the Entry of Some of the Fathers of the Company of Jesus into China; Pantoja 1606). Eventually it was translated into French, German, Latin, Italian, and Spanish, and ten editions had been published by 1608; it stayed in print until superseded by Ricci's narrative.

Son of a poor Italian nobleman, Matteo Ricci entered the Jesuits at seventeen and went to Macao in 1582 at age thirty. Nineteen years later he established a mission at the court in Beijing. Known as Li Matou, Ricci became arguably the most learned European of his day regarding China. Ricci's journal traced the history of the Jesuit's China mission from 1582 to 1610, the year of Ricci's death. Ricci also included chapters reviewing Chinese religion, customs, government, trade, and other topics. Flemish Jesuit Nicolas Trigault (1577–1628) arrived in China in 1610, succeeding Ricci. He edited, updated, and translated Ricci's text into Latin when he returned to Europe in 1613. He also added material from other Jesuits about their China experiences. First published in 1615 in Augsburg, the book was translated into French by Trigault's nephew, physician Riquebourg-Trigault, and published in Lyons in 1616. It quickly achieved international fame—translated into multiple European languages and published throughout Europe. Later Purchas published an abridged English version, together with selections from Polo, de Rada, Pantoja, Mendoza, and others.

Late in the Ming, some of the Chinese ruling family converted to Christianity. Faced with Manchu incursions, in 1650 the empress Yongli dispatched Jesuit Michael Boym (Michal Piotr Boym, 1612–1659) to seek papal assistance. Boym, son of the physician to the king of Poland and himself interested in medicine, entered the order in 1629. Sent to China in 1645, he wrote *Flora sinensis, fructus floresque humillime porrigens* (Chinese Flora, or a Treatise on the Flowers, Plants, and Animals Particular to China, 1656) and *Clavis medica ad Chinarum doctrinam de pulsibus* (Medical Key to the Pulse Doctrine of the Chinese, 1686). Thwarted by the Portuguese, the lengthy journey, and time spent gaining a new pope's ear, Boym began his return to China in 1656, with eight companions. Three reached China, including Fr. Philippe Couplet. Arriving too late to aid the former ruling family, Boym went to Vietnam and died shortly thereafter (Chabrié 1933; Zhang 1996).

The Jesuit Martino Martini (1614–1661) first encountered China through his birthplace, Trento, Italy—a way station for Chinese goods. Inspired by Ricci's example, he joined the Jesuits at seventeen and arrived in Macao at age twenty-six. He spent years traveling through China, studying classical and contemporary Chinese. In 1651 he went to Rome to defend the Jesuits in the Rites Controversy, returning to Macao in 1658. Such books as *De bello Tartarico historia* (History of the Tartar War, 1654), *Novus atlas Sinensis* (New Atlas of China, 1654), and *La Sinicae historiae decas prima* (History of China from the Beginning, 1658) qualified him, too, as a leading early sinologist, though some of his evidence eventually was questioned.

No Western physicians reported entering China during this period, but two recorded Chinese herbs they encountered in India, and one described acupuncture. García d'Orta was the son of Spanish Jews who emigrated to Portugal during the 1492 expulsion from Spain. In 1534 he went to India as physician to his friend and patron Martim Afonso de Sousa. D'Orta aspired to learn the names and uses of indigenous medicinal drugs and remedies (Boxer 1963). In Goa, he wrote *Coloquios dos simples, e drogas he cousas medicinales da India* (Colloquies on Simples and Drugs and Medical Things of India, 1563), including some Chinese herbs.

Cristóvão Acosta (d. 1594/1596?), a North African whose family may have been Portuguese Jews, went to Goa in 1568 to serve the Portuguese armada. He never met d'Orta but did read the *Coloquios.* He, too, studied medicinal plants. He returned to Portugal in 1572 and from there went to Spain. His *Tratado das drogras e medicinas das Índias Orientais* (Treatise on the Drugs and Medicines of the Oriental Indies; Acosta [1582]1964) included discussions of Chinese herbs. Flemish botanist Charles de l'Écluse published Acosta's and d'Orta's works together in Latin in 1593, with illustrations based on products available in Antwerp markets. The third physician, Dane Jakob de Bondt (1592–

1631), was surgeon general for the Dutch East India Company. He wrote the first notice about acupuncture.

Thanks to movable type, invented during the mid-fifteenth century, such publications spread throughout Europe, reaching many readers through institutional, princely, and private libraries. Donald Lach's survey of printed inventories from the second half of the sixteenth century shows that sixty of the extant lists included at least one of the twenty-four key titles on China (O'Neill 1986). Some American colonists, like Puritan Cotton Mather (1663–1728), owned such works as Purchas's *Pilgrimes* (Isani 1970).

Mental Maps of the West

Time, space, and humankinds remained organizing frameworks into which Western observers inserted the Chinese, asking: Are the Chinese the lost tribe of Israel? Had there been more than one Creation? Some intellectuals, exploring ancient Greece and Rome for models of philosophy, art, governance, and medicine, posited Chinese analogies.

Mapping Time and Space

Early explorers still believed that China lay across the Atlantic. Reaching Cuba, Colón wrote, "I thought this must be the mainland, the province of Cathay . . . I have taken possession of a large town which is most conveniently situated for the goldfields and for communications with the mainland both here, and there in the territories of the Grand Khan, with which there will be very profitable trade" (Phillips 1994, 24–25). Europeans had no grasp of the scale of the Americas. In 1634 explorer Jean Nicolet stood in Chinese robes on the shores of Lake Michigan, hoping to encounter the Khan (Phillips 1988). Moreover, in their maps both Europeans and Chinese expressed their perceptions that their lands were the center of the world. Trigault commented, "Today we usually call this country Ciumquo or Ciumhoa [*Zhongguo*] . . . When put together the words are translated, 'To be at the center.' . . . Due to this idea, when they first saw our geographical maps, they were somewhat puzzled to find their empire placed not in the center of the map but at its extreme eastern border" (Ricci and Trigault 1616, 7). Ricci's world map laid out the relationship between the five continents. From Manila galleon exchanges and such maps, the Chinese became well aware of lands to the west and east.

Well Proportioned and Gallant Men

Renaissance writers struggled with how to categorize new groups, focusing on physical appearances, or on "'types,' 'varieties,' 'peoples,' 'nations,' and 'species'" (Smedley 1993, 162). Sometimes "race" (Spanish, *raza*) served as a generic synonym. Giordano Bruno and Jean Bodin, for example, drew on skin color, "duskish colour, like roasted quince," "black," "chesnut," and "farish and white" (162). Northern Europeans considered Spaniards and Portuguese browner than themselves, reminding us of the complex classifying among Europeans themselves. Spanish and Portuguese categories, based in *limpieza de sangre* (purity of blood), reflected the stigmatizing of Jewish or Muslim ancestry. In the Americas such "purity" contrasted with *mestizaje* (mixed ancestry) involving Spaniards, Africans, and Indians (Klor de Alva 1996). The term *chino* in this connection referred not only to Chinese immigrants, but also to descendants of multiple combinations of Africans, Indians, and a single Spaniard.

Physical descriptions of the Chinese arose in such contexts. Pantoja (1606) observed, "The Chinese commonly have sparse beard, small eyes and noses, and all of them have dark eyes" (107). Lorenzo Corsalis wrote to Lorenzo de'Medici in 1515 that the Chinese "are people of great skill, and of our quality, though of uglier aspect with little bits of eyes" (Honour 1961, 16), reflecting a complex assessment. The words "of our quality" acknowledged Chinese civilization; "uglier" functioned as a qualifying detail. Da Cruz drew equally mixed comparisons: "The women commonly, excepting those of the seacoast and of the mountains, are very white and gentlewoman, some having their noses and eyes well proportioned. From their childhood they squeeze their feet in cloths, so that they may remain small, and they do it because the Chinas do hold them for finer gentlewomen that have small noses and feet" (Boxer 1953, 149).

Color, region, and class intersected, whiteness linked to breeding, and "gentlewoman" to foot binding—a practice described solely by its mechanics. Descriptions of men were similarly mixed. Da Cruz wrote,

"Although the Chinas commonly are ill-favoured, having small eyes, and their faces and noses flat, and are beardless, with some few little hairs on the point of the chin, notwithstanding there are some who have very good faces, and well proportioned, with great eyes, their beards well set, and their noses well shapen. But these are very few, and it may be that they are descended from other nations which of old times were mixed up with the Chinas" (Boxer 1953, 137). The moral valence of "good" faces reflected Renaissance aesthetics. Giovanni della Casa wrote that a gentleman should be "very desirous of beautiful things, well-proportioned and comely" (Plumb 1961, 314–315). Those among the Chinese who were "well-proportioned," da Cruz speculated, descended from non-Chinese. According to de Rada, "The people of Taybin are all, on the one hand, white and well-built, and when they are small children they are very fair, but when they grow up they become ugly" (Boxer 1953, 282).[1]

Mendoza recognized greater variety: "Those of the province of Canton . . . be browne in colour like to the Moores, but those that be farther within the countrie be like unto Almaines, Italians and Spanyardes, white and redde, and somwhat swart."[2] Mendoza, a Spaniard, compared certain "swarthy" Chinese with himself, drawing additional parallels with Muslim groups and other Europeans. He added, "Both men and women of this countrie are of a good disposition of their bodies, well proportioned and gallant men, somewhat tall, they are all for the most part brode faced, little eyes and flat noses" (Mendoza 1588, 19). Mundy, who had read Mendoza, commented that "swart coullour" derived from living "allmost under the tropicke of Cancer (allthough there bee amongst them many handsome Faces and proper men)"—"swart" otherwise suggesting unattractiveness (Mundy 1919, 261–262). He sketched some of the people he observed (see Figure 4). Like Mundy, Ricci attributed differences in Chinese skin color to sun exposure, and he cataloged the shape of the head and face, the color of hair and eyes, and the structure of people's features. Such descriptions gradually became formulaic.

The nearest even the most elite Europeans came to embodied Chinese were painted figures, like Henry VIII's "Cup of Purselaine glasse fation with two handles" (Honour 1961, 37) or Queen Elizabeth's breakfast set. The first Chinese porcelain shop in London opened by 1609, selling blue-and-white trade ware manufactured for overseas markets, and influencing ceramic design in Europe and Mexico. Representations of the Chinese turned theatrical, as when English king James I sponsored a masque to entertain the French ambassador in 1604. One eyewitness wrote, "On New Yeares night we had a . . . maske brought in by a magicien of China. There was a heaven built at the lower end of the hall, owt of which our magicien came down and after he had made a long sleepy speech to the king of the nature of the cuntry from whence he came comparing it with owrs for strength and plenty, he sayde he had broughte in cloudes certain Indian and China Knights to see the magnificency of this court" (Appleton 1951, 65). Freighted with heavy costumes and jewels, the actors could barely move, illustrating China's imagined wealth. Everything about the Chinese was fabricated, evident in the manifestation of "China Knights" through magic arts.

Occasionally Chinese converts accompanied Jesuits to Europe for further education. Some, like Zheng Manuo (renamed Emmanuel de Seuqera, d. 1673), became fluent in European languages. He traveled with Fr. Alexandre de Rhodes to Rome, becoming a novice in 1651.

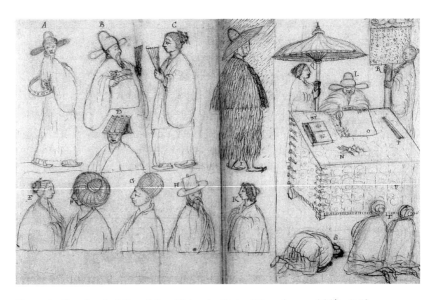

Figure 4. Sundry habits of the Chinois. Peter Mundy, ca. 1637. (MS Rawl.A315, between fol. 144ᵛ and 145ʳ.) Courtesy of the Bodleian Library, Oxford University.

After studying rhetoric, logic, natural theology, and metaphysics, he taught grammar and human letters to European students for three years. After fifteen years in Europe, he returned to China, serving as a missionary until his death. Zheng embodied Jesuit objectives of the Christianized *literatus* (Rouleau 1959).

Zheng Mane, a Chinese protégé, accompanied Martini to Rome. They met astronomer Jacobus Golius (1596–1667) in Leiden, and discussed the Chinese "twelve branches" and "twenty-four seasons" that Golius had encountered in the work of Arabic alchemists (Needham 1954, 38). Zheng studied at the Collegium Romanum in Rome, becoming a Jesuit. Boym also brought to Rome two young Chinese men, Andreas Xu and Joseph Ko; he and Xu returned to China (Zhang 1996; Xu 1996). Yet such encounters were so infrequent that most Europeans met the Chinese only through accounts by foreign observers, including representations of bodies, healing, and medicine.

The Medical Marketplace

European medical books included *practica* that critiqued learned physicians and provided easy-to-use diagnoses and treatments. Reformer-physician Nicholas Culpeper (1616–1645) advocated writing in the vernacular, as he did in his own *Directory for Midwives* (1651a), *Astrological Judgment of Diseases* (1651b), and *Pharmacopoeia Londinensis* (1653). Nor were physicians the only healers. There were "wise women, astrologers, herbalists, uroscopists, empirics, apothecaries, barber-surgeons, physicians, or specialists like tooth-drawers" (Wear 1995, 232). Itinerant vendors sold medicines, removed cataracts, or cut out tumors, some vending in public markets with hired street performers. The "mountebank" recited a cure's virtues, sometimes swallowing poison and then curing himself (Cook 1997).

Europeans in China witnessed analogous pluralism, set amid expanding urbanization and transportation networks. The printing of Chinese vernacular literature had exploded. Anyone who wished to become a physician could claim that status, provided he could attract patients (Cullen 1993). Some learned through state-sponsored programs, some through family lineages, and some as autodidacts. Women generally acquired medical knowledge through their families (Leung 2003). Some physicians wrote case histories, drawing attention to their authors' expertise (see Furth 1999; Grant 1998). Men sometimes became doctors after failing civil service examinations. Ricci observed,

> There are no public schools for this art, rather each person is individually taught by whatever master he chooses. In both courts [Beijing and Nanjing] after an examination degrees are granted in medicine, but as if in passing, and without conferring any advantage, since one who is honored with a degree in medicine acquires no greater authority or reputation than one who is not, because no one is prevented from treating the sick, whether he be knowledgeable or ignorant of medicine. Finally, it is known by all that no one studies mathematics or medicine who believes he can excel in moral philosophy. (Ricci and Trigault 1616, 48–49)

This statement reflected the diminished status of physicians, related to reduced state support during the Ming. Patients sought opinions not only from literati physicians, but also from illiterate ambulatory practitioners and diviners, who also healed sores, practiced acupuncture and moxibustion, and made mannequins for sympathetic magical use (Cullen 1993).

Transmission of Western medical practice was limited. The Jesuits sent few physicians, because they did not view medicine as a vehicle for missionizing. One exception—the Santa Casa da Misericórdia's St. Raphael Hospital, founded in Macao in 1569 by Mgr. Melchior Carneiro (ca. 1519–1583)—included a leprosy ward. The hospital integrated Chinese medicine into its practice early on, possibly due to the Jesuits' having been impressed by Chinese pulse diagnosis and extensive herbal repertoire (Standaert 2001). Generally, however, Portuguese missionaries provided care primarily for other Portuguese. One lay brother, who worked in the *botica* (pharmacy) of the Jesuit College of Macao in 1625, complained that he did not have medical training but was expected to care for the six hundred Portuguese citizens. He complained, too, that many of the Chinese or part-Chinese wives of the Portuguese preferred their own healing systems (Boxer 1974).

Fr. Giulio Aleni (1582–1649) described European medical training and charitable institutions, such as hospitals and orphanages, in his *Zhifang waiji* (Chronicle of Non-Tributary Countries, 1623), *Xixue fan* (Summary of Western Learning, 1623), and *Xifang dawen* (Questions and Answers Regarding the West, 1637). Ricci converted official Xu Guangji, baptizing Xu's daughter as Candida (1607–1680). Widowed at thirty, Candida took up charity work and established a foundling hospital and orphanage, both of which were in keeping with Chinese traditions.

Preservatives against All Sicknesses and Infirmities

Ricci compared Chinese *materia medica* with Europe's: "They use medicines, simples, herbs, roots, and the like. In fact, the whole of Chinese medicine is almost contained in the precepts of our own botanicals" (Ricci and Trigault 1616, 48). In Europe, Dioscorides remained influential, even as travelers collected plants, raising the number of known herbs from several hundred in the late fifteenth century to thousands a century later. Travel narratives provided descriptions of Asian plants. New herbal works appeared, like Otto Brunfel's *Herbarum vivae eicones* (Living Images of Plants, 1530), distinguished by Hans Weiditz's detailed woodcuts. Much as Reformation theology stressed direct access to God's Word, and anatomists stressed direct observation of the body, so botanists strove for fidelity to nature, seen as God's work (Stannard 1999).

The Jesuits collected Chinese books, including medical works like those brought by de Rada to Manila and cataloged by Mendoza.

> Manie herbals or books of herbes for phisitions, shewing how they should be applied to heale infirmities.
>
> Manie other bookes of physicke and medicine, compiled by authors of that kingdome, of antiquitie and of late dates, containing in them the maner how to use the sicke, and to heale them of their sicknes, and to make preservatives against all sicknesses and infirmities. (Mendoza 1588, 104)

Mendoza added that such books had been "interpreted by persons naturally borne in China, and brought up in Philippinas with the Spaniardes that dwell there" (105). Still, not everyone supported the value of Chinese medicinal learning. De Rada conceded that Chinese practitioners knew the properties of herbs, but said that "there is nothing to get hold of, since they have nothing more than the smell or shadow of the substance" (Boxer 1953, 295).

Production of Chinese *materia medica* texts flourished during the fifteenth and sixteenth centuries. Many such texts were produced by private individuals distilling content from earlier *materia medica,* transmitting home remedies, or writing about the fruits of fieldwork. A few resulted from governmental initiatives, although these were not considered authoritative. Encyclopedic works, like naturalist Li Shizhen's (1518–1593) *Bencao gangmu* (The Systematic Materia Medica, 1596), impressed foreign observers, but the shorter, eclectic works were more convenient and popular among Chinese practitioners (Unschuld 1986a). Michael Boym may have drawn on such works, merging them with a new European genre, the *flora* (works cataloging plants from particular regions). Boym's brief *Flora sinensis* (1656), for example, described and illustrated selected Chinese plants and animals, including their medicinal uses.

A few Jesuits prepared tracts for the Chinese about drugs and practices used in Europe. Sabatino De Ursis (1575–1620) wrote about distillation mechanisms for preparing aromatic essences for medicines. Giulio Aleni's *Xifang dawen* (1637) described other Western methods. Ricci also communicated with well-known physician Wang Kengang (1553–1612), and discussed European diagnostic uroscopy with physician Cheng Lun (fl. 1621), who then wrote about it (Standaert 2001).

Noble and Delicate Medicines

Although Chinese physicians like Wang Ji (1463–1539) commonly used more than 120 drugs (Grant 1998), Europeans generally recognized only a handful—primarily those, like camphor, also used in Europe. D'Orta (1563, 60) characterized camphor as "noble and delicate" and as generally unknown to the ancient Greeks, "except Aetius among the moderns, although the vulgar and common examples of Serapion allege, falsely, the authority of Dioscorides of which there are two species." The Chinese sort, shipped to Europe in small cakes, he added, was inferior.

D'Orta fretted over whether "canella," "cinnamon," or "cassia" was the true cinnamon, turning for advice to Chinese and Persian traders. Boym simply extolled its virtues: "It cures colic and winds, provokes urine, fortifies the heart, liver, spleen, nerves, brain, and even serves against the bites and poison of serpents, excites the appetite, preserves one from epilepsy; from its fruit they make an unguent for cold fluxions; when one burns it, it renders a very agreeable odor, cinnamon powder drunk with water cures the bites of vipers, extinguishes kidney inflammations, and being used with things that soften, it removes spots from the face" (Boym 1656, R). D'Orta also described Chinese galangal, "lavandou," a small aromatic shrub with leaves like a myrtle, propagated from roots. "If you find anything written to the contrary," he cautioned, "don't you believe it. For Avicenna, Serapion, and other Arabs only had confused accounts" (Boxer 1963, 16).

Europeans began cultivating ginger as far north as Paris. In 1530 the Spanish introduced it to Mexico, where it so flourished that by the end of that century Mexico exported ten times what Asian countries shipped to Europe (Lach 1977). Ricci described ginger's aromatic properties, availability, and quality in China, while Boym explained that Chinese doctors administered a strong decoction to induce a sweat. Ginger treated gout, and those who took it in the morning could not be poisoned that day. Some made a preserve, a proven remedy against cold-damage stomach disorders (Boym 1656).

Da Cruz described tea, "a kind of warm water which they call *cha,* which is somewhat red and very medicinal . . . made from a concoction of somewhat bitter herbs; with this they commonly welcome all manner of persons . . . and to me they offered it many times" (Boxer 1953, 140). Ricci speculated that ancient Chinese could not have known the drink, because he found no character for it in old books, and that it might be native to Europe. "It is not unpleasant to the taste," he added, "being somewhat bitter, and it is usually considered to be wholesome, even if taken frequently" (Ricci 1942, 17). Mundy (1919, 191) also described *chaa,* "which is only water with a kind of herb boyled in itt. It must bee Drancke warme and is accompted wholesome." Dutch physician Nicolas Tulpius (1593–1674) wrote about tea's medicinal qualities; in 1648 Jean-Armand de Mauvillain (dates unknown)—Richelieu's godson, Molière's friend, and professor of botanicals on the Faculty of Medicine of Paris—wrote the first medical thesis on tea, *An the chinesium menti confert* (Huard and Wong 1966).

Rhubarb, a purgative, addressed humoral imbalances. European traders sought seeds or plants, especially the "true" Chinese rhubarb described by Polo. Boym included it in his *Flora sinensis* (see Figure 5). D'Orta (1563) commented, "This drug, which is produced only in

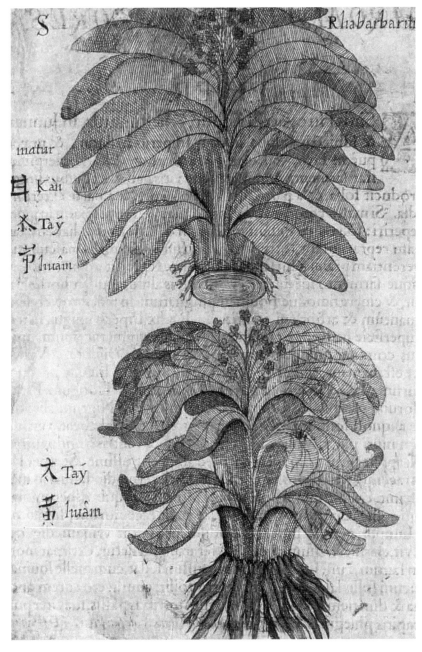

Figure 5. Rhubarb. Michael Boym, *Flora sinensis,* 1656. Courtesy of the
Boston Medical Library in the Francis A. Countway Library of Medicine.

China, is shipped thence in Chinese vessels to India. But rhubarb is also conveyed from China overland through Tartary to Ormuz and Aleppo from whence it reaches Alexandria and Venice. When coming this way the drug is less subject to become wormeaten" (207). Sixteenth-century herbals generally concurred that the best rhubarb originated in China, even as they realized there were multiple types (see Foust 1992).

One drug in particular—"China root" or "China"—drew attention in 1535 when Spain's Carlos V recovered from gout after taking some brought by the Portuguese. D'Orta described it as a remedy for syphilis, as did physician Amato Lusitano when Portuguese sailors brought him a specimen in 1549 (Lach 1977). Yet two drugs were often called by this name, complicating the identification. D'Orta may have been thinking of either a fungus called *fuling* or a plant called *Smilax China*. Ricci (1942) described "that famous remedy for many diseases, called Chinese wood by the Portuguese and Sacred Wood by others. It grows freely in barren parts and without cultivation, and may be exported at high price" (16). Boym called it *pe-fo-lim* (possibly *fuling*). The Chinese preferred the white to the red, he wrote, eating the pulp in meat broth, and using it to treat sciatica, kidney problems, paralysis, and sore bones, and to dry all sorts of humors. "They believe that the powder of this root, with sugar, is good for the chest, and that the conserve has the same effect" (Boym 1656, T).

"China wood" entered European *materia medica*. The *Pharmacopoeia Londinensis Collegarum* (Royal College of Physicians of London 1655), for example, listed it along with galangal and rhubarb. Robert Burton (1577–1640), author of *The Anatomy of Melancholy*, recommended it. "China, saith Manardus, makes a good color in the face, takes away melancholy, and all infirmities proceeding from cold" (Burton [1621]1977, 257).[3] Culpeper (1653) observed that it "wonderfully extenuateth and drieth, provoketh sweat, resisteth putrification, it strengthens the Liver, helps the Dropsie and malignant Ulcers, Leprosie, Itch, and French-pocks, and is profitable in Diseases coming of fasting" (5). Small wonder that Ricci characterized it as "famous."

Boym's *Flora sinensis* also included date palms, areca, and pepper. The first counteracted snake venom and was the greatest of cardiac remedies if drunk with water in which it had steeped. Areca, or betel, strengthened the stomach. (Boym said he had omitted images of both because they were in most European herbals.) "Pepper," he wrote, "is hot, and provokes urine. It helps digestion, is a resolvent, clears one's vision, and is good against the bite of savage beasts. Mixed with laurel leaves, it helps women deliver their fruit when it has died . . . taken with raisins, it gently purges the water from the testicles" (Boym [1656]1730, 1, 24).

The first observer to mention ginseng appears to have been Alvaro de Semedo (1643, 1655), who also discussed camphor, China root, and rhubarb. In *Atlas sinensis*, Martini mentioned "the most celebrated ginseng, the most noble root in all of China" (Bretschneider 1881, 18–19). There is some speculation that the Dutch may have identified a North American version and shipped it down the Hudson to Amsterdam and then London, selling it to the British East India Company "at a 500-percent profit" prior to 1664 (Goldstein 1978, 22).

Ricci (1942, 11) noted those who ate no meat, "either because they are forced to do so by reason of poverty or because they embrace this course of life for some religious motive."[4] He had in mind Buddhist vegetarianism, although he was right that vegetables were the primary dietary option for the poor. Yet vegetables were also included among medicines. Li Shizhen, for example, attributed restorative, calming effects to the fragrant leek, which he also said eliminated stomach fevers (Mote 1977). European herbals, too, commonly listed vegetables like asparagus, useful as a diuretic.

Although specific Chinese animal-based medicines might have been unfamiliar to Europeans, they would have appeared conceptually comprehensible. European *materia medica* included "worms, foxes' lungs, lozenges of dried vipers, oil of wolves, moss from the skull of a victim of a violent death, and crabs' eyes" (Margotta 1967, 193). Few European physicians would have questioned Chinese uses of insects, snakes, and fish. "Dragon" bones—fossilized bones of prehistoric animals—were roasted, powdered, and used for "gaseous distension of the stomach and abdomen, for stoppage and alterations of the bowels, for paralysis of the extremities, for night sweats and frightening dreams, to contract the penis . . . quiet the mind and . . . dispel noxious influences, such as devil possession and spells" (Read 1977, 8). Boym's *Flora sinensis* (1656) described musk, which facilitated delivery, benefited the chest, and cleansed bad humors. "I have drawn these properties and what I have said here from Chinese books themselves, and their dictionaries" (27).

Then there was *lo-meo-quei,* a crab found principally in Hunan; when drunk powdered with wine, it stopped stomach flux, and with vinegar, the bloody flux. It cured eye problems, eased fevers, and countered poison (27). *Gen-to,* a large serpent, devoured whole deer. Its skin was prized for treating eye afflictions. The head of another serpent contained a stone that cured otherwise deadly bites from that same serpent. "This stone is round, white in the middle, and outside is blue or green, as soon as one applies it to the bite, it attaches itself, and does not fall until it has drawn out the poison. One washes it afterwards in milk, and leaves it for some time, to cause it to recover its natural state" (29). A third, highly poisonous, snake was put, still alive, in a vessel of wine. Only the head protruded, to make it vent its venom. One then removed the head, boiling the body in the wine for an excellent remedy against poison.

Hearbs Medicinable and Profitable

Diplomats, traders, and missionaries sought trade openings, promoting the cross-fertilization of medicine traditions. Some European observers gave readers glimpses into the commerce of Chinese medicines. Mendoza (1588) wrote: "Such merchants as do keepe shoppes . . . they have a table or signe hanging at their doore, whereon is written all such merchandise as is within to be sold . . . The Apothecarie that selleth simples, hath the like table" (22). Sometimes, the sign was a dried calabash—also the crucible of Daoist elixirs. There were fortunes to be made, Mendoza suggested. "There are also many herbs for medicines, as very fine Reubarbe, and of great quantitie, and wood called Palo de china [China wood] . . . I do leave to speake of many other hearbs medicinable and profitable for the use of man, for that if I should write the particular vertue of everie of them, it would require a great vollume" (9). Ricci (1942) located rhubarb in the context of history and economics, assigning it Western origins: "China is rich in medicinal herbs which are known elsewhere only as importations. Rhubarb and musk were first brought in from the West by the Saracens, and after spreading throughout the whole of Asia, they were exported to Europe at an almost unbelievable profit. Here you can buy a pound of rhubarb for ten cents, which in Europe would cost six or seven times as many gold pieces" (16).

As the collection and study of plants flourished, so did great gardens of living specimens. Hérouard, First Physician to Louis XIII, founded Paris's "Jardin des Plantes" (Garden of Plants) in 1626 as an educational resource. In 1640 Louis XIII appointed three professors from the Faculty of Medicine to lecture at the garden on botany, pharmacology, and chemistry, renaming it the "Jardin Royal des Plantes médicinales." Jesuits were among the most active collectors.

Of Vitalisms, Spirits, and Souls

Some Chinese herbal medicine drew on empirical experience without explicit theory, but much of what literate practitioners used was rooted in the *qi* paradigm. One could argue that parallel developments in European vitalism might have disposed foreign observers to be curious about Chinese theories, were it not for reactions from the Catholic Church, which informed Jesuit understandings of *qi*. So how did the foreign observers interpret Chinese theories, and in relation to which Western medical and religious constructs?

Sixteenth-century European vitalist theories existed in tension with the growing power of the anatomically read body. The strongest challenge to Galen came from Flemish researcher-physician Andreas Vesalius (1514–1564). Vesalius's *De humani corporis fabrica libri septem* (Seven Books on the Structure of the Human Body, 1543) acquired renown almost immediately because of its detailed observations and the precision of its woodcuts. The very materiality and replicability of anatomical dissection made its observations seem indisputable, overshadowing the reality that Vesalius had studied physical structures to understand the enlivened form and the soul. Chinese models, based in *qi*, would suffer by comparison.

William Harvey's (1578–1657) work would exercise an equally disproportionate influence on European judgments about *qi* and meridian theory. In 1628, Harvey, a reader in surgery and anatomy at London's St. Bartholomew's Hospital, published *Exercitatio anatomica de motu cordis et sanguinis in animalibus* (An Anatomical Exercise on the Motion of the Heart and Blood in Animals). Having studied with renowned anatomist and surgeon Hieronymus Fabricius of Aquapendente (1533–1619), Harvey shared Aristotle's interest in the animal (as in *anima*) soul, whose central organ was the heart. *De motu cordis* detailed how blood flowing through the heart became, alternately, venous and arterial. Harvey's work also explored *spiritus,* arguing that blood *is* spirit: "So there is a spirit, or a certain force, inherent in the blood . . . and the nature, yea, the soul in this spirit and blood is identical with the essence of the stars" (Hay 1993, 192).

Some of these formulations entered China. Physician-turned-Jesuit Johann Schreck (1576–1630) wrote *Taixi renshen shugai* (Abstract of the Western Theory of the Human Body, ca. 1625), summarizing recent Western ideas, possibly informed by Vesalius. Physician Bi Gongchen (d. 1644) published it in around 1634. Of the few Western anatomical tracts prepared for Chinese readers, most remained in manuscript form, but Jesuit religio-philosophical works discussing human physiology in relation to the soul, to Galen, or to the nervous system, were more often published (see Standaert 2001, 790–791).

The impact of Western theory on Chinese thinking about blood and *qi* was minimal. As early as Confucius it was held that blood and *qi* converge, constituting one's *shen,* or mind-spirit—the life in a person. Meridian pulses manifested the state of one's *shen.* As Shigehisa Kuriyama (1999) observes, "In Chinese medicine, blood and *qi* were essentially the same. Doctors did, to be sure, occasionally spotlight distinctions . . . But all these represented differences in aspect, not essence. Ultimately, blood and *qi* were complementary facets of a unique vitality, its yin and yang manifestations" (229). Neither Galenic notions of *aer* permeating the blood or of *pneuma/spiritus,* nor Harvey's equating blood with spirit, was identical to Chinese blood and *qi.* Yet superficial resemblance would persuade European observers that they knew what the Chinese meant; the underlying differences would generate lasting, and sometimes willful, misinterpretation.

The Jesuits, for example, first equated *qi* with *aer,* only gradually realizing that *qi* "constituted the very core of Chinese medical, cosmological, metaphysical, and moral discourses" (Zhang 1999, 76). Ricci (1942, 95) wrote, "The doctrine most commonly held among the Literati . . . asserts that the entire universe is composed of a common substance; that the creator of the universe is one in a continuous body . . . together with heaven and earth, men and beasts, trees and plants, and the four elements, and that each individual thing is a member of this body." Ricci was recalling the "Western Inscription" of Zhang Cai (1020–1077): "Heaven is my father and Earth is my mother, and even such a small creature as I finds an intimate place in their midst. Therefore that which fills the universe I regard as my body and that which directs the universe I consider as my nature" (Chan 1963, 497). The Jesuits rejected this perspective, which contradicted the doctrine of a Creator distinct from Creation. Humans were made in the *image* of God, *not* of a common substance, except through the person of Christ. Church authorities who suspected Galen of denying the soul's immortality resolved the issue by redefining the soul as the driving force behind the *pneuma/spiritus*. The Jesuits rendered *qi* in corresponding terms. Ricci, borrowing Aristotelian notions of air, made *qi* one of the four elements composing the material world. It was, he then argued, the immortal soul that caused *qi* to circulate (Zhang 1999).

Ricci translated *wuxing*, or "Five Phases," as "Five Elements," criticizing the Chinese for adding an element. He blamed the Buddhists, claiming they had borrowed the Western theory of four but had erroneously omitted air while adding metal and wood. Moreover, only in alchemy did one element become another. He ignored *wuxing* "elements" as metaphors for different aspects of change, the transmutation of one into another being intrinsic to the paradigm. Herein lay critical barriers to Europeans' ability to grasp the inner logic of Chinese medical thought, as both *qi* and Five Phase models provided conceptual frameworks for determining the causes and stages in illness.

Other developments in European vitalism would repeatedly inform later Western readings of Chinese vitalism. Reflecting religious loyalties, René Descartes (1596–1650) critiqued the argument that the soul died with the body, a position also opposed by the Lateran Council, which "expressly enjoined Christian philosophers to refute their arguments" (Michael 2000, 157). To prove the soul's immortality, Descartes insisted on its qualitative difference from the body. Instead, he imagined the body as a "machine" directed by the immortal, nonmaterial soul (French 1989)—a position congruent with Ricci's differentiation of *qi* and the soul. By "machine," Descartes meant that the body's "nature can be characterized mathematically, so that the laws that govern it are mathematical" (Voss 2000, 179). Such laws were imprinted in both human souls and the natural world, unifying all reality. This radical body/soul differentiation supported Church teachings. Neither could accommodate a *qi*-based paradigm.

Moreover, Christian doctrine required a single immortal soul, whereas the Chinese held that, as an expression of *yin* and *yang*, a person consisted of corporeal and ethereal aspects. Souls followed suit. *Po* souls were corporeal, *yin* in nature and present in the body from birth. They entered the ground with the corpse. Should they not receive correct burial, food, or grave maintenance, they became hungry and disturbed, afflicting the living as *gui*—ghosts or demons. Ethereal *hun,* or *yang,* souls entered the body after birth. Following death, *hun* souls both ascended to Heaven and entered ancestor tablets on a family or clan altar. One honored the *hun* souls, represented by the tablets, inviting their help and protection as *shen,* or kindly spirits, with *shen* also referring to the essential quality of all deities. Between *po* and *hun,* a person possessed ten souls. No amount of Christian revisionism could accommodate this anthropology.

Still other European thinkers investigated vitalist forces that were understood to be both supernatural and natural, including holy powers, the stars, witchcraft, and other forces hidden or "occult." Natural forces included magnetism, which physician William Gilbert (1540–1603) discussed in his *De magnete* ([1600]1958, 160). Gilbert concluded that the earth is a great magnet, "endowed with a primordial and . . . an energic form" (105). Magnets, he argued, are animate, like a soul, as are the world, the planets, and the stars. He cited magnets' medicinal virtues, emphasizing those from China: "Gartias ab Horto [Garcia d'Orta] does not think [magnets] injurious or unwholesome . . . Pure loadstone may also be harmless; and not only that, but many correct excessive humors of the bowels and putrescence of the same, and may bring about a better temperature, such loadstones are the Oriental ones from China" (3, 18, 52–53). Western theorists began to imagine magnetism as a subtle, vital fluid. Over time, as they struggled to understand how practices like acupuncture worked, "magnetic fluid" would provide a persisting analogy, gaining particular currency in the nineteenth century.

On Systems of Circulation and Needling

Assessing a person's *qi* could entail reading different meridian pulses, as part of a larger diagnostic repertoire that included the art of looking *(wang)*, listening and smelling *(wen)*, asking *(wen)*, and touching *(qie)*. Looking examined someone's physical condition, coloring, and tongue. Listening and smelling involved the patient's voice and odor. Asking elicited the illness's symptoms and phases. Touching involved pulse taking. Ricci wrote, "The precepts of medicine in China are in no small way different from our own," quickly adding, "but they do not feel the pulse or beating of the veins [differently] than we do. And certainly they are equally felicitous in medicine" (Ricci and Trigault 1616, 48–49).

As we have seen, earlier versions of the meridians provided the foundation for bloodletting and acupuncture. Yet knowledge of this network did not derive from anatomical dissection, which would have violated the Confucian prohibition against harming the body bestowed by one's parents. In his *Zhenjiu wendi* (Questions and answers on acupuncture and moxa, 1530), physician Wang Ji criticized his contemporaries for their ignorance of both acupuncture and bloodletting: "Physicians of old gave first place [in their therapies] to the needle, the stone, and to moxa. Drugs were secondary. Nowadays . . . acupuncture is used in less than one case in a hundred. As for the stone, the tradition is quite lost" (Cullen 1993, 120). Yet even Wang critiqued acupuncture as potentially depleting.

In 1628, Jacob de Bondt, Danish surgeon general of the Dutch East India Company, also commented on the practice. His notes (published as *Historiae naturalis & medicae Indiae*, 1658) read: "The results (with acupuncture) in Japan . . . surpass even miracles. For chronic pains of the head, for obstructions of the liver and spleen, and also for pleurisy, they bore through (the flesh) with a stylus made of silver or bronze and not much thicker than the strings of a lyre. The stylus should be driven slowly and gently through the above-mentioned vitals so as to emerge from another part, as I myself have seen in Java" (Lu and Needham 1980, 270). Yet de Bondt said nothing about *qi* or pulse diagnosis.

Wang Ji had also alluded to moxa, or moxibustion: "Nowadays, moxibustion is only applied in *fengbi* 'Wind [Heteropathy] Blockage' . . . or in *urgent* cases" (Cullen 1993, 120).[5] Wang's case reports included patients treated with acupuncture or moxa by other practitioners, who, he argued, worsened their conditions. Wang told one patient that the combination had "scorched the bones, harmed the muscles, and contributed to the depletion of the blood" (Grant 1998, 60). In Europe, cautery and therapeutic heat remained common. Fabricius of Aquapendente (1649) commented, "Masué and Albucasis consider this remedy particularly suited for cold and moist illnesses of the head, such as headaches, vertigo, dizziness, cephalalgy, limpness, paralysis, and other similar ills proceeding from the retention of said humors in the head" (505). Over time, Western surgeons would take an interest in moxibustion.

The absence of acupuncture and moxa from most reports prior to 1660 may be related to acupuncture's increased identification with illiterate, lower-class practitioners in China. Ricci did not mention it, leaving us to wonder whether he witnessed it or, if he did, whether he thought it beneath mention. In the popular 1618 erotic novel *Jinpingmei* (The Plum in the Golden Vase; Roy 1993), Liu Pozi, "Old Woman Liu," used acupuncture and moxibustion. One male character called her an old whore who would "stick in needles and cauterize you at random." Learning that she had treated his son with moxibustion, he threatened her with "the finger squeeze torture." Liu Pozi also practiced pulse reading, prescribed medications, and sometimes provided diagnostic spirit mediumship. It is noteworthy that the women of the household preferred her to a local scholar physician (Cullen 1993, 127–128).

One episode suggests that Europeans might have encountered Chinese acupuncture in Mexico. In 1635, Spanish barbers petitioned Mexico City's municipal council, protesting the "excesses" of Chinese competitors. The *cabildo* proposed that Chinese barbers relocate to the suburbs to reduce competition (Dubs and Smith 1942). Ambulatory practitioners in China, like barbers, practiced minor surgery, for which some used the nine needles. Given the presence of Chinese barbers in Mexico, it is probable that they and like practitioners provided such therapies.

Dressed in Chinese Robes

The Jesuits initially assumed that Buddhist monks occupied the role closest to their own, and donned Buddhist robes—only to discover that many literati despised the monks. The priests quickly adopted scholars' robes. Boym reflected the strategy, writing, "Here I am, dressed in Chinese robes, in the same manner that our Fathers appear in public" ([1652]1694, 1). Indeed, Christian priesthood intersected with different religious categories in China, confusing prospective converts. Erik Zürcher suggests that, as scholars and moral teachers, Jesuits resembled literati. Yet they were also technological experts. The Chinese viewed these two roles as incompatible. Priests looked like charismatic preachers, instructing followers in how to live. When they marked converts' doors with texts or symbols, they resembled sectarian leaders who throughout Chinese history had led popular uprisings. Finally, they looked like *daoshi* (masters of the Way), who transmitted sacred power, commanded esoteric rituals and texts, dispensed protective and healing spells and amulets, and exorcised demons. Fr. Étienne Faber, for example, "possessed the gift of healing; succeeded in warding off an invasion of grasshoppers by sprinkling them with holy water; exorcised haunted houses; foresaw the precise date of his own death; his corpse did not decay, his tomb was spared by a river in flood and after his death he was transformed into a god of the Local Soil" (Zürcher 1990, 425). Christian priests condemned Buddhists as superstitious, but then donned vestments, performed rites before an altar, and worked wonders and exorcisms.

Churches contributed to the confusion, as many were former mansions of wealthy donors and some were converted temples. Trigault wrote of one such site:

> In the main hall there was a very large altar, made of stone and of brick
> . . . As is customary in the temples, the color of the altar was red . . .
> Over the middle of the altar there was seated a horrible looking monster in clay, but gilded all over from head to foot . . . After removing them from their altars in the former temple, the clay idols were reduced to dust and the wooden ones consigned to flames . . . The altar of the gods was dismantled and the pictures on the wall were whitewashed. A place was then prepared, above a new altar, for a picture of Christ the Saviour, beautifully painted by one of the [Chinese] Lay Brothers . . . Beside the public church and the funeral chapel, the Fathers erected another altar, dedicated to the Blessed Virgin . . . [and] had two Chinese written characters inscribed on the architrave of the main entrance . . . reading, "Royal Munificence," a title held in high esteem by the Chinese. (Ricci and Trigault 1616, 489–502)

The ambiguities were patent. Dust from the "idols" was eventually used to make cement for Ricci's tomb, encasing the body of the priest. Although hidden, the older pictures on the walls remained. Titles with prior religious associations were applied to the Virgin. The church retained its former structure, making it potentially difficult to draw absolute distinctions between older practices and Christian ones, even as the missionaries imposed a supersessionist message by converting the site.

Not surprisingly, hybrid practices emerged among Chinese Christians. Zürcher (1990) describes Jesuit Giulio Aleni (Ai Rulue), who reached Fuzhou in 1625, converting a circle of literati. They in turn illustrate six aspects of local acculturation, many related to healing. The first involved the "appearance and strange qualities of auspicious objects," as when the Holy Name, written on a piece of paper, cured smallpox, or a Christian book emitted light and toppled idols—stories with Buddhist and Daoist parallels. Second, Chinese converts sometimes had visions while ill, in coma-like states, or dreaming, of texts predicting someone's death or providing visions of God. Third, converts claimed to have been rescued by prayer or reliquaries from otherwise fatal sicknesses and disasters. The fourth included revivals from temporary death, followed by descriptions from beyond the grave (a popular narrative device in Chinese religious and fictional literature). The fifth involved miraculous healings attributed to prayers, holy water, scripture chanting, reliquaries, and destroying paper gods. The patient had generally exhausted other possibilities, only to find efficacy in Christian strategies—even Christian versions of Chinese practices, like burning paper figures. The final type involved exorcism. Usually the local exorcist had proved unable to expel the demon. The patient's Christian relatives, friends, and neighbors assembled crucifix, candles, holy water, reliquaries, and the Holy Name written on paper, instructing the afflicted in how to pray, confess sins, and be healed. The victim then converted. Trance, possession, and spirit writing—staples in stories of mediums—were reconfigured, the converts' deity proving stronger than the demons. Such stories explain why some local authorities suspected missionaries of fomenting heterodox cults and sowing seeds of rebellion.

In turn, missionaries drew artificially absolute boundaries between what the Chinese called *sanjiao,* or "three teachings," reifying these as

Confucianism, Buddhism, and Daoism. Ricci construed them as three distinct cults, with literati primarily involved in the Confucian cult (Paper 1995). Claiming that Chinese classics showed evidence of monotheism, the missionaries invented an early Christian religious impulse in China that they said had been lost due to book burnings during the Qin (221–207 BCE) and to Buddhist corruptions. The missionaries failed to grasp the interconnectedness of the three teachings, arguments from the Chinese notwithstanding. Ricci (1942) complained, "The most commonly accepted opinion of those who are at all educated among the Chinese is, that these three laws or cults really coalesce into one creed and that all of them can and should be believed. In such a judgment of course, they are leading themselves and others into the very distracting error of believing that the more different ways there are of talking about religious questions, the more beneficial it will be for the public good" (105). By honoring "three laws," he thought, the Chinese could not follow any of them authentically and could only fall "into the deepest depths of utter atheism" (105). Chinese scholars found this perspective difficult to fathom. Thinker Li Zhi (1527–1602) wrote of Ricci, "He is an altogether remarkable man . . . But I do not know why he has come here . . . I considered that he wanted to take his learning to transform our teachings of the Duke of Zhou and Confucius. But that would be too foolish—that surely can't be it!" (Waltner 1994, 422–423).[6] Yet this was precisely the missionaries' objective, and it biased every observation of Chinese healing practices that stood outside of what they narrowly classified as "religion" and "medicine."

The Idols They Do Worship

Mendoza (1588) wrote, "I do prosecute . . . the idols they do worship" (39). The Catholic Church viewed Christian iconography as consistent with the incarnation of God. The issue lay with how "idol" was defined. Biblical prophets had described idolatry as worship where the image itself becomes the object of devotion. For the Jesuits, God had taken a single form, in the person of Jesus. Referring to any other image in relation to God could only be false. In contrast, from the Chinese perspective, if Heaven and Earth are of a single substance, then one can encounter the Way of Heaven, the Dao, in anything from a figurine to the most mundane reality.

Gods populated China's landscape. Tombs of local worthies sometimes became shrines. If healings and other miracles ensued, regional magistrates might declare the deceased divine. If his fame spread, he might come to the emperor's attention, receiving further honors. Chinese gods, that is, had at one time been humans. Their shifting status reflected a fluid reality, permitting transformations from human to ancestor, and from ancestor to ghost or to god, as in the story of the young drunkard Liulang.

Liulang drowned while inebriated. His ghost met a fisherman who, not recognizing his companion's real nature, shared wine with him each night. In return, Liulang drove fish into the fisherman's nets. Eventually Liulang worked off his unfortunate karma, becoming ready for rebirth. He alerted the fisherman that a woman would replace him when she drowned while crossing the river. The woman appeared as anticipated, but carried a baby. She began to drown, then suddenly she pulled herself out and walked away. The following night, Liulang returned. He confessed to having spared the woman to prevent her baby's death. He would remain. Days later, however, he returned to announce that the Emperor of Heaven had rewarded his compassion by making him a local deity. Over time, he worked many miracles, including healings (P'u [1740]1925, 380–385).[7]

Local gods protected particular cities, which was especially important during epidemics. Although Chinese illness categories differed from those of Europe, it appears the Chinese suffered smallpox, pulmonary diseases, malarial fevers, other febrile illnesses, dysentery, and possibly the plague, along with scarlet fever, cholera, diphtheria, and syphilis (Leung 1993). The etiologies assigned to epidemics varied. Sometimes "noxious qi" was blamed, sometimes fears of demonic contagion, to the government's dismay, particularly when the sick turned to shamans—a widespread phenomenon during the Song dynasty. Some epidemics were explained by zhu, "the invasion of the body by one or more demons; these demons' transformation into or manifestation as worms; the transmission or sequential infestation of these demons, usually from corpse to living person; and in later accounts the contamination or infestation of not only the body, but the clothing, food, personal belongings, and surroundings of the victim. Zhu disorders['] . . . wide range of symptoms often include chills and fever, spitting up blood, confusion, wild speech or speechlessness, weakness, and a cumulative decline over some years leading to death" (Hinrichs n.d., 2–3). During the Song and Yuan periods, the state published pharmaceutical works, established infirmaries, distributed free medicine, set up charity pharmacies, and appointed medical staff. During the Ming, medical relief received less support, although the state recognized epidemics as public health crises. Local officials distributed medicine, or money to purchase it.

During the Qing, the Manchus set up "smallpox secretariats," banishing symptomatic individuals thirteen miles outside city walls (Leung 1987). The city god might also be processed through the streets, armed with charms, thunderous noise, and smoke to expel demons. In south China, "pacification of plagues" rituals involved sending miniature dragon boats onto rivers and streams and invoking spirits to receive offerings, capture plague deities, and force them onto the boats, which were then burned (Katz 1995). People also turned to deities identified with specific illnesses. Crossroad shrines were sometimes shared by the Princess of Multi-Colored Clouds, her son the God of Black Smallpox, and the two goddesses of measles. Because gods could both afflict and protect, people sought their help prophylactically and therapeutically. They also turned to the Buddha and bodhisattvas.[8] Both da Cruz and de Rada (Boxer 1953), for example, remarked on devotion to the bodhisattva Guanyin and other "Omitoffois."[9] Besides condemning such practices as idolatrous, the missionaries were mystified when Chinese supplicants vilified gods who failed to address petitions. Mendoza (1588, 32–33) reported worshippers "calling them dogs, infamous, villains, and other names like in effect." He did not understand that gods—as former human beings—worked within a celestial bureaucracy, where they petitioned superiors to get the ear of Heaven. Gods unable to fulfill requests were subject to dismissal (Hymes 2002).

Public religiosity as a response to epidemics was not unique to China. In Europe, civil authorities and the churches organized relief for the poor, sometimes providing physicians to visit the sick at the parish level. The Catholic Church sometimes provided hospitals, similar to hospices for the poor. As epidemics were still thought to signal a people's sinfulness (Protestants threw in popery and atheism), governments supported communal religious responses. Catholic communities processed saints' relics through their city and held public prayer. Protestant communities might dedicate themselves to days of prayer and self-mortification. Structurally, Chinese public religiosity so strongly resembled such practices that the missionaries could only lament what they viewed as further evidence of idolatry.

The Question of Immortality

Popular stories of *xianren* (immortals) reported transmuted earthly bodies overcoming death, with bones of gold and flesh of jade, feeding on air and dew in a celestial realm. The Jesuits viewed related practices as contaminated by association with the Daoists, whose teachings Ricci attributed to "the original parent of falsehoods, the father of lies." He described exercises aimed at extending life, "such as definite sitting positions accompanied by particular prayers and medicines, by use of which they promise their followers the favor of the gods and eternal life in heaven, or at least a longer life on earth" (Ricci 1942, 102–103).

Such exercises had a long history. A late fifth-century BCE jade pendant referred to *xingqi,* or "moving *qi.*" Mengzi (Mencius, 371–289 BCE) discussed cultivating his "floodlike *qi,*" while Zhuangzi said that "huffing and puffing, exhaling the old and inhaling the new, the bear pull and the bird stretch, is for long life and only that" (Holcombe 1993, 12). By the Han, these exercises appeared in silk-scroll paintings like those excavated at Mawangdui. They were still advocated by neo-Confucian Zhu Xi (1130–1200) during the Song dynasty.

Ricci also noted alchemical "medicines," or elixirs, aware that Europe had its own versions of alchemy. Intellectuals like the physician Theophrastus Aureolus Bombastus von Hohenheim (1482–1546) merged botanical, medical, religious, and alchemical interests. Styling himself "Paracelsus"—which means "exceeding" the Roman medical author Celsus—he viewed the world as replete with spiritual and vital forces, and explored alchemy for ways to treat illness and prolong life. In the American colonies, alchemy and astrology were technically illegal, which was no deterrent to their widespread use (Butler 1990). The problem for the Jesuits was that Chinese approaches to immortality lacked even a tenuous connection with Christian eternal life in Heaven. Ricci disagreed not with "immortality" itself, but with the form being pursued. It didn't help that court eunuchs lodged charges of espionage against him in 1598, after realizing he would not teach them alchemy.

Pantoja (1606) observed that, for extending life, "they take many medicines . . . there are many teachers and books about this error, that ordinarily are serious and wealthy people. There are many who pretend to be very old, whom people follow as they would saints to learn some prescripts for living" (121–122). Some people refused to believe the priests were as young as they claimed to be, convinced they were actually centenarians. The reason? "That we do not marry, because we would live long" (Purchas 1625, 382). In Daoist longevity practices, conserving semen preserved one's vital essence—the presumed rationale for Jesuit celibacy. In turn, Jesuits like Ricci voiced frustration that longevity practices engaged the literati. "This upper class . . . get the idea that there is nothing to be added to their perfect beatitude but the means of rendering their present state unending and themselves immortal. Therefore, they devote themselves entirely to the study of discovering the necessary means to this vainly coveted end. Here in the province of Pekin . . . there are few, if any, of the magistrates, of the eunuchs, or of others of high station, who are not addicted to this foolish pursuit" (Ricci 1942, 91). The deadlier outcome of such pursuits resulted from ingredients like cinnabar—a salt of mercury—in the elixirs. In theory, longevity disciplines refined the body beyond the need for earthly sustenance; in reality, reports of adepts' demise numbered emperors among the casualties.

Buddhism introduced yet another approach to transcending death. It taught that nothing about reality is unchanging or permanent, but that clearly something persists from one life to another, even if only the accrual of residual desires and unexpiated misdeeds. When the effects of such desires and misdeeds—one's karma—go unaddressed during one's lifetime, they pull one into another birth, its nature determined by the previous life. Elaborate paradises, purgatories, and hells resulted, ghostly judges assigning the dead to await rebirth. Some Buddhist sects expressed devotion to a particular version of the Buddha and his or her paradise. Few expected to escape the cycle of rebirth altogether, making such paradises the best interim alternative. The Jesuits rejected such teachings altogether.

Expelling the Supernatural

It both amused and annoyed the Jesuits that the Chinese called them *fangui,* "foreign demons." Things foreign (*fan*) were not Chinese, and therefore were barbarous. Sometimes the term referred to tribal peoples at the empire's margins. It also referred to what entered from outside—by definition strange and therefore possibly dangerous. *Gui,* as we have seen, referred to ghosts and demons. The compound for "foreigners" could thus mean "outsider ghost." Others' ghosts were a threat, as one could mollify one's own. The word targeted Europeans as questionably human and potentially dangerous.

Physician Xu Qunfu (fl. 1570) considered demons figments of the imagination; other Chinese doctors discussed them as pathogens. Yu Bo (fl. 1515) acknowledged in *Yixue zhengquan* (The Correct Tradition of Medicine) that demons existed. It was the shamans and sorcerers claiming to exorcise them who were fraudulent. Li Ting (fl. 1570), in *Yixue rumen* (Introduction to Medicine), wrote that demonic influence entered through the victim's nose and mouth, causing him to fall in pain. One assembled relatives to beat drums, light fires, and burn incense, and administered a medicine of ground rhinoceros horn, cinnabar, and musk. To treat the pain, one placed peach skin on the sore point, and then a walnut-size ball of rolled mugwort on the bowl of a spoon, burning the mugwort to warm the spot (Unschuld 1985). For that matter, Li Shizhen accepted that patients could be afflicted by corpse-spirits and demons, and he provided related prescriptions (Unschuld 1986a).

The Jesuits never doubted the presence of demons. After the Council of Trent (1545–1563), the Catholic Church taught the need to be perpetually on guard against demonic possession. Both Catholics and Protestants saw such possessions increasing toward the end of the sixteenth century (Midelfort 1999). What the Jesuits did reject was other traditions' authority to expel them. Ricci (1942) described Daoist exorcists: "The special duty of the ministers of this group is to drive demons from homes by means of incantations. This is done in two different ways; by covering the walls of the house with pictures of horrid monsters drawn in ink on yellow paper and by filling the house with a bedlam of uncanny yelling and screaming and in this manner making demons of themselves" (103). Yet the Jesuits themselves exorcised ghosts. A literati friend built a palace, which was soon invaded by ghosts and demons. Would the Jesuits like it for their mission, at half price? Trigault described setting up an altar, praying, and processing through the house, sprinkling holy water. After that, "the evil spirits made no further appearance. He to whom all beings are subject had permitted the evil spirits to inhabit this house in order to prepare it for the coming of His servants, and when they came, the spirits were driven out of it. This story was spread through the whole city, and afterwards throughout the kingdom, with the result that respect for the faith was greatly increased" (Ricci and Trigault 1616, 347). The Jesuits, that is, did not hesitate to promote themselves as religious wonder-workers, thereby exhibiting the power of their teachings.

What the Jesuits did not do was practice spirit mediumship, a form of popular religiosity involving trance possession and consultation with deities or the dead, based on the premise that the world of the living is not separate from the realms of the dead or of the gods. Spirit mediums, as Stephen Teiser (1996, 22) observes, were and are called in "to solve problems like sickness in the family, nightmares, possession by a ghost or errant spirit, or some other misfortune." The deity possessed the medium, providing spoken and sometimes written answers and solutions. Ricci (1942, 84) condemned the practice, writing, "It is a common practice also to consult the demons, the family spirits, as the Chinese call them, and there are many of them . . . In such consultations, oracles are received through the voices of little children and from the sounds of brute beasts, revealing the past and the absent, as proof of the truth of what they foretell in the future." Chinese medical literature often characterized women healers as *wu*, or mediums, and criticized those who turned to them (Cullen 1993). Nevertheless, Wang Ji described a physician who recommended treating a girl, depressed by her mother's death, by hiring a medium to tell the girl that her mother, now in the *yin* realm of the underworld, was angry with her. The therapeutic rationale involved treating strong emotion with another strong emotion, in this case by angering the girl herself and curing her (Grant 1998).

A Horde of Deceitful Directors

Just as the Jesuits objected to mediumship, so they condemned the many popular forms of divination, often used diagnostically and to determine appropriate remedies. Ricci (1942, 83) described "a horde of deceitful directors" who advised on such matters as when to begin a journey or construction of a building. When the time arrived, if weather or other conditions militated against the undertaking, one enacted it symbolically—taking only four steps, turning over two shovels full of earth—so as not to lose benefits accruing to the designated time. Whether practitioners read the future through the stars, numerology, physiognomy, palmistry, dreams, the cackling of birds, or shadows cast on a roof, such phenomena disclosed webs of connection with one's fortunes. Rada's collection of books included texts on "how to devine upon dreames, and cast lottes when they beginne any journey, or take any thing in hande, whose end is doubtfull" (Mendoza 1588, 105). Ricci (1942) protested, "The streets and the taverns and all other public places abound in these astrologers and geologists, diviners and fortunetellers, or, to group them all in one class, in these imposters. Their business consists in making vain promises of prosperous fortunes at a given price. Some of them are blind men, others of low station in life, and at times, women of questionable character" (84). Future-readers claimed to predict illness, although Ricci thought the prediction precipitated the affliction. "If, for example, they are told that they will fall sick on a certain day," he complained, "when that day comes they will actually persuade themselves that they are sick and will fight against the imaginary sickness in fear of impending death" (84–85). People cast divinations in temples for prescriptions or other remedies. Participants included not only the poor, but "the high and the low, the noble and the plebeian, the educated and the illiterate . . . the magistrates, the dignitaries of the realm, and even the King himself" (Mendoza 1588, 105).

The Jesuits also targeted geomancers. Within the Confucian tradition, one transcended the finality of death as an ancestor honored by one's descendants. Such measures included recruiting a divinatory specialist with a *luopan*—a special compass—to align the grave within the interplay of *yin* and *yang* at a site, avoiding an incompatible convergence of influences. Otherwise, the deceased person would rest badly, afflicting the descendants until they rectified the problem. This assessment of a site's *yin* and *yang*, called *fengshui*—literally (the forces of) wind and water—was also used to position buildings and furnishings, ensuring prosperity, luck, and health. What the missionaries failed to credit was the degree to which *fengshui* embodied filial devotion, as expressed in the Song dynasty by Cai Fa, who wrote, "Regarding sons, none should be ignorant of medicine or the science [of choosing burial] sites" (Huang 1993, 89).

Ironically, after Ricci's death two companions remained in Beijing to attend his tomb—in the Chinese context, implying the appropriate rites and sacrifices owed to the dead. Trigault explained, "The Chinese frequently keep the bodies of the deceased in the home, hermetically sealed in a coffin, and sometimes for years, until they have built or discovered a suitable place for burial" (Ricci and Trigault 1616, 588). Because the former temple was still being remodeled, Ricci's casket was sealed in this way, remaining unburied for almost a year. To local Chinese, it must have looked like Christian *fengshui,* with disciples awaiting a properly aligned grave site.

The priests' reactions occurred against a backdrop of movements in Europe to "purify" the faith from pervasive lay interest in magicians, wizards, occult healers, soothsayers, fortune-tellers, "cunning persons," "wise men," and "wise women" (Butler 1990, 9). Rome viewed astrological prediction, for example, as a threat to religious faith. In 1586 Pope Sixtus V prohibited astrology and forbade the faithful to use books on the topic. In 1631 Pope Urban VIII reiterated the decree, although the Church could not enforce it. Fr. Schall, made director of the Imperial Bureau of Astronomy, had little influence over the traditional Chinese almanac, but he tried to introduce a "new method" based on European astronomy. He also took advantage of his position to interpret sunspots that appeared before the Dalai Lama's visit to Beijing in 1652 as a warning from Heaven. Following the visit, Schall blamed a smallpox epidemic and recent military reversals on the respect accorded the Buddhist leader (Huang 1993, 101).

The Jesuits failed to understand that the prevalence of divination in China indicated a worldview according to which an underlying order structured events. As J. P. Vernant observes, "Divinatory rationality does not form, in these civilizations, a separate sector, an isolated mentality, opposed to the modes of reasoning that govern the practice of law, administration, politics, medicine, or daily life; it is inserted in a coherent way into the whole of social thought" (Vernant 1974, 10; Keightley 1984). The deeper workings of all things, that is, were knowable through divination.

In addition to mapping the human body, Europe had engaged in mapping the world, in a vast comparative project in which commercial, cultural, and religious powers were at stake. For thinkers like Francis Bacon (1561–1626), knowledge seemed potentially limitless. Against an ideal of unlimited knowledge, all other ways of knowing would be measured and assessed. During the period discussed in this chapter, the question of how the Chinese were like, and different from, Europeans was asked in every conceivable way.

New China narratives emerged, providing more detailed descriptions than those of earlier reporters, and some with more explicit discussions of Chinese healing practices. Observers elaborated on the reading of Chinese bodies. Although no longer linked with monstrous regions, the Chinese were further pulled into typologies based on color, infused with moral, aesthetic, and class-based overtones. Missionaries like Ricci exhibited a rudimentary awareness of Chinese approaches to reading the body in the light of *qi,* but resisted its challenges to Western religious paradigms. No one had yet attempted to explain Chinese physiological theory. Nor, with the exception of Boym's *Flora sinensis,* had the reporters begun the project of relaying the content of Chinese medical texts.

The missionaries drew increasingly absolute lines between medicine and religion, showing some understanding of the social role of Chinese physicians and discussing herbs in more detail, with an eye to trade possibilities. Other healing practices were categorized as idolatry or superstition, given missionary condemnation of Chinese gods, divination, mediumship, exorcism, geomancy, and alchemy. It was Chinese Christian converts who blurred those boundaries, overt similarities informing their hybrid initiatives, even as they slid into practices considered illicit by the priests, who themselves contributed to the confusion.

CHAPTER 3

Model State, Medical Men, and "Mechanick Principles": 1660–1736

Empires were expanding. China's Kangxi emperor ascended to the throne at age seven in 1662, ruling until 1722. He incorporated Taiwan into China's administrative structure and in the late 1690s repelled Mongol invasions. In 1720 he made Tibet a protectorate. Britain seized New Amsterdam from the Dutch in 1664, renaming it New York. France's Louis XIV reorganized New France, following Jacques Marquette's and Louis Joliet's exploration of the Mississippi in 1673.

In 1684 the British East India Company secured permission to trade through Canton. Until the 1710s, company ships were each directed by a supercargo—an agent who oversaw arrangements for a given port. The supercargoes, in turn, could trade only with the "Co-Hong," Chinese merchants authorized by the Chinese government to serve as liaisons. The *hong* merchants rented out warehouse spaces (factories) in segregated neighborhoods at the edges of Canton and prohibited Westerners from interacting with the general population (Rubinstein 1996; Gibson 1992).

Jesuits during the previous period had largely been Italian, Portuguese, Spanish, German, Swiss, or Belgian. In 1685 France's Louis XIV dispatched six French Jesuits, initiating the French Beijing mission. In 1692 the Jesuits won toleration for Christianity throughout China, even as they came under growing fire in Rome. Dominican Domingo Navarrete (1618–1689) targeted Jesuit tolerance of Chinese ancestor rites. Complicating matters, when the Manchus seized power in 1644, the Jesuits had to decide whether to ally with the Chinese literati or with the Manchu court. They chose the latter, destabilizing their position with the literati.

Pope Clement XI ruled against the Jesuit order in 1704 and again in 1715 and 1742. When he sent a legate to Beijing to convey the ruling, the Kangxi emperor pointed to two pieces of cloth, saying, "If anyone should maintain that this red cloth is white, and that the white one is yellow, what would you think of it?"—a commentary on conflicting edicts from successive popes. When the legate tried explaining papal infallibility, the emperor replied, "Is it possible that the pope can judge of the nature of the rites of China, which he has never seen, or had any knowledge of, any more than I can judge the affairs of the Europeans, who are unknown to me?" (Twitchett 1989, 35).

With the Kangxi emperor's death in 1722, his fourth son, Yongzheng (r. 1722–1736), forced his way to the throne, uninterested in relations with Europe. Many missionaries retreated to Canton or Macao. Information about other parts of China diminished. Chinese reservations regarding the "sea barbarians" found corroboration when British traders entered the opium trade, which the Manchu government outlawed in 1729. Although the British East India Company prohibited using company ships to run opium, the trade grew alongside European expansion.

The Reporters

Again, merchants, missionaries, and physicians generated so many accounts of their observations that they required anthologizing. Not all reports were given equal credence, as the cumulative knowledge about China gained in sophistication.

Merchants produced few reports. Johannes Nieuhof (1618–1672), steward to a China delegation of the Dutch East India Company, published a report that was later translated as *An Embassy from the East India Company of the United Provinces, to the Grand Tartar Cham, Emperour of China* (Nieuhof [1665]1669). Nieuhof padded his narrative with excerpts from Martino Martini's 1654 *Atlas sinensis*. Unfortunately, many of Nieuhof's observations were flawed, as were some of Martini's. Navarrete described a dinner party where guests debated whether Marco Polo or Martini had been the more uninformed about China. As Martini had, on occasion, cribbed from Polo, they concluded that "both of them had writ many mere chimeras" (Spence 1998, 41).

Among priestly narrators, Count Lorenzo Magalotti (1637–1712) published a 1665 interview with Fr. Johann Grueber (1623–1680) about Grueber's three years in China (Magalotti 1676). The interview included Grueber's experience with a Chinese physician. Fr. Gabriel Magalhães (1609–1677) traveled throughout China from 1640 to 1648, then lived in Beijing until his death. His *Doze excelencias da China* was translated into English (*A New History of China*, Magalhães 1688) and French. Fr. Louis le Comte (1655–1728), a mathematician sent to China by Louis XIV in 1687, arrived in Canton and traveled north to Beijing. Letters from his two-year sojourn, published as *Nouveaux mémoires sur l'état présent de la Chine* (1696), were almost immediately translated into English (*Memoirs and observations . . . Made in a late Journey Through the Empire of China*, 1698). Le Comte's encyclopedic concerns rested on an epistemological assumption that the world was "(like a Machine) being best understood, and manag'd, by taking it to pieces, viewing and comparing the several parts together" (le Comte 1698, A3). These parts included approaches to healing.

From 1702 to 1776, anthologies of Jesuit letters were published as *Lettres édifiantes et curieuses concernant l'Asie, l'Afrique et l'Amérique* (Edifying and Curious Letters about Asia, Africa, and America). Some pertained to China, and included observations about Chinese healing practices. The Jesuit procurator for the China mission in Paris edited nine of these anthologies; Fr. Jean-Baptiste Du Halde (1674–1743) edited the other twenty-five. German Jesuit Athanasius Kircher (1602–1680) received voluminous correspondence from Jesuits overseas. His *China monumentis, qva sacris qva profanis, nec non variis naturae & artis spectaculis, aliarumque rerum memorabilium argumentis illustrata* (China Illustrata: With Sacred and Secular monuments, Various Spectacles of Nature and Art and Other Memorabilia, [1667]1987) distilled the writings of Martini, Grueber, and Boym, among others. Du Halde produced a similar work—*Déscription géographique, historique, chronologique, politique, et physique de l'empire de la Chine et de la Tartarie chinoise* (1735), drawing on twenty-seven Jesuit authors. Its English translation, *The General History of China* (1736), became a leading eighteenth-century source and included discussions of Chinese pulse taking, herbal medicine, and other healing practices.

The Jesuits shipped Chinese books to European kings and to Rome.

Historian Michel Baudier (1682, 80) alluded to "the many fair *Chinese* volumes" in the Vatican library, "whereof some treat of . . . the Secrets of Physick." Louis XIV received fourteen crates in 1708. Royal librarian Abbé Bignon added eight hundred volumes from the Seminary for Foreign Missions. Jesuit Fr. Fouquet transported four thousand volumes to Paris. The Bodleian Library in England also began building a collection (Spence 1988). Information about China abounded, and into it was mixed the matter of healing.[1]

Among medical writers, Andreas Cleyer (1634–1697), German surgeon general with the Dutch East India Company, lived in Batavia (Jakarta) from 1665 to 1697. In 1682 he edited and published *Specimen medicinae sinicae* (Examples of Chinese Medicine) on Chinese pulse theory. The treatise inspired *Physician's Pulse-Watch* (1707) by Sir John Floyer (1649–1734), a British physician who attempted to integrate Chinese and European systems, having read both *Specimen medicinae sinicae*, sent to him by Charles Hatton, an antiquarian, and selections translated by William Wotton (1660–1726), chaplain to the Earl of Nottingham (Wotton 1694).

Dutch physician Willem ten Rhijne (ca. 1647–ca. 1700) went to Japan intending to study acupuncture and moxibustion, which he did for two years; then he proceeded to Batavia, where he spent twenty-four years. Ten Rhijne wrote the first medical essay on acupuncture, "De acupunctura" (On Acupuncture), including it in his *Dissertatio de arthritide* (Dissertation on Arthritis, 1683). The German naturalist Engelbert Kaempfer (ca. 1651–1716) received medical training in Sweden. He accompanied the Swedish embassy to Persia for four years, next traveling through India and Ceylon. The Dutch East India Company sent him to Japan from 1690 to 1692. His 1694 dissertation *Amoenitatum exoticarum politico-physico-medicarum* (Charming Political, Natural Science, and Medical Exotica) contained a section on acupuncture. It was published in 1712 (Kaempfer [1712]1996). The work of these three doctors would be quoted and paraphrased for generations.

Imagining China and the Chinese

Some European writers perpetuated endeavors to insert Chinese history into their own temporal frameworks. Kircher believed the Chinese were postdiluvian, assigning them Egyptian origins based on superficial similarities between hieroglyphs and Chinese characters and both cultures' multiple deities. He designated Ham as China's ancestor, arguing that he had brought idolatry and pictorial writing to the East (Godwin 1979).

The Jesuits and other observers did not understand that, in China, studying history constituted a sacred project. It was no accident that the five classics included two histories. The ideal human order enacted the Dao, or Way, of Heaven. To cultivate oneself as a profound person, or sage, was to learn the nature of the Dao so deeply that one's own actions spontaneously articulated it. History provided human exemplars who embodied the Dao and others who served as vilified object lessons. "Didactic history," like divination, foretold the future as "a record of pre-facto portents" (Keightley 1984, 21). There was no exact equivalent in Christian history. True, the Jesuits observed *imitatio Christi* (imitating Christ's example) and had a memory bank of Church martyrs who had died in obedience to that principle. But the primacy of salvation history left no room for alternate relationships between humans, time, and the sacred.

A Material Space

An imagined China became the space where well-to-do Europeans lived. Manufacturers copied Chinese technologies, modified for European tastes. During the 1680s, chinoiserie designs adorned British pottery and Chinese porcelain painters produced designs appealing to a European audience. A craze emerged for lacquer furniture, decorated with Chinese landscapes through which Chinese figures moved. French rococo chinoiserie shaped and was shaped by Jean Antoine Watteau (1684–1721), who painted "solemn priests and pagods [figures of gods], obsequious courtiers and devout worshippers, parasol canopies suspended in mid-air . . . and temples open to the sky" (Honour 1961, 90).

In 1735 Christophe Huet (1700–1759) painted mandarins *with* monkeys (*singes*) and *as* monkeys, a genre known as *singerie*. (Monkeys parodying humans originated in medieval manuscripts.) One scene depicted a Chinese herbalist with monkey assistants. A self-styled act of whimsy, identifying human groups and apes had its shadow side, interrogating the humanity of another people. Gardens and pavilions also fell sway to a fashion that identified irregularity and a cultivated sense of wilderness with the Chinese. Sir William Temple (1628–1699), British diplomat and essayist, preferred this style over the symmetry of British landscaping.

The wealthy wore Chinese brocades and silks. Englishmen sported waistcoats embroidered with dragons and chrysanthemums. French and British weavers protested, seeking protectionist measures. France imposed tariffs, banning imported silk and painted cloth in 1714. England weavers rioted, and in 1721 Parliament extended an earlier ban to include all Eastern cottons—a measure that only fueled smuggling.

Pseudo-Chinese fiction like Thomas-Simon Gueullette's *Chinese Tales, or the Marvellous Adventures of the Mandarin Fum-Hoam* (1723) and *The Thousand and One Quarters of an Hour (Tartarian Tales)* (1724) became popular, jumbles of mock-Chinese, Indian, and Middle-Eastern narratives. China entered the fantasy space of theater in Elkanah Settle's *Conquest of China*—a hash of details about the fall of the Ming culled from Mendoza, Martini, and Nieuhof. China became the stage set, too, for *harlequinades,* plays involving "Harlequin," the masked buffoon from Italian *commedia dell'arte.* In France there was the *Arlequin pagode et médecin* ("The Harlequin 'Pagod' and Physician"). Popular French theater developed a stock character in the Oriental buffoon, some twenty-one plays appearing between 1715 and 1775 lampooning the peoples of Asia. Daniel Defoe, author of *Robinson Crusoe,* was the most virulent anti-Chinese author, deriding China fanciers for stacking their collections "upon the tops of cabinets, scrutoires, and every chimney piece to the tops of the ceilings . . . [until it] was injurious to their families and estates" (Dawson 1967, 110).

Model States of Mind

Early cartographers had located monsters and paradise in the East. Mental mapmakers now peopled China with Confucian philosophers. Magalhães (1688) explained Confucian self-cultivation: "Unfold the Rational Nature, . . . reform Mankind, . . . and stop at the sovereign good." Drawing on Mencius, he equated rational nature with "the Heart of Man, for the *Chineses* make no distinction between the Understanding and the Will; but attribute to the Heart what we attribute to those Faculties" (84). He meant *xin* (heart-mind), which endowed one with the capacity for human-heartedness *(ren)*, defined by Mencius as the inability to encounter others' suffering without feeling moved. Neither term was related to European conceptions of Reason, the foundation of science and, by extension, of medical inquiry—although, ideally, *ren* inspired medical practice. Still, le Comte pointed to Confucianism's "degeneration." The early sage kings, he argued, had understood the true God, as evidenced by references to *tian,* Heaven. Such insights, however, had suffered corruption, particularly by Buddhist monks. Given that many literati also blamed Buddhism for undermining Confucian thought, the Jesuit condemnation entailed complex cross-fertilizations.

Nevertheless, praise for Confucian government inspired sinophiles like Temple, who viewed China as the model state where the learned held public office. Unlike le Comte, however, he believed he had found Deist principles in Confucius, also because of the sage's allusions to *tian.* Both le Comte and Temple illustrate the transposing of Western religious frameworks onto a Chinese concept through the skewed equating of terms. Temple acknowledged that some Chinese practiced "idolatry," but assumed they were only commoners and women. The learned "adore the Spirit of the world, which they hold to be eternal, and this without temples, idols, or Priests" (Temple 1814, 344). Years of European religious warfare, absolute monarchs, and excesses of the nobility facilitated projecting onto China the opposite of such failings. Temple did not understand that the Confucian tradition was religious as well as moral and political, with emperor and local officials conducting state rites and sacrifices. Indeed, the Chinese term for ritual *(li)* applied equally to state and more overtly "religious" rites.

Most Deists preferred religion's rational dimensions, some arguing that knowledge of God could be achieved through reason alone, making it universal. Such claims challenged biblical claims to authority based on revelation—which the Jesuits had never foreseen Chinese thinkers being used to critique. The Church proposed a universal religion in Christianity, arguing that regardless of who received Christian revelation first, it was now available to everyone. The antiquity of the Chinese empire meant that its intellectual and religious traditions could not be easily dismissed, opening new questions about Christianity. Moreover, by linking the Chinese with the privileged faculty of Reason, and by pointing to the apparent success of Chinese religio-political teachings, European intellectuals found themselves wondering whether they themselves stood in need of tutelage.

They Are Naturally as Fair as We

In 1677 the Royal Society of London instructed travelers to document the skin color of peoples they encountered. Even before that, however, foreign observers had recorded such details. Most Chinese, wrote Nieuhof (1669, 208), "are almost as White of Complexion as the People of Europe." "As for their Colour," added le Comte (1698, 124), "they are naturally as fair as we, especially toward the *North*." Locating the Chinese as white, the observers emphasized similarity, attributing differences to external influences. Le Comte noted that "[because men in the south] wear on their Head nothing but a little Bonnet very improper to defend their Face from the Sun-beams, they are commonly as Tawny as the *Portuguese* in the *Indies:* The People also of the Provinces of *Quantum* and *Yunnan,* by reason of the excessive Heat, and working half naked, are of a Dun Complexion" (124). Whiteness coincided with privilege; brownness, with peasant status. Poorer Chinese sometimes resembled Mediterranean peoples. Only François Bernier suggested, in 1684 and again in 1688, that humans could be divided into four color groups, one of them yellow (Huard and Wong 1968).

Nieuhof (1669, 208) thought that "in other parts of the Face, they differ very little or nothing from those of Europe." Le Comte (1698, 124) cautioned that figures on dishes and furniture from China, drawn by the Chinese, "make them maimed and ridiculous. They are not so ill-favored as they make themselves." Du Halde proved the point with an engraving of graceful figures in different styles of "Chinese and Tartar" dress (see Figure 6).

The Chinese, Magalhães observed, had a book explaining three thousand forms of civility. Within Confucian tradition, learning how a profound person acted came, in part, through schooling one's body in ritual behaviors appropriate to different contexts. Le Comte (1698, 123) noted, "That curious Feature, that lively Aspect, that stately and noble Gate and Deportment the *French* so much esteemed does not at all please them." Du Halde (1736, 2:128–129) added, "The Genius of the Country requires that we should master our Passions, and act with a great deal of Calmness; the *Chinese* would not hear patiently in a Month what a *Frenchman* can speak in an Hour."

European writers tried to define a Chinese national character, much as the British and French typed one another. Nevertheless, such differences merged into homogeneity as "European," when compared with "Chinese." This does not mean that observers failed to propose similarities: "They Cozen and Cheat in Traffick; Injustice reigns in Sovereign Courts; Intrigues busie both Princes and Courtiers. In the mean time Persons of Quality take so many measures to conceal Vice; and the Out-works are so well guarded, that if a Stranger be not careful to be instructed concerning Affairs to the bottom, he imagines that ev-

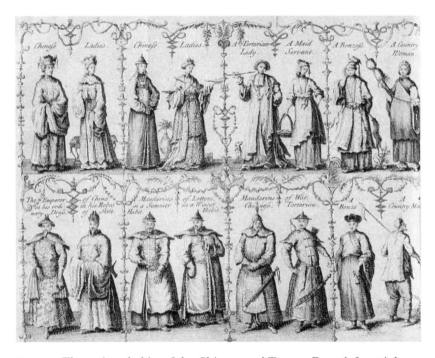

Figure 6. The various habits of the Chinese and Tartars. From left to right: Chinese ladies; a Tartarian lady; a maid servant; a bonzess [Buddhist nun]; a country woman; the emperor of China in his ordinary dress, in his robes of state; mandarins of letters in a summer habit, in a winter habit; mandarins of war—Chinese, Tartarian; a bonze [Buddhist monk]; a country man. Fr. Jean-Baptiste Du Halde, *The General History of China,* 1736. By permission of the Houghton Library, Harvard University.

ery thing is perfectly well regulated. Herein the *Chinese* resemble the *Europeans*" (le Comte 1698, 123). Both groups engaged in their share of dishonesty, dissembling virtue—a resemblance to neither group's credit. Chinese self-containment aroused ambivalence, because Europeans could not interpret its meanings. It became easy to assume malice and project danger. Du Halde (1736) wrote, "They detest every Action, Word, and Gesture that seems to betray Anger, or the least Emotion, and know perfectly how to dissemble their Hatred" (2:137). Renaissance Europe idealized courtly manners, as in Count Baldassare Castiglione's *Libro del cortegiano* (Book of the Courtier, 1528). However, courtesy provoked unease. Was it artifice, concealing treachery? The presumption of concealed vengefulness became a trope, as European writers overdetermined meanings assigned to appearances.

Du Halde (1736) noted Chinese merchants' disposition to swindle foreigners and, if caught, to apologize for having been clumsy at deception: "There are some who, being catch'd in a Fault, are impudent enough to apologize their want of Dexterity; *I am but a Blockhead, as you perceive,* say they, *you are more dexterous than I, another time I shall have nothing to say to an* European; and in reality it is said that some *Europeans* have taught them their Trade" (2:132). That the Chinese both cheated and had learned to cheat from Europeans became further tropes, some observers claiming that Chinese merchants were dishonest primarily in the trade ports. Still, feelings persisted that Chinese and Europeans did not define honesty in quite the same ways.

Chinese in Europe

Chinese protégés continued to visit Europe with Jesuit mentors. Fr. Philippe Couplet (1624–1692) brought Shen Fuzong (Michael Alphonsus Shen, 1658?–1691), son of a Christian physician, reaching Europe in 1684. In Paris, Shen met Louis XIV, who invited the party to dine. Over dinner, "le jeune Indien" (the young Indian) was asked to recite Christian prayers in Chinese and to demonstrate eating with chopsticks. Sources from the period periodically referred to the Chinese as "Indian," with "Indies" referring to countries east of the Near and Middle East, analogous to later uses of *Oriental.*

The king agreed to establish a scientific mission and to send Jesuit mathematicians—including le Comte—to China. In 1685, Couplet and Shen met with Pope Innocent XI and gave him a library of Chinese books. Shen received permission to become a Jesuit. During the return to France, he taught a Jesuit companion Chinese, assisted Couplet with the Chinese in his own work, and helped Magalhães with linguistic sections of his book (Foss 1990). In London, he met King James II, who had a full-length portrait painted of him by Sir Godfrey Kneller (see Figure 7). He also met Thomas Hyde at the Bodleian Library; he helped him catalog the Chinese books and introduced him to rudimentary Chinese phrases, which Hyde recorded as: "'Na li kiu *(quo abis)*?' 'Kia li kiu *(domum sane)*' [Where are you going? I'm going home]" (Ch'ien 1940, 383). During the spring of 1691, Shen left for China, but he died in a shipboard epidemic.

Fan Shouyi (Louis Fan, 1682–1753) left Macao in 1707 and entered a European Jesuit theological school for young Chinese men. After ten years he returned to China with his mentor, Fr. Francesco Provana, with whom he had twice met the pope. On the voyage back, Fr. Provana died; it was Fan who insisted his body be taken to China. To the consternation of other Jesuits at court, the emperor interviewed Fan in 1720. Fr. Carlo Amiani wrote, "We are very fearful what he [Fan] might say to the Emperor to whom the mandarins have sent him, not to mention the dangers to which he as a priest will be exposed, and the contempt our religion may be placed in" (Rule 1995, 287). The emperor retained Fan as an interpreter for about a year, after which Fan returned to pastoral work for the next thirty years.

Arcadio Huang (d. 1716) went to France with Bishop de Lionne in 1714, thinking to become a Jesuit but then changing his mind. Abbot Jean-Paul Bignon, director of the king's libraries, hired him as royal interpreter of Chinese language. Huang worked on a Chinese-French dictionary and on the library's Chinese collection. He met Louis Secondat, Baron de Montesquieu; the two discussed Chinese government, social customs, language, and religious traditions. Huang married a Frenchwoman, with whom he had a daughter. The three died in 1716. Then there was Jean Hu (Spence 1998), a barely literate custodial worker for the Jesuits in Canton. Fr. Fouquet brought Hu to Paris to help with his four thousand Chinese books—an endeavor that proved an abject failure. And in 1732, painter and engraver Fr. Matteo Ripa established a college in Naples to train Chinese youth for evangelical work.[2]

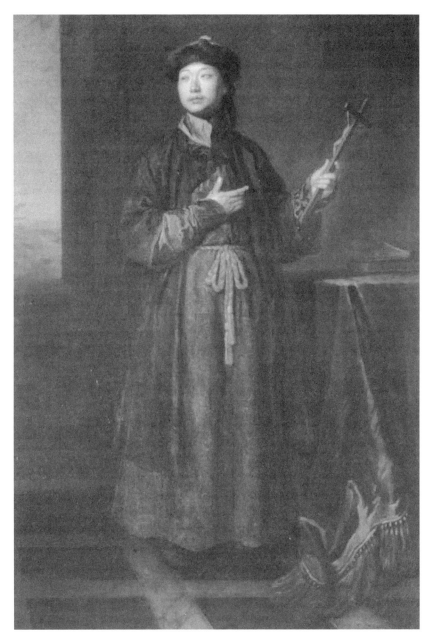

Figure 7. Michael Alphonsus Shen-Fu-Tsung. The Chinese Convert. Sir
Godfrey Kneller, ca. 1685. (Kensington Palace.) Courtesy of the Royal Collection. © 2004, Her Majesty Queen Elizabeth II.

In 1720 the *Journal historique* described a Chinese prince baptized in France, relocating possibly in 1697 to Danzig. A letter from a Fr. "Sirmond" written in 1718 mentioned having been received by this prince—the problem being that there is no other record of a priest by that name in Dantzig at that time. (It may have been a Fr. François Simonelli.) No additional details are available (Duhergne 1964, 395). Yet even cumulatively, none of these encounters could balance impressions generated through print and material culture. Nor did they occur free of the motives of others, particularly the Jesuits, for whom Chinese converts served as walking notices of the mission's self-proclaimed success.

Medical Learning

Foreign observers continued to compare Chinese social roles with those of Europe. Nieuhof (1669) paraphrased Ricci, reminding his readers that a medical degree did little to advance the recipient, "and for this cause it is probable that few or none study Physick but the meaner sort of people" (163). Le Comte complained that one only had to study a medical text for a few months to set oneself up as a physician.[3] He observed the combining of physician and apothecary roles, and cited Chinese acquaintances who questioned the European differentiation. "They think it strange that the *Europeans* . . . commit the principal point of the Cure to Men that are not concerned in curing them; and are not solicitous about the goodness of the Drugs, provided they get rid of them to their advantage" (le Comte 1698, 227). He also portrayed physicians as false prophets. "'You were never troubled with the Head-ach,' say they, 'but with an Heaviness that hath made you Drowsie . . . This evening, about Sunset, your Head will be freer, your Pulse indicates Pain in the Belly, unless you have eaten such and such Meat; This Indisposition will last Five Days, after which it will cease'" (217).

The honor of operating with little training was not exclusive to Chinese physicians. While new centers of medical education had emerged in Leiden, Halle, London, and Edinburgh, a plethora of self-styled doctors continued to practice. In the colonies, most physicians were self-taught or learned through apprenticeship, relying on Galenic therapies—blistering, purging, vomiting, sweating, and bloodletting.

People frequently received care from women in the family, bonesetters and herbalists supplementing such services. Land grant companies, missionary groups, and governments sometimes sent doctors, but well-educated physicians had little incentive to emigrate.

Parts and Wholes

Chinese and Western practitioners learned radically different and even incommensurate ways of reading the body, the disparities rooted in different cosmologies. "Things have their roots and branches [*benmo*]," observed the *Daxue* (Great Learning; third or second century BCE).[4] "Affairs have their beginnings and their ends. To know what is first and what is last will lead one near the Way [*Dao*]" (Chan 1963, 86).

Roots and Branches

The metaphor of roots and branches signified the ability to recognize organic relationships between parts and to discriminate between essential and secondary aspects. "There is never a case when the root is in disorder," added the text, "yet the branches are in order" (Chan 1963, 86–87). *Benmo* had nothing to do with "mechanickal" orientations to parts and wholes, or with European interest in identifying natural laws articulated through mathematics. Western dissectors, for example, focused on fine anatomical structures to learn their function in the "animal economy." This structure-function model presupposed an ideal baseline condition, allowing one to recognize changes in structure and corresponding problems in the mechanism's capacity to function.

Chinese thinkers focused, instead, on "substance" *(ti)* and "function" *(yong)*. *Ti* referred to "body," whole person, trunk, or limbs. It also signified a thing's core substance or essence. The "substance" of a human being was human nature, which in its natural state was quiescent. Because all humans shared this substance, one could speak of a universal human nature, whose essential quality *(ren)* combined compassion, benevolence, and human-heartedness. *Yong* meant either the *use* to which something could be put, or the *action* of using it. The term was charged. Confucius criticized the person who functioned as a "vessel"—who was defined by "use," by what he or she *did,* rather than by the cultivation of *ren.*

Tiyong referred to essence put into action, no longer a quiet, hidden state.[5] For example, one could recognize enacted *ren* in expressions of love, compassion, or benevolence. *Ti* was quiescent; *yong* was manifest. Results and effects followed from *yong,* because *yong* participated in change. *Tiyong,* therefore, had no connection with the European project of knowing physical structures and their respective functions. Dismantling a whole into its parts afforded one no greater comprehension of the whole. The *Laozi* said, "Enumerate all the parts of a chariot as you may, and you still have no chariot" (Chan 1963, 160). The very conceptual foundation of anatomical dissection, therefore, had little match in Chinese thought.

A few Jesuits attempted to introduce European anatomical models; a few Chinese used them. Fang Yizhi (1611–1671), for example, incorporated Galenic humoral theory and a discussion of anatomical structures into reflections on structure and function—*ti* and *yong*—in his *Wuli xiaoshi* (Notes on the Principles of Things, ca. 1664). Fang also drew on earlier, more theologically oriented anatomical work by Jesuit Adam Schall (1592–1666). The Kangxi emperor took an interest in Western anatomy. He involved Fr. Joachim Bouvet (1656–1730)—sent by Louis XIV and serving as professor of chemistry and anatomy—in drafting an anatomical work based on Pierre Dionis's (1643–1718) *L'anatomie de l'homme, suivant la circulation du sang* (Human Anatomy, Following the Circulation of the Blood, 1690). Bouvet's work included ninety anatomical plates, copied primarily from Thomas Bartholini's (1616–1680) *Anatomia renovata* (Anatomy Renewed, 1673). Bouvet characterized Chinese anatomical knowledge as "very confused," despite Chinese physicians' being quite able.

Fr. Dominique Parennin (1665–1741), who arrived in China in 1698, continued Bouvet's project, translating it into Manchu. (Parennin may have previously performed dissections himself.) The emperor read and corrected each page and considered permitting dissection of criminals condemned for capital crimes (Huard 1968). (He decided against the idea.) The project reached completion around 1710, remaining in manuscript form in Beijing, where only a small number of individuals had access to it (Walravens 1996). Written in Manchu, it exercised no influence on Chinese physicians. Parennin sent one copy to the French Academy in 1723.

The impact of Western anatomical models thus remained nominal. Du Halde (1736) described Chinese knowledge as "depending upon a doubtful System of the Structure of the Human Body"; moreover, he argued, the Chinese seemed "not to have made the same Progress in this Science as our Physicians in *Europe*" (3:356). This early coupling of "progress" and "science" equated the increase of knowledge with breaking new ground, rather than with revisiting and rethinking the ancients. That these terms entered discussions of Chinese healing in 1735, in relation to readings of the body, did not bode well for European efforts to understand Chinese systems.

Qi, Blood, and Spirits

Still, some writers attempted to explain core Chinese concepts to European audiences. Ten Rhijne translated *qi* as "Spirits," equating it with Galen's "animal spirits." Yet while both terms involved vital force and blood—making the connection natural—it was still wrong. Ten Rhijne's misunderstanding surfaced in his statement that Chinese doctors, although "ignorant of anatomy, nonetheless . . . have perhaps devoted more effort over many centuries to learning and teaching . . . the circulation of the blood, than have European physicians individually or as a group" (Carrubba and Bowers 1974, 375). Le Comte (1698, 215) also leapt to Galenic conclusions, describing *qi* as "a Circulation of the Blood and Humours." Du Halde (1736) translated *qi* as "Spirits," coupling it with blood. He noted that the Chinese had known about their circulation "since about four hundred Years after the Deluge" (3:358).

Developments in European thinking about blood exacerbated the misunderstanding, particularly with William Harvey locating life in the blood. Oxford's Richard Lower (1631–1691) demonstrated that blood leaving the lungs through the pulmonary vein took on the bright redness of arterial blood prior to reaching the heart. The demonstration tightened connections between blood, air, and the lungs, challenging conceptions of blood as a humor. Blood became a "mechanical" fluid that circulated essential components deriving from food and air. Disease, in this connection, was "an uncertain irregular motion of the Fluids of the Body" (Browne 1703, 103). European doctors like renowned physician Hermann Boerhaave (1668–1738) emphasized "hydrostaticks"—the part of mathematics dealing with the properties of fluids. Yet this fascination with fluids, directly linked to a disease model, did not translate into an active interest in Chinese notions of *qi*. Therefore, to European eyes the Chinese seemed to be saying more or less the same thing and contributing nothing novel.

Jing, Qi, and Shen

Du Halde included a longevity text, the *Tchang Seng* [*Chang Sheng,* or Longevity], wherein a Chinese physician described how he overcame poor health: "Our Life depends upon the regular Motion of the Spirits: There are three sorts . . . the Vital Spirits, which we call *Tsing* [*jing*]; the Animal Spirits, which we call *Ki* [*qi*]; and a third degree of Spirits, much more noble, more free from matter, and to which the Name of Spirit does much more properly agree, which is called *Chin* [*shen*]" (Du Halde 1736, 4:72).

Jing, the most refined cosmic *qi*, was fluid, underlying all organic life. "The Particles which compose the Animal Spirit [*qi*] are much smaller, and more subtle than those which compose the Vital [*jing*] . . . The Particles of the Animal Spirit move in every sense unmix'd and unblended as the Particles which compose the Air: This is the *Chinese Ki.* The Particles of the Vital Spirit creep and glide the one over the other, as the Parts of Water: This is the *Chinese Tsing*" (4:72). One inherited prenatal *jing* from one's parents, deriving postnatal *jing* from food. Prenatal *jing* was fixed, in quantity and quality, and was revitalized by postnatal *jing. Jing* endowed an organism with the innate capacity for organic change. Likewise, one's *qi* came from one's prenatal *jing,* enabling one to act and move, and transform food into postnatal *jing.* "The Animal Spirits, according to the Antients, are nothing but a subtle Air, a very fine Breath, and this exactly answers to the *Ki* . . . These Spirits, according to the Moderns, are nothing else than a subtle Moisture, which runs from the Brain into the Nerves with such an impetuous force, which if open'd, are very difficult to be stopt" (4:73– 74). While retaining Galenic overtones, the explanation better approximated Chinese understandings than did ten Rhijne's translation.

The third "Spirit," *shen,* was the conscious vitality underlying *jing* and *qi.* "The Particles of the Animal Spirit are so rapid that they are imperceptible to all the Senses; and 'tis the finest part of these Spirits which is called *Chin*" (4:72). *Shen,* Stephen Teiser suggests, is central to

Chinese cosmology and anthropology, particularly through three of its meanings. The first pertains to the "spirit" of a person, as in "human spirit" or "psyche." It is the inner force that enables one to be and to do, and requires cultivation to fulfill its potential. Where it differs from "spirit" as often used in English is that, like *qi*, it has a subtle material aspect. The second meaning translates as "spirits" or "gods," associated with stars, mountains, and streams, as opposed to *gui*, or demons. The third meaning can be rendered as "spiritual" in the sense of being numinous, or inspiring awe and wonder. As Teiser notes, that these three meanings ("spirit," "spirits," and "spiritual") converge in a single word "indicates that there is no unbridgeable gap separating humans from gods or, for that matter, separating good spirits from demons. All are composed of the same basic stuff, *qi*, and there is no ontological distinction between them" (Teiser 1996, 34–35). *Jing, qi*, and *shen* came together, too, in relation to longevity. As the *Tchang Seng's* physician author explained: "If the Vital Spirits come to fail the Animal must also fail; and this second sort of Spirits being exhausted the third cannot subsist, and the Man must die: It is therefore of importance not to dissipate idly these three Principles of Life, either by an immoderate use of sensual Pleasures, or by violent Labour, or by too intense and too constant Application of the Mind" (Du Halde 1736, 4:72).

The nearest Western parallels appeared in European vitalism. For example, Friedrich Hoffmann (1660–1742), professor of medicine at Halle, was struck by living organisms' capacity for self-renewal. He posited three souls—one immortal, one of fine matter, and the third gross and material. Hoffmann's colleague Georg Ernst Stahl (1659–1734) argued that *anima* distinguished living from lifeless matter. He conceptualized it as a substance that was both rational and spiritual. Where matter was passive and inert, the soul communicated the "spiritual act" of movement, resulting in physiological development. Stahl suggested that the living organism should be conceptualized as a unity, rather than as a material mechanism knowable through dissection. His argument for a "vital principle" would identify him as the originator of a vitalist approach to biology.

Such ideas illustrate that a Cartesian approach coexisted with alternative conceptions in the West. By the 1730s even the mechanical metaphor had undergone modulation. Medical theorists remembered

Newton's also positing *aether,* "a most subtle spirit." Newton had wondered whether it resembled the animal spirits in the nerves, or even the vibration of nerves, which early on had been identified with volition, the disposition to act. *Aether* began with the will, in the brain, and from there moved through the nerves and into the muscles.[6] As Andrew Wear (1995, 358) observes, "Spirit had been brought back into physics and into physiology." Still, these theories remained unconnected with Chinese thought.

Yin, Yang, and the Jingluo

With nothing quite like *yin* and *yang,* Europeans resorted to the familiar. Ten Rhijne translated *yin* (coolness, darkness, and dampness) as Galen's *humidum radicale*—radical, or root, moisture. *Yang* (heat, light, and dryness) became *calidum innatum*—innate heat. The mistranslation further embedded the Chinese concepts in a humoral framework, erasing *qi* and uprooting *yin* and *yang.* Floyer (1707, 256) perpetuated the error: "The *Calidum Innatum* of the Greeks, and the *Calor Primagenius* of the *Chinese,* is the Animal Spirits, which by the help of different Organs, produces all the Natural, Vital and Animal Actions." Du Halde (1736, 3:357) concurred: "They give the Name of *Yang* to the vital Heat, and that of *Yn* to the radical Moisture." He included a pulse manual translated by Fr. Julien Hervieu, who explained, "*Yang* and *Yn* are . . . applied by the *Chinese* in almost every Distinction of two things, wherein one gives place to the other in some particular manner" (Du Halde 1736, 3:382). The treatise added, "There is often in the *Yn* a little of the *Yang,* and in the *Yang* a little of the *Yn*" (3:402). Although accurate, the explanation was insufficiently illustrated to enable Western readers to understand it.

Like Ricci, Cleyer and Du Halde equated the Five Phases (*wuxing*) with Aristotle's "elements." It was, Cleyer (1682) noted, necessary to balance them; otherwise, a "morbid state," or illness, resulted. Quoting Cleyer, William Wotton (1694, 148) wrote, "Out of the Eastern Region arises the Wind, out of the Wind Wood, or Plants, out of Wood Acidity, from thence the Liver, from the Liver the Nerves, from them the Heart." The sequence merged elements/phases and anatomical parts, obscuring the principle of correspondences. In contrast, Du Halde (1736) explained that the phases were the "natural

Seats of Vital Heat and radical Moisture"; he added: "Thus Fire reigns in the Heart, and the chief Viscera, which lie near it; and the South is the Part of Heaven which has the principal Reference to these Parts, because Heat is chiefly situated there, and it is in Summer that they observe the Affections of the Heart" (3:360–361). Fire, the south, summer, and heart interfaced through *yang,* although not in ways that would have seemed self-evident to Western readers.

By "heart" (*xin,* heart-mind), kidney, liver, spleen, lung, stomach, intestines, and gallbladder, the Chinese did not exactly mean anatomical organs. Although the *Nanjing* (Canon of Difficult Issues) provided some results from dissection, interest in anatomy did not outlast the Han. Instead, the body was envisioned as a network of organ-related *processes,* described as "storage facilities" or "depots" *(zang),* and "grain collection centers" or "palaces" *(fu).* Half were predominantly *yin,* the other half primarily *yang.* The *yin* organ-functions produced, transformed, and stored *qi,* blood, *jing, shen,* and bodily fluids. The *yang* ones changed food into *qi,* blood, *jing,* and the rest. The first set lay deeper within the body, making them *yin,* relative to the more external, *yang* functions. Even so, each organ function had both yin and yang aspects (Unschuld 1985).

Connections between *zangfu* occurred through the twelve meridians *(jingluo),* as pathways of *qi.*[7] The meridians connected all "six depots" and all "six palaces," forming a circuit. The *luo* connected the *jing,* like the mesh of a net. Cleyer (1682) provided Chinese drawings, illustrating each of the twelve "*viis,*" or "Ways," but unfortunately he called them "anatomical" (see Figure 8). Du Halde's discussion, although flawed, remained the most accessible. "The radical moisture *(Yn)* and the vital heat *(Yang)* are conveyed from the six members and the six intestines to the other parts of the body by means of twelve ways, or Canals" (Du Halde 1736, 3:360).

In contrast, Floyer (1707) invented anatomical meridians, positing that these originated in physical organs and proceeded to anatomical sites. He styled them *Hepatis, Cordes, Pulmonum, Stomachi,* and *Vesicae* (liver, heart, lungs, stomach, and bladder). Although he argued, "The best Method I know is that mixed of the *European* and the *Chinese*" (272), it did not catch on, probably because there were no actual physical channels to which anatomically oriented practitioners could relate. Despite strong correlations between the different translations

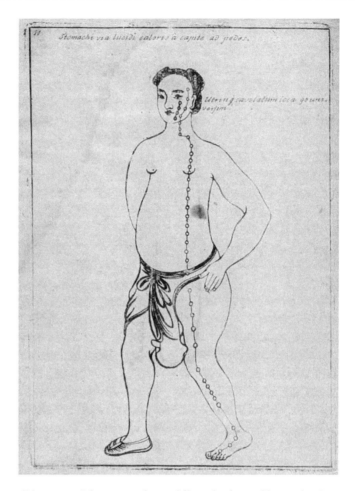

Figure 8. Diagram of the stomach meridian. Andreas Cleyer, *Specimen medicinae sinicae,* 1682. Courtesy of the Boston Medical Library in the Francis A. Countway Library of Medicine.

and explanations, even Floyer could not escape the pull of material anatomy, convinced that one could not do without it.

Perfect Knowledge of the Pulse

Confusions notwithstanding, Chinese pulse taking developed a reputation for sophistication. The more comprehensive China narratives at least mentioned it. In 1671 an anonymous French missionary wrote *Secrets de la médecine des Chinois*. A preface explained that the writer had been expelled from Beijing and sent to Canton. Grmek (1962) argues that thirty missionaries were expelled from Beijing in 1665, four of them French (Jean Valat, Adrien Greslon, Humbert Angery, and Jacques Le Favre), and one a "Mechlin Francophone," who would have been Couplet.[8] The work, published in Grenoble—although translated into Italian in 1676 and English in 1707—drew little notice. The first section presented general rules of pulse doctrine; the second, rules for discerning what pulse differences disclosed, with a focused discussion of women and children; and the third, prognostics, especially of impending death. The author concluded by questioning Chinese medical doctrines because they were not grounded in an anatomical foundation.

In 1680 Cleyer published *Clavis medica ad Chinarum doctrinam de pulsibus* (Key to the Medical Doctrine of the Chinese on the Pulse) and in 1682 *Specimen medicinae sinicae sive opuscula medica ad mentem sinensium* (Specimens of Chinese Medicine, or Medical Treatises according to the Spirit of the Chinese), with parts added by "an *eruditus Europaeus* living in Canton." Both works appear to have drawn heavily on translations and writings by Boym, whose *Clavis medica* was published posthumously in 1686.[9]

European authors faced major challenges in trying to explain Chinese pulse theory. Nieuhof (1669, 105) wrote that each pulse had "some secret Coherencies with certain parts of the Body; as that of the first, to the Heart; of the second, to the Liver; of the third, to the Stomack; of the fourth, to the Spleen; of the fifth, to the Reins, &c." He assumed that these terms referred literally to physical organs. Cleyer (1682) reiterated the relationship between pulses and *zangfu*. Six pulses lay along each wrist—three deeper, three closer to the skin. The text diagramed each variation, along with diagrams of different states of the tongue (see Figure 9). Le Comte (1698) understood the pulses as registering alterations of the blood, facilitating detection of humoral "distemper":

> . . . an Undulation or Trembling, caused by the Ebullion of the whole Mass of the Humours; which may be perceived like to a Bell that trembles after it hath been rung; sometimes also the Artery will not bear a

stroke, but will swell by little and little. By pressing it, one will moreover be able to perceive several Effects that do not declare themselves to the bare touch; for at that time the Course of the Circulation, which is suspended or lessened, which begins again immediately after with more force, will give occasion to judge variously and differently of the Disposition of the Heart, . . . of the Quality of the Blood there prepared, of the Obstacles that impede its passages, of Gross and Crude Matter that

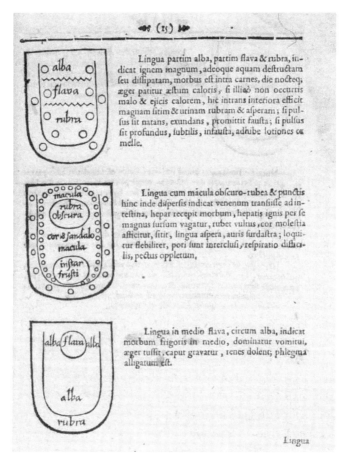

Figure 9. Tongue diagrams. Andreas Cleyer, *Specimen medicinae sinicae*, 1682. Courtesy of the Boston Medical Library in the Francis A. Countway Library of Medicine. *Alba* meant white; *rubra,* red; and *flava,* yellowish.

over-charges it, of the Nature of the Spirit that too much rarifies it, and precipitates Transpiration. (216–217)

This description suggested a subtle practice requiring the physician to visit and revisit specific sites. For European readers, however, references to heart and blood superimposed anatomical frameworks upon references to obstacles in the flow of *qi*/blood.

Hervieu's translation in Du Halde pointed to the third-century *Mai-jing* (Classic of Pulses) by Ouang chou ho (Wang Shuhe, 265–316):

> It is Motion, say they, that makes the Pulse, and this Motion is caused by the Flux and Reflux of the Spirits, which are carried to all Parts of the Body by the twelve Passages before mentioned.
>
> Every thing that gives Motion, add they, thrusts forwards some moveable Body, and every thing that is moved either gives place easily, or makes resistance; thus as the Blood and Spirits [*qi*] are in a continual Motion, strike against, and press the Vessels [*jingluo*] in which they are conveyed, there must necessarily arise a Beating of the Pulse . . . 'Tis by these Beatings that one may know the Nature of the Blood and Spirits, as likewise what Defects and Excesses may be found therein, and it is the part of skilful Physicians to regulate and reduce them to their first Temperament. (Du Halde 1736, 3:361–362)[10]

After cataloging the pulses, the author reviewed signs of disorder:

> The Pulse of the Liver in its usual and healthy Condition is long and tremulous; when it is superficial and short the Liver undergoes an Alteration, and one is subject to Emotions of Anger.
>
> When the Pulse of the Liver is full one dreams of Mountains, Trees and Forests; when it is empty one dreams of Herbs and Bushes . . .
>
> When the Pulse is long and tremulous in the three places of the left Arm, where it is usually felt, the Liver . . . is faulty thro' excess; upon which is generally felt a Pain in the Eyes, and large Tears are shed by intervals: The Patient is fretful, easily provoked, and very subject to be clamorous. (3:420–421)

To treat imbalances of *qi* was to address affective states, which were analogous but not identical to the humoral temperaments and their imbalances.

Among such details, a musical trope surfaced. Du Halde (1736) wrote, "They likewise suppose that the Body is . . . a kind of a Lute or musical Instrument, whose Parts render diverse Sounds . . . and it is by this means that the different Pulses, which are like the various Sounds, and diverse Touches of these Instruments, are Marks whereby to judge of their Disposition" (3:358–359). The analogy entered specific pulse descriptions: "*Kong* is when we distinguish, as it were, two Extremities, and an empty Space in the middle"; it was "as if the Finger was put upon a Hole of a Flute; this Comparison is taken from the *Chinese* themselves" (3:385). What would often strike Europeans as imprecise metaphors were attempts by generations of Chinese physicians to equate precise experiences with sensations generated by specific pulses. Such descriptions corresponded to drawings, some of which Cleyer reproduced (see Figure 10).

Only one European, Fr. Grueber, described having his pulses read:

> [The physician] caused me to sit down and suffered me to rest quietly a while. Afterwards he uncovered both my Arms as far as the Elbows, placing them upon a Table, and felt the Pulses of both Arms, one after another; pressing the Arteries sometimes hard, sometimes softly, sometimes equally; and at other times he prest hard upon one Arm, leaving the other free: Sometimes he prest hard upon one Pulse, and softly upon another; he continued to feel it a long while, anon he felt it but by turns; sometimes he caused me to hold my fist closed, anon he made me open it. In short, he felt and examined my Pulse, as it did beat in every posture of my Arm and Hand, which lasted a long while, about three quarters of an hour. After all this, I had almost a mind to discover to him my disease, but Father *Adam* [Schall] interrupted me, and told me, that he knew it better than I did. When the Physitian was sate down, he described with a wonderful majesty my disease, and all its properties and circumstances, assigning to them the time of their first beginning, in such an exact manner, that I was strangely surprised. (Magalotti 1676, 75–77)

Such descriptions contributed to the general, albeit contradictory, impression that the Chinese knew little about anatomy and yet were superb diagnosticians.

A handful of Europeans struggled to figure out how to apply the practice. David Abercromby (1685), for example, experimented without great success. Floyer's integrative model included tables correlating European with Chinese pulses. While acknowledging his inability to formulate absolute correspondences, Floyer remained convinced that Cleyer's descriptions involved arteries and veins. Because some

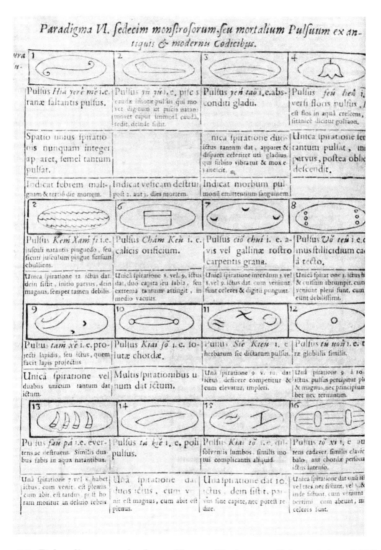

Figure 10. Pulse diagrams. Andreas Cleyer, *Specimen medicinae sinicae*, 1682. Courtesy of the Boston Medical Library in the Francis A. Countway Library of Medicine.

European medical authors argued that if one's observations were imprecise, one's diagnosis inevitably entailed conjecture, Floyer invented the "Pulse Watch," a mechanism that ran for sixty seconds, making him the first physician to document applying a watch in this way.[11] It illustrated enhanced attention to precise observations and the use of mechanisms to accomplish them. Yet although pulse measurement gradually became a routine practice, explicit inclusion of Chinese theory did not.

Discussions of Chinese anatomical models filtered into European works. Wotton, who had translated sections of Cleyer, wrote:

> The Chinese divide the Body into Three Regions: First is from the Head to the Diaphragm: The Second from thence to the Navel, containing Stomach, Spleen, Liver and Gall, and the Third to the Feet, containing the Bladder, Ureters, Reins [kidneys] and Guts. To these Three Regions, they assign Three sorts of Pulses in each Hand. The uppermost Pulse is governed by the radical Heat, and is therefore in its own Nature overflowing and great. The lowermost is governed by the radical Moisture, which lies deeper than the rest, and is like a Root to the rest of the Branches: the middlemost lies between them both, partakes equally of radical Heat and Moisture, and answers to the middle Region of the Body, as the uppermost and lowermost do to the other Two. (Wotton 1694, 151–152)

The description, although accurate, was undercut by Wotton's calling it "tedious" and the anatomical diagrams in Cleyer "so very whimsical, that a Man would almost believe the whole to be a Banter, if these Theories were not agreeable to the occasional Hints that may be found in the Travels of the Missionaries" (Wotton 1694, 152). Wotton concluded that the Chinese, although "sagacious and industrious," had yet to apply themselves to "learning in good earnest." Consequently, even a relatively "small Skill in Physick and Mathematicks" on the part of the missionaries positioned them as "the greatest Scholars" (147) in the Chinese court. Floyer (1707) also criticized the Chinese "want of anatomy." Still, their pulse taking dazzled him. "The great excellency of the *Chinese* Art is, That they can by feeling of the Pulse, discern the Part affected; but the *Europeans* are forc'd to inquire after it by its Qualities, Actions or Excretions. I cannot but particularly esteem the

Chinese Art, because they have discover'd by their Touch more than any *European*" (354–355).

Yet even Floyer ultimately dismissed Chinese meridian theory, writing: "We must reject it, and stick to our Anatomy, which has discovered the true Circulation to us, and by that we find how a Disease may circulate from the Head to the lower Circulations" (322). Still, he acknowledged, his judgment might reflect insufficient knowledge. He conceded that if Europeans had a fully translated *Neijing*, "it might have prov'd like *Hippocrates*, more clear and true than any of his Commentators, who, by their extreme Niceties and symbolical Argumentations, have obscured the Sense of the Author" (325). Caught between European rationality and a Chinese worldview he only dimly discerned, he, too, did not understand that Chinese pulse descriptions were more than fanciful metaphors.

Hervieu argued that "defective" anatomical knowledge did not invalidate Chinese diagnoses. In hindsight, Du Halde's texts could have been joined with ten Rhijne's and Cleyer's diagrams to yield an overview of connections between Chinese theory and practice. The problem was timing. Responding to Boym's *Clavis medica,* Pierre Bayle (1647–1706) noted: "It is easy to see from what he says that the physicians of China are rather clever men. True, their theories and principles are not the clearest in the world, but if we had got hold of them under the reign of the Philosophy of Aristotle, we should have admired them much, and we should have found them at least as plausible and well based as our own. Unfortunately, they have reached us in Europe just at a time when the mechanick Principles invented, or revived, by our Modern Virtuosi have given us a great distaste for . . . the *calidum naturalis* and the *humidum radicale* too, the great foundations of the Medicine of the Chinese" (in Lu and Needham 1980, 286). Translators' use of humoral vocabulary irreparably linked the Chinese system with Galen, who was steadily being marginalized. There simply was not intellectual room left for what seemed, at best, variations on a waning paradigm.

The Vertues of All Kinds of Herbs

The intellectual community of Europe remained interested in foreign plants, for both intellectual and commercial reasons. Members of the

Imperial Academy of Sciences of St. Petersburg, for example, sent questions to Jesuit missionaries, concerning illnesses of the Chinese, vaccination, and the cultivation and preparation of rhubarb, ginseng, mugwort *(Artemesia vulgaris)*, tobacco, tea, and other plants used medicinally. Some missionaries engaged in botanical work. Fr. Parennin sent samples of Chinese medicines to the Académie des Sciences in Paris; Antoine de Jussieu (1686–1758) and Bernard de Jussieu (1699–1777) examined these. A perennial problem involved whether—contingent on political and economic circumstances in Europe—to send plants by sea via Canton, or overland, through St. Petersburg, to ensure their safe arrival in Europe (Dumoulin-Genest 1995).

Fr. Bouvet researched Chinese *materia medica,* although his work has been lost. Fr. Le Chéron d'Incarville (1706–1757), trained as a botanist, sent details to Jesuits in France. Yet foreign reporters did not necessarily write about Chinese herbs from direct observation. Parennin, in a 1723 letter, mentioned hearing of botanists and druggists sent from Paris to Canton:

> I can scarcely believe that they would have been able to make a considerable collection. The good plants are only found in the provinces . . . where doubtless they will not be able to go: for some time there have not been missionaries established in these provinces, and when there were, they would have had to be botanists and had the time and the facility to look for plants and study their properties. If one knew how they travel on their missions, one would hardly complain about the little knowledge that they give about simples that are found in their district. The missionaries, especially in the South, ordinarily go by boat from one mission to another: if there are roads . . . they make go in closed chairs, and do not have the ease to stop in the countryside, nor the liberty to go walking by foot, outside of the city walls where their churches are. The only thing possible to them is to make some version of Chinese herbals, whose drawings scarcely resemble the plants from which they have been made. (Rochat de la Vallée 1980, 185)

Not surprisingly, le Comte (1698, 220) characterized Father Visdelou—a member of the 1687 team—as "intent upon the Translation of the *Chinese* Herbal; wherein are all the Vertues and Qualities of all those Plants explained" to enrich Western botany.

Ten Rhijne described several herbs, but employed Chinese terms that have proved difficult to identify. Kircher reprinted Martini on rhubarb, telling the story of Martini's visit, while in Europe, to a Dutch mayor's garden. There Martini noticed a tall, white plant with full, round leaves and identified it as true rhubarb. Kircher also included Boym's discussion of the serpent whose venom was used for rabid-dog bites. Fr. Grueber described "Tigers Milk," a plant gathered from ground moistened by the milk of a tiger "when they are furious and inraged by the pursuit of Huntsmen" (Magalotti 1676, 78). It induced sweating. John Evelyn, who recorded witnessing Eastern rarities, included, "Divers Drougs that our Drougists & physitians could make nothing of: Especialy, one which the Jesuite called *Lac Tydridis* [Tiger's Milk] it look'd like a fungus, but was weighty like metall: yet was a Concretion or coagulation of some other matter" (Spence 1998, 63–64). Fr. François Xavier d'Entrecolles (1663–1741), who arrived in China in 1698, discussed how the Chinese produced mercury ([1734]1843a). Le Comte (1698, 220–221) praised tea, claiming the Chinese did not suffer "Gout, Sciatica, or Stone," and that some found it "good for the Gravel, Crudities, [and] Head-aches."

Du Halde (1635) dedicated three sections to herbs, the first in an essay on geography; the second, excerpted from Li Shizhen's *Bencao gangmu* (1684 printing); and the third, herbal formulas, also from the *Bencao.* One of his correspondents, Fr. d'Entrecolles, detailed the description and uses of *foulin* (the fungus sometimes called China root), *Ko-Ken, Thi-fiao-Téou, Cho-Yo, Kin-Inhoa, Tcha-cha,* sea horses, tea, and ginseng—none of them indigenous to Europe (see Figure 11). D'Entrecolles also provided a remedy for night blindness, using a decoction of sheep's liver cooked with the leaves of water lilies. One put one's head under a linen cloth with one's eyes open. The steam bathed one's eyes, dissolving the morbid humor (Thomaz de Bossièrre 1982). Du Halde presented examples of Li's classificatory schema, without grasping that, for the Chinese, the analysis of plants at this time came under the neo-Confucian heading of *gewu zhizhi,* or "extending one's knowledge." The objective derived from the *Daxue*'s encouragement to put oneself in order by extending knowledge through "the investigation of things." Teacher Zhu Xi (1130–1200) interpreted this to mean exploring, or investigating, the workings of *li,* or "principle"—the patterned working of the *Dao* expressed through human affairs and natural phenomena.

Chinese social order provided metaphors for organizing *materia medica* within therapeutic formulas. The *Bencao,* for example, equated the highest class of remedies with the sovereign. No matter how long or in what quantities one took them, they would do no harm. Some in the second class, however, might have "a malignant Quality," offset by herbs functioning as "Servants or domestick Officers." The third and lowest class had "great Malignity, or some poisonous Quality." As "Officers not belonging to the House," they could not be used together, their worst effects requiring neutralization by other ingredients. Such relational language provided structures for balancing ingredients, as did family-based metaphors:

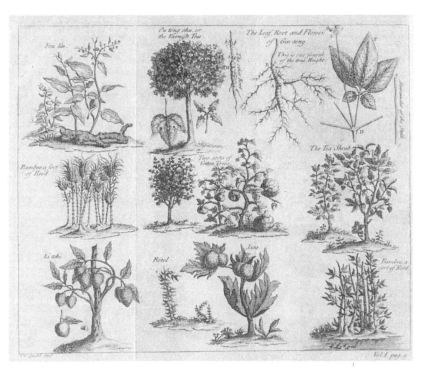

Figure 11. Medicinal plants. From left to right: *Fou lin; Ou teng chu,* or the varnish tree; the leaf, root, and flower of ginseng—"This is one fourth of the true height"; remainder of the stalk; bamboo, a sort of reed; two sorts of cotton trees; the tea shrub; *li tchi;* betel; java; bamboo, a sort of reed. Fr. Jean-Baptiste Du Halde, *The General History of China,* vol. 1, p. 9, 1736. By permission of the Houghton Library, Harvard University.

The *Kiun,* or Sovereign, ought to be chief; there should be two *Tchin* or domestick Servants; three *Tso,* or general Officers; one *Kiun,* three *Tchin,* and nine *Tso cê,* is likewise a just Proportion.

Among the Remedies there are some which partake of the Nature of *Yn,* and others of *Yang,* to which great regard should be had when they are mixed together: Certain Remedies have likewise Relations among themselves like that of the Mother and Child, and the eldest Brother and younger. (Du Halde 1736, 3:469–471)

Correct herbal balances had political and familial equivalents, and vice versa. In every sphere of life, one attended to connections between things. At the same time, Du Halde (1736) quoted Li's critique of his contemporaries: "In the first Age the Ancients prepared the Medicines, but seldom used them their Health was so perfect: That in the middle Age Virtue being degenerated and Strength decayed, when any Disease arose, of ten thousand Persons who took Medicines, there was not one that did not recover his former Health: And that as for the present time Medicines are used, which are of a malignant and poisonous Quality, for the Cure of Diseases when they lurk within the Body" (3:478). This comparison of past and present paralleled missionary criticisms. However, for Li the past of the ancients remained a standard of inspiration. European writers resorted to such comparisons to represent the ancient Chinese as having understood things significant to eighteenth-century Europeans, in ways that latter-day Chinese supposedly did not. The critiques sounded alike but represented different agenda.

The *Bencao* excerpts explained how and when to gather various herbs and how to understand the five tastes and various smells. They instructed the reader how to assess the soil where an herb grew, as this would affect the herb's quality, and whether an herb or formula was best encapsulated, powdered, or boiled, detailing actual preparation. They addressed connections between herbs and food. In short, they gave a rich overview, accompanied by instructions and examples. The difficulty for European readers was that Du Halde's selections rarely went beyond generalization. Moreover, illustrated discussion of specific drugs—rhubarb, China root, *Fen se, Ti hoang, San sti,* and cinnamon—were limited to substances relatively more familiar to Europeans. Only a few European physicians corresponded with Jesuits in

China, as did Jean Astruc (1684–1766) with Frs. Parennin and Étienne Rousset (1639–1758), sending them questions in 1721 about Chinese therapies for venereal diseases. He included material from their reply in the fourth edition of *Traité des maladies vénériennes* (Treatise on Venereal Diseases, Astruc 1777; Standaert 2001).

The Remedy That Dispenses Immortality

Semedo (1655) described ginseng, as had Martini and Cleyer. Christian Mentzel (1622–1701) wrote about it in a 1686 issue of *Miscellanea curiosa,* the journal of the German scientific society Academia Naturae Curiosorum. During the 1680s, Fr. Etienne de Fèvre called it the Chinese elixir of life. Melchisédec Thévenot (1620–1692) cited Martini's explanation that "ginseng" derived from *ren* (person): like mandrake root, it resembled a body with arms and legs. Le Comte (1698) rhapsodized about "the *Panacea,* and the Remedy that dispenses Immortality," adding, "Its Colour inclines to yellow, and when it is kept any time it grows wrinkled, and dry'd like Wood." Its taste "is sweet and delightful, altho' there be in it a little smack of bitterness: Its effects are marvellous; it purifies the Blood, fortifies the Stomach, adds motion to a languid Pulse, excites the Natural Heat, and withal augments the Radical Moisture" (226). He included three remedies for faintness, one instructing the user to "take a Dram of this Root . . . dry it before the fire in a Paper, or infuse it in wine, till it be Sated by it; then cut it in little pieces with your Teeth (and not with a Knife, Iron diminishing its Virtue) and when it is calcined, take the Poder in form of a Bolus, in warm Water or Wine, according as your Distemper will permit" (127).

Philosophical Transactions reviewed Thévenot, and Dr. Andrew Clench presented the Royal Society with ginseng wrapped in Chinese paper, along with a discussion of his own experiments (Appleby 1983). Dr. Robert Wittie of Yorkshire wrote to the Society about treating a relative of poet Andrew Marvell "who was . . . reduced unto a perfect Skeleton, a meer Bag of Bones, by a long Hecktick Feaver, joyned with an Ulcer of the Lungs." After administering ginseng in warm milk, Wittie found the patient's "lost Appetite restored, and his natural Ruddy Complexion revived in his Cheeks, to the Amazement of his desponding Relations, that he was called *Lazarus the Second*" (Wittie 1680, 3–4). He observed that popes—often elderly—"do make great use of this

Root, to preserve their Radical Moysture and natural Heat" (4–5). Having cited successful applications, he concluded, "Mr. *Boyle* once told me, he thought it was a Medicine sent from Heaven, to save the Lives of Thousands of Men, Women and Children" (7). (Boyle directed the British East India Company.) After reading Cleyer, John Locke commented in his journal about ginseng. Kaempfer cited Cleyer, and members of the Royal Society cited Kaempfer. At Kaempfer's death, Hans Sloane, president of the Royal Society, purchased his collection—including Japanese ginseng.

In 1711, Jesuit Pierre Jartoux described an imperial mapmaking expedition during which he observed four ginseng plants. Curious, he took his own pulse, ate a piece of the root and an hour later felt hungry and vigorous, with an enlivened pulse. He repeated the experiment days later when, so tired, he could "barely mount a horse," with identical results. The emperor, he added, dispatched herbalists to gather ginseng. One simmered it in a glazed ceramic pot, reducing the water to a goblet-full. After straining and reserving the liquid, one repeated the process for morning and evening doses. He posited "that in the hands of Europeans who understand pharmacy, this would be an excellent remedy, if they had put it to the necessary tests, to examine its nature in view of chemistry, and to apply it in the appropriate quantity, according to the nature of the illness to which it might be helpful" (Jartoux [1713]1762, 426). His letter, which included a drawing, originally appeared in anthologized Jesuit correspondence—the *Lettres édifiantes et curieuses* (Edifying and Curious Letters, Jesuits 1717). The Royal Society translated it that same year (Jartoux 1713).

Montreal-based Jesuit Joseph François Lafitau read Jartoux's letter. Speculating that Canadian terrain resembled northern China, he spent months talking with local Mohawks and searching the woods. In 1715 he located a plant matching Jartoux's description and took it to a Mohawk woman, who recognized it immediately (Lafitau [1716]1858). French botanists concluded there were two species, one from northern China and Korea, the other from Canada. French traders recruited Native Americans to gather the root, purchasing it at the exploitative price of two francs per root in Quebec and selling it for twenty-five francs in China (Nash 1898). East India traders also shipped it to Europe, where it appeared in herbals like *Pharmacopoea Amstelaedamensis renovata* in 1726 (Rutten 2000).

William Byrd Jr. corresponded with Sloane about surveying Virginia and North Carolina, commenting that he chewed ginseng root against fatigue:

> It gives an uncommon Warmth and Vigor to the Blood, and frisks the Spirit, beyond any other Cordial. It chears the Heart even of a Man that has a bad Wife, and makes him look down with great Composure on the crosses of the World. It promotes insensible Perspiration, dissolves all Phelgmatick and Viscous Humours, that are apt to obstruct the Narrow channels of the Nerves. It helps the Memory . . . 'Tis friendly to the Lungs, much more than Scolding itself. It comforts the Stomach, and Strengthens the Bowels, preventing all Colicks and Fluxes. In one Word, it will make a Man live a great while, and very well while he does live. And what is more, it will even make Old Age amiable, by rendering it lively, chearful, and good-humour'd. (Byrd 1929, 272–274)

Ginseng, he added, did not have the aphrodisiac qualities sometimes attributed to it, and appeared to lose some of its properties when shipped overseas. Still, Britain's Charles II and France's Louis XIV sampled it.

Du Halde explained how to preserve the root, detailing its taste, virtues, properties, and effects, and providing seventy-seven formulas from Li Shizhen. One patient, for example, following a debauch, suffered fainting, unconsciousness, numbness in his hands, sweating, and incontinence. With multiple draughts of ginseng tonic and applications of moxibustion, his symptoms gradually disappeared. There followed decoctions for building appetite, dissolving phlegm, counteracting vomiting from decay of the stomach, treating shortness of breath in women with childbed asthma, treating melancholy, and other complaints. The translator fretted over translating unfamiliar Chinese illness names, such as "dreaming of a ghost sitting on one's chest." His translations, he asked readers to understand, were intended to provide only a "Notion of the Sentiments of the Chinese with regard to Physick, and the manner in which they make up their Medicines" (Du Halde 1736, 4:19), with no expectation that Western practitioners would necessarily adopt Chinese formulas. A persistent gap therefore remained between European interest and the applicability of available Chinese knowledge.

Medical Exchanges

On occasion, Jesuits recorded observations of Chinese physicians at work. Du Halde (1736), for example, included the description of a man who fell ill while in a Nanjing prison. A physician provided three medicines. "The Patient found himself worse the following Night, lost his Speech, and they believed him to be dead, but early the next Morning there was so great a Change that the Physician, having felt his Pulse, assured him that he was cured" (3:363–364). Jesuit Jean de Fontaney recorded a similar story: "We thought to lose Father Gerbilon," he wrote. Sent with an imperial team by the Kangxi emperor to map Mongolia, Fr. Gerbilon fell so ill that his brethren administered last rites. They returned to Beijing, with Fr. Gerbilon in a cart that overturned several times on the rocky roads. "He would most certainly be dead, were it not for the care he received from a man who is now the first *colao* of China." Fr. Gerbilon slowly recovered, only to suffer a stroke. Then, "a Chinese doctor saved him" (de Fontaney 1843, 112–113).

Fr. Bernard Rhodes (1645–1715) related his experience of a physician in Vietnam when he had contracted a violent fever: "After having taken my pulse quite leisurely, [he] said to me, smiling, do not fear, Father, your illness has no malignancy; were you to leave it alone, you would surely be cured, but you would be cured much sooner if you took [medicine]. I wish to take it, I said to him, and to pay well for it; he then drew certain simples from his bag, he made various packets, then he told me the way to prepare and take the medicine in two doses. I took it for the two following days, and the third, I was without fever, shortly after I was entirely restored to health" (Grmek 1962, lviii). One suspects that missionaries who were in China for long periods of time routinely went to Chinese doctors.

Just as Europeans were unfamiliar with many Chinese medicinal plants, some common European medicinal plants were unknown in China, although the Kangxi emperor dispatched missionaries with Chinese botanists to seek them. Fr. Parennin wrote, "In vain did we seek for gentian, master-wort, juniper and the ash-tree: we found nothing that had the least resemblance to them" (Grosier 1788, 1:557). The presence of Jesuit doctors, surgeons, and apothecaries in these expeditions hints at ongoing medical cross-fertilization.

By 1685 the Kangxi emperor had asked for European physicians at his court—a request that Fr. Ferdinand Verbiest reported—and for current European medical works. The Jesuits themselves sometimes hesitated to provide the emperor with medical care, aware of Chinese physicians in Beijing who had been flogged after treating members of the imperial family unsuccessfully. (When subsequently summoned to treat another relative, the physicians performed better and were released, but they were ordered to wear a small chain around their necks as a warning.)

Despite such reservations, Jesuits Jean-François Gerbillon (1654–1707), who had come to China in 1687, and Tomé Pereira (1645–1708) treated the emperor for a fever in 1692 with medicinal lozenges prepared for France's Louis XIV. When symptoms recurred, they treated him with quinine brought from India by Fr. Claude de Visdelou (1656–1737). (Before taking it, the emperor had "outsiders" and "members of the Imperial clan" taste it, as a precaution; Spence 1974, 98). In 1709 Rhodes applied a plaster to a boil on the emperor's face, and on another occasion he treated him for cardiac palpitations. The emperor wrote, "Western doctors have their own special lore and skills: their wine is a tonic, Rhodes' brandy and cinnamon stopped my heart palpitations as his scalpel removed the growth on my lip. I keep him nearby and take him on my tours, together with Baudino the botanist and Viera the pharmacist, to complement Doctors Ma Chih-chün and T'ang Yü-chi" (Spence 1974, 99).[12]

Portuguese Jesuits continued to operate a pharmacy in Macao, a French doctor arriving in 1673 to work with lay brother Fray Braz García, providing free care for the poor. The Frenchman died a year later, but left Fray Braz his *materia medica* (Boxer 1974, 7). The Spanish Franciscans maintained an infirmary in Canton from 1678 to 1732, when they relocated it to Macao. Brother Antonio de la Concepción (ca. 1667–1749) served there as physician and surgeon; he treated two Guangdong governors and discussed a book of Western anatomy with one of them, Nian Xiyao. From 1715, Fr. Joseph da Costa (1679–1747) maintained a dispensary in Beijing, paid for by patients. The staffs of Russian missions generally included doctors. The emperor requested a good physician and "serviceable physic for pleasure" (probably an aphrodisiac). British Dr. Thomas Garwin reached Beijing in 1716 but apparently did not engage with the emperor (Wu 1931, 7). Beginning in 1719, Fr. Rousset continued da Costa's work, also accompanying the emperor as a physician and apothecary. Other Jesuits—Emmanuel de Mattos (1725–1747) and Louis Bazin (1712–1774)—practiced medicine as well (Wu 1931).

During a widespread illness in 1716, Fr. Ripa (1855) reported, the Jesuits in Beijing were ordered to visit the sick, as were court physicians and Buddhist priests. The missionaries did so but, not being doctors, refused to prescribe medicines. Ripa, however, let slip that he knew remedies for constipation. "I told them of a mechanical one," he wrote, "which, on being explained to the Emperor, amused his imperial Majesty amazingly" (91). In general, in direct encounters there appears to have been appreciation for the diagnostic and therapeutic skills of the other system, without extensive incorporation of its methods.

The Physic Gardens

Part of the transmission of herbal knowledge included shipments to Europe of Chinese medicinal plants. Parennin, for example, when accompanying the Kangxi emperor on expeditions, gathered specimens from different regions. He sent samples to the Académie Royale des Sciences in Paris, including *hiacao dongzhong*, or "plant in summer, insect in winter"—a medicinal fungus he himself had tried; *sanci*, of unknown origin; and an aromatic root that was probably *danggui*. Moravian Fr. George Joseph Kamel (Camellus), when sent to the Philippines, opened an herbal shop to distribute medicines to the poor, including some Chinese herbs. He sent specimens and drawings to British botanist-collectors John Ray (1627–1705) and James Petiver (1663?–1718). A network of correspondents around the world also sent Petiver specimens and descriptions of local flora. James Cunningham—a British East India Company surgeon in Amoy—provided the bulk of Petiver's Chinese samples. When Petiver died, his collection went to Hans Sloane.

British botanist and physician Leonard Plukenet (1642–1706) oversaw the Royal Garden at Hampton Court, building a botanical garden in Westminster. He and Petiver wrote about some six hundred of Cunningham's plants. His *Amaltheum botanicum* described roughly four hundred Chinese specimens, including some herbs. After his death, his collection of eight thousand plants was incorporated into the British Museum's Sloane Herbarium, most registered under "China" (Bretschneider 1881). The Physic Garden of Chelsea regularly exchanged seeds with Leyden's botanic garden, and developed a Garden of World Medicine that included Native American, Maori, Australian Aboriginal, ayurvedic, South African, and Chinese medicinal plants, along with samples from the Mediterranean and northern Europe. Some European physicians may have experimented with them therapeutically.

Cauterization and Needling

As Europeans encountered Chinese therapies applied externally, they drew parallels with humorally based surgical interventions and in some cases attempted to translate the underlying theory and rationale. The two modalities that most attracted their attention were moxibustion and acupuncture.

An Indian Moss

In 1674, Dutch Reformed minister Hermann Buschof published *Erste Abhandlung über die Moxibustion in Europa* (First Treatise/Disquisition on Moxibustion), following treatments by a woman in Batavia for gout and arthritis. (He sent samples of moxa to his son at Utrecht to sell.) In 1676, Bernhard Wilhelm Geilfus wrote a related dissertation, *Disputatio inauguralis de moxa* (Inaugural Discussion of Moxa). Buschof's experience added to Willem ten Rhijne's resolve to study acupuncture and moxibustion, informing his eventual dissertation on the subject (1683).

In 1676, afflicted by gout at a Dutch diplomatic conference, Sir William Temple resigned himself to waiting six weeks for it to heal, when a friend, Monsieur de Zulichem, explained "the Indian way" of curing it with a kind of moss: "to take a small quantity of it, and form it into a figure broad at bottom as a two-pence, and pointed at top; to set the bottom exactly upon the place where the violence of the pain was fixed; then with a small round perfumed match . . . to give fire to the top of the moss; which burning down by degrees, came at length to the skin, and burnt it till the moss was consumed to ashes" (Temple 1814,

254–255). Sometimes one cone sufficed; sometimes more proved necessary. Having rejected the alternatives—purging, poultices, plasters, and patience—Temple reviewed what he knew of therapeutic fire among Egyptians, "Moors," and Incas. After reading Buschof, he applied moxa. The pain disappeared. His story circulated throughout the conference; at de Zulichem's urging, shortly thereafter he wrote "An Essay upon the Cure of the Gout by Moxa."

It is not clear whether Temple identified moxa as Chinese. In a later essay, "Of Health and Long Life," he wrote, "For in China, though their physicians are admirable in the knowledge of the pulse, and by that, in discovering the causes of all inward diseases, yet their practice extends little further in the cures beyond the methods of diet, and the virtues of herbs and plants either inwardly taken or outwardly applied" (Temple 1814, 297). The "outwardly applied" may have meant moxa. Still, he apparently admired Chinese medicine, criticizing European physicians for "the various and fantastical changes of the diseases generally complained of, and the remedies in common vogue," which "among the Chinese would pass for mists of the mind or fumes of the brain" (299).

In the early 1680s Abraham Janusz Gehema (1647–1715) identified moxa as Chinese. In 1683 ten Rhijne's dissertation discussed both moxa and acupuncture as primary Chinese and Japanese pain therapies, which he traced to the *Sin non Hongteé*—presumably "Shennong" and "Huangdi" (Carrubba and Bowers 1974, 382). Le Comte learned about moxa as "Buttons of Fire" for dissipating winds. He was told, "Here they Martyr us by Fire; this Mode will probably never alter, because Physicians feel not the Mischief they do us, and are not worse paid for tormenting us, than for curing us" (le Comte 1698, 218). He did not know whether the practice originated with the Chinese or the Indians. Yet Kaempfer, pointing first to Western precedent among Arabs, Egyptians, and Greeks, linked the practice to China, Japan, and Korea (Kaempfer [1712]1996).

Le Comte (1698) was told that, for acute colic, "they lightly apply an Iron peal red hot to the Soles of the Feet; if the Patient shews any signs of feeling, they pass no further, and he is cured" (219). Kaempfer (1996), in contrast, argued that "the kind of fire that savagely attacks and eats away the skin and flesh," and that was applied with "glowing iron," characterized "Occidental surgery, with its grim attitude toward human beings" (110). The Chinese method involved the application of "gently glowing and slowly burning fire" (120). Ten Rhijne listed substances used in Western cauterization, tight cylinders of cotton in particular. He contrasted these with burning the down from dried mugwort leaves. Detailing how to hang, dry, and store the leaves, he noted that the Chinese and Japanese sometimes stored them for ten years before use. Preparing the down took no great skill. One ground the leaves in a mortar and pestle, then rubbed them between one's hands to remove the tougher fibers (Carrubba and Bowers 1974). Pressing the down into small cones, one placed these on selected points of the body.

Ten Rhijne, himself a surgeon and former anatomy instructor, attempted to explain the Chinese paradigm governing the placement of moxa cones, anticipating potential objections. Skilled anatomists would probably belittle the meridian diagrams he had included, particularly if they tried to match them with the blood vessels. But, he admonished, "we must not on this account casually abandon our confidence in experiments undertaken by the very great number of superb and polished intellects of antiquity" (Carrubba and Bowers 1974, 377). Those reluctant to accept the Chinese points could, through experimentation, propose their own. He then identified each meridian, explaining its related *yin* and *yang* characteristics and its beginning and end points in the body, matched to his four diagrams. Determining the point for burning moxa, he wrote, was like steering a navigational course through familiar waterways. One had to know the movements of the minuscule streams of blood as defined by the Chinese. At the same time, one could also resort to Hippocrates, who had directed the physician to burn wherever pain had set in, particularly where the arteries beat more strongly.

Kaempfer (1996) raised the issue that, in Chinese and Japanese practice, treatment points did not necessarily correspond to sites of pain:

A European is likely to judge as most appropriate for withdrawing vapors (since this is the sole purpose of burning) a location closest to the afflicted part. For the most part, however, the practitioner selects a remote location, often one not related to the troubled part by any known anatomical connections except through the common integument of the whole body. For just as a certain Lithuanian nobleman considered it absurd that an enema was prescribed when his head ached, so, too, do foreigners think that instant successes by moxibustion are illusory when cauteries are applied to a member and a location that are remote and completely free from pain. (128)

Kaempfer himself seemed open to the Chinese alternative, even though the prevailing European assumption was that one treated the afflicted point. Yet such assumptions had not always been operative. Galen had wondered whether bleeding specific veins yielded better results for specific conditions. To address a liver condition, one bled the right elbow. Back pain required bleeding inside the ankles, because *phleps* (vein, pl. *phlebes*) referred not to veins, as distinct from arteries, but to a network of blood-carrying tracts that were relatively unrelated channels (Kuriyama 1999).

Phlebes, observes Kuriyama (1999, 201), "were not just anatomically indiscriminate; they were anatomically false." One bled the vein thought to serve a specific part of the body, however far or near. Sometimes, points selected to treat more distant sites of pain actually resembled Chinese versions.[13] Exposure to anatomical structures undermined the theory of *phlebes* in the West. By the time Kaempfer wrote his dissertation, *phlebes* were a thing of the past, even though the therapeutic commitment to topological bleeding persisted. Otherwise, meridian logic might have looked more familiar to him and to other European surgeons.

Kaempfer contrasted moxibustion, as a preventive practice, with drugs, whose function was to cure. Preventive burning entailed smaller cones; curing required more and larger cones. Moxibustion could be used for all conditions "in which the imprisoned vapor [*qi*] causes the dissolution of solids, pain, and an impairment of proper functioning"—in short, "for almost the entire list of illnesses" (Kaempfer 1996, 125). At the same time, Kaempfer suggested that Buschof had exaggerated moxa's infallibility in curing gout.

Some European surgeons picked up on ten Rhijne and Kaempfer. Johann Pechlin (1646–1706) included a section on moxa in *Observationum physico-medicarum* (1691). He cited Buschof and ten Rhijne and identified moxibustion as Chinese, while also citing Hippocrates among the Greeks and Prosper Alpini's discussion of Egyptian methods in *De medicina aegyptiorum* (On the Medicine of the Egyptians, 1591). Moxa also found an advocate in Matthias Gottfried Purmann (1649–1711), former military surgeon and later chief surgeon of Breslaw, in his *Chirugia curiosa* (Purmann 1706), under the section on cauterizing. Purmann, too, linked moxa with the Egyptians. In Europe, he added, "Bishhof" (Buschof), Gahema (Gehema), Ericus Mauritius, and a Dr. Eltzholtz had transmitted the practice. But it was "Dr. *Cleyer* coming out of *India*"—"Indians" being "chiefly the inhabitants of China and Japan"—who had specified the use of mugwort (Purmann 1706, 246). Purmann also explained moxa's preparation and application.

Thomas Sydenham (1624–1689), a widely admired physician, in his treatise on gout and dropsy discussed "a certain Indian moss, called *Moxa,* which has, of late years, got a great name in the cure of gout" (Sydenham 1850, 156). He argued, however, that the remedy is "older with us," dating it to Hippocrates, and that consequently "no one can think that the difference between the flame excited on common flax and the flame excited on this Indian moss is of a specific kind: so that the one should be a bit more useful in the cure of gout than the other. This would be like thinking that a fire made of oaken was different from the one of ashen billets" (157). He saw no need to look to the Chinese.

Initially, Purmann (1706) observed, moxa's efficacy seemed quasi-miraculous, leading to correspondingly high prices. "I gave twelve Crowns for half an Ounce of it . . . I have sold to some Chirurgeons a small top of it for half a Crown, and that esteemed a favour also, it was so dear" (246). As it grew more common, prices dropped, and it was used indiscriminately "[by] the Confident and Ignorant [who] seeing that it would not Cure all Diseases whatsoever, they thought it good for nothing, and so the Noble *Moxa* lost its Reputation by the Silly Applications of Chirurgeons, that knew not where to place it, how to manage it, or repeat it in contumacious cases" (246). To correct such errors, Purmann provided detailed instructions. After the burning, one applied garlic and "some other Mollifying Plaister" to the point (247).

Purmann's application appeared deceptively Chinese. However, he did not adopt the Chinese diagrams, instead relocating moxa under methods related to Galenic cautery. More specifically, one opened any resulting blister, or created an irritation by putting the rough side of a plantain leaf against the burn, keeping the wound open to generate pus. Moxa "not only exhales Vapours and Humours from the affected Parts, but also strengthens them to resist the further Assaults of any Humour." "Vapor" was easy to equate with "Malignant, Acrid, and soure Humours" instead of *qi*. Following Hippocrates, one applied moxa "to the place where the Patient feels most Pain, except it is in the Eyes, Nose, Ears, and Privy Parts, which must be carefully avoided least you raise a Spirit you cannot easily lay again" (247). Purmann narrated his own experience of a painful left hip, which he successfully treated by requesting applications of moxa.

The only "Chinese" aspect entailed the use of mugwort. As would often happen, even when European physicians identified a practice with the Chinese, they did not necessarily view themselves as practicing Chinese medicine. For Purmann, for example, Chinese use became a detail equivalent to Prosper Alpini's having discovered moxa among the Egyptians. Over time, a litany of names emerged: Hippocrates, Alpini, Purmann, ten Rhijne, Cleyer, and Kaempfer. Eventually others were added, none of them Chinese.

The Famous Needling of the Chinese

Kaempfer summarized Chinese illness-producing factors as "winds and vapors" (Bowers and Carrubba 1970, 120). One perforated afflicted parts to release both. In northern China and the steppes beyond, winds had long been included among serious causes of illness. One finds them in Shang divinations—not as mere meteorological variables, but as spirits coming out of the four cardinal directions, each with particular influences. Wind, suggests Kuriyama (1999), was the conceptual ancestor of *qi*, although the two never quite meant the same thing. By the Han dynasty, winds were identified as originating from eight directions. Just as winds—some evil or empty—could stream through openings in rock or the ground, so they could penetrate the body's unprotected orifices and pores. Acupuncture, wrote ten Rhijne, conquered "corrupted and corrupting wind" (Carrubba and Bowers 1974, 391).

Fr. Hervieu's work on Chinese pulse-taking included a section on acupuncture, describing "large needles of silver, slightly blunted at the end . . . rolled between the fingers, to achieve effects in depth" (Lu and Needham 1980, 285). Ten Rhijne provided additional details. Needles had to be long, sharp, and round, with a spiral-grooved handle, and made of gold (or, more rarely, of silver). One inserted them either by rotating them between the index finger and thumb, or with gentle taps from a small hammer. Sometimes a small guide tube was used to prevent the hammer from driving the needle in too far. One left the needle in for the duration of thirty breaths, repeating the process as many as five or six times. (Kaempfer provided a similar description.) Ten Rhijne explained how practitioners learned the courses, locations, and pulses of the "arteries" with the aid of "hydraulic machines" and figures, referring to figurines for practicing needle insertions into preformed holes representing treatment points (Carrubba and Bowers 1974, 393). Kaempfer, who like ten Rhijne related acupuncture to a form of "colic" *(senki)* prevalent in Japan, also described nine abdominal punctures, in three parallel rows of three insertions each. One could use acupuncture to treat "headache, vertigo, lippitude, cataracts, apoplexy, spasmodic distortion, emprosthotonos, opisthotonos, tensions, nervous convulsion, epilepsy, catarrh and rheum, intermittent as well as continuous fevers, hypochondriacal melancholia, intestinal worms and pain arising from them, both diarrhea and dysentery, cholera, but above all for colic pain and other intestinal ailments produced by winds, spontaneous weakness also created by winds, swelling of the testicles, arthritis, and lastly for gonorrhea" (Carrubba and Bowers 1974, 395).

More dramatically, according to ten Rhijne, needles were sometimes supposedly inserted into the uterus of pregnant women, into the head of the restless fetus, to quiet it. Sinophile and classical scholar Isaac Vossius, in reviewing ten Rhijne, wrote uncritically: "Not less to be wondered at is that Surgery which they have cultivated in practice for so many centuries, especially in that perforation of all parts of the body which they do, even of the very brain itself, transfixed from one side of the head to the other with a metal bodkin a cubit in length or longer. Such things have often been seen by us [Europeans], either greatly mitigating or even totally removing by these means those pains to which the flesh is heir" (Vossius 1685, 76).

Like moxa and cautery, acupuncture was loosely grouped with Western surgical practices like bloodletting. Le Comte (1698) was told that the Chinese applied "red hot Needles." When he questioned the practice, a local pointed to European bloodletting "with the Sword" (scalpel) (218–219). Ten Rhijne insisted that both Chinese and Japanese "detest phlebotomy because, in their judgment, venesection emits both healthy and diseased blood, and thereby shortens life. They have, accordingly, attempted to rid unhealthy blood of impurities by moxibustion and to rid it of winds, the causes of all pain, with moxibustion and acupuncture" (Carrubba and Bowers 1974, 375).

And yet, as we have seen, Chinese practice did include bloodletting. Du Halde—apart from mentioning that Li Shizhen had used "sharp Instruments" to expel distempers—included only a discussion of Chinese bloodletting. Hervieu elaborated: the practice was common, but the Chinese drew only small amounts of blood. He presented a case: A Chinese Christian man suffered "gravel."[14] The person sent to treat him "tied the Patient's Arm above the Elbow, washed and rubbed the Arm under the Ligature, and then with a Lancet, made upon the Spot with a bit of broken *China*, he opened the Vein in the usual Place, that is at the bending of the Arm; the Blood spurted out very high, upon which the Ligature was untied, and the Blood suffered to run and stop of itself, and . . . instead of binding up the Orifice made by the Lancet, they generally apply a grain of Salt; the Patient was cured, and the next Day in the Evening he came to the Church" (Du Halde 1736, 3:427–429). Examining the site, Hervieu observed that it was "the same where it is generally done by Europeans." The operator was neither a physician nor a surgeon. Nor did he use a specialized implement. No one objected, suggesting a routine practice. Still, witnesses like Fr. Grueber commented, "They never let any man's blood, as we do, but instead of that, they make use of Cupping Glasses in the Shoulders" (Magalotti 1676, 77). Le Comte (1698) qualified the stereotype, writing, they "do not let Blood nor know the Clyster [enema] but since they have had Correspondence with the Physicians of *Macao*. They do not disapprove the Remedy, but name it *The Remedy of the Barbarians*" (218). Nevertheless, the trope that the Chinese rejected bloodletting took root, resisting Hervieu's qualifications.

Ten Rhijne reminded his readers of existing Western uses of needles in removing cataracts, sewing up wounds or harelips, sucking out harmful fluids, or perforating nasal polyps. Prior to its association with the Chinese and Japanese, "acupuncture" had referred to "tapping"—puncturing dropsical, or edematous, areas to expel fluid. Sydenham

(1850, 182) believed acupuncture useless for that purpose, although the issue was revisited for years. Neither ten Rhijne nor Kaempfer mentioned the nine needles of the Chinese. Yet analogous surgical applications using "needles" had long pertained in China. Some acupuncturists—many of them Daoists—used needles for eye surgery. Infections were also lanced (Leung 2003). Sewing up harelips was part of Chinese surgical tradition, dating back to the Han dynasty (Ma 2000). Literate elite physicians disdained such practitioners, whose techniques were often kept as family secrets.

Only one missionary recorded a surgical experience. Ripa, while accompanying the Kangxi emperor on an expedition in Tartary sometime in 1711, fell from his horse, injuring his head and other parts of his body. A Manchu surgeon poured ice-cold water on his neck to staunch the blood and restore his senses. The surgeon then bound Ripa's head with a cloth band, the ends of which two men held taut while the surgeon struck the cloth with a piece of wood to "set the brain, which he supposed had been displaced." Finally, Ripa was instructed to walk outside without his shirt. The surgeon threw a bowl of freezing cold water on his chest, forcing him to inhale abruptly, repositioning possibly dislocated ribs. He was not allowed to sleep until that evening, but was to walk as much as he could, supported by two people. "These remedies," concluded Ripa, "were barbarous and excruciating; but I am bound in truth to confess that in seven days I was so completely restored as to be able to resume my journey into Tartary" (Ripa 1855, 66–68). In turn, the Kangxi emperor remarked on the skills of Western doctors. They sewed up one of his generals who had been shot through the stomach. "The 'Ripped-Belly General' he was called," wrote the emperor. "When we met on the southern tour I made him loosen his clothes so that I could see the scar myself and touch it with my own hands" (Spence 1974, 99).

Although the meridian-based application of acupuncture had no direct match among surgical practices in Europe and China, there were discernible parallels. However, European surgeons were also building on knowledge acquired from anatomical dissection in ways that would dramatically reconfigure their self-understanding, practice, and views of the Chinese. As we shall see, these factors would engender growing biases against Chinese surgical methods.

Of Epidemics and Etiologies

The study of physiology and the pursuit of effective therapies in both China and Europe were related not only to lesser illnesses, but also to large-scale epidemics and the need to determine their causes and cures.[15] In Europe, the microscope, invented in 1590 and refined by Marcello Malpighi (1628–1694), allowed researchers to see "worms" and speculate about their role in disease. Sydenham tracked disease histories, mapping symptoms over time, along with recovery and mortality rates. In the colonies, Cadwallader Colden (1688–1776) recorded climate data, comparing it with epidemic patterns. William Douglas (ca. 1700–1752), a Scot, followed the scarlet fever epidemic in Boston in 1735. Such efforts coexisted with humoral models.

This interest in epidemics and illness histories appeared in Du Halde's excerpting from Zhang Ji's *Treatise on Cold-Damage Disorders (Shang-hanlun)*. A leading Chinese source on epidemics and infectious diseases, it addressed conditions attributed to cold, dampness, and sudden disturbances (see Ågren 1986). Zhang focused on common sequences of symptoms instead of individual constitutions (Epler 1988). Hervieu, the translator, explained: "*Chang* [*shang*] signifies to wound, to hurt; and *Han*, cold; as if one should say a malignant and dangerous Cold: This Distemper is very frequent in China; it is a malignant Fever to which they give the Name of *Chang han* in Winter, and which has other Names in the other Seasons of the Year" (Du Halde 1736, 3:451–452). The text provided examples of how to track exact times of onset, with interventions calibrated to each illness phase. Zhang classified disorders, not as "diseases," but by symptom clusters and related pulse patterns. The word for "disorder," *bing,* applied to chronic and acute illnesses, wounds and lesions, general discomfort, and serious or fatal conditions. It also referred to underlying physiological states, as when *zangfu*—the organ processes—exhibited deficits or plethora of *qi*. Therefore *bing* could mean "symptoms," "diseases," and "syndromes" (Epler 1988). Zhang explained what one could accomplish in relation to each variation. Seventeenth- and eighteenth-century Western physicians also focused on physical manifestations of sickness, clustering them, not as diseases, but as types of fever: smallpox was fever with eruptions; malaria, intermittent fever; and typhoid, continuous fever.

However, the *Treatise on Cold-Damage Disorders* represented a level of analytical sophistication regarding the treatment of epidemics that European and American doctors had yet to match.

Heavenly Doctors, Graves, Mountains, and Worms

Some reporters wrote about Chinese longevity practices. Magalhães (1688) criticized practitioners who cheated people "by means of their Chymical Operations, and their Gorgeous and Glorious Promises of . . . Life almost Eternal, and to Empower them to flit from one Mountain, City, or Province to another in a few Minutes" (110). The Kangxi emperor voiced similar complaints, characterizing many Daoist adepts as "boasters." Despite their claims to special powers, he had seen them age like other men. "If they were immortal why should they bother to descend to our humble world?" he asked sarcastically (Spence 1974, 101). Le Comte (1698) called Laozi a charlatan who

> did at length fancy, that by a certain sort of Drink, one might be Immortal. To obtain which his Followers practice Magick, which Diabolical Art in a short time was the only thing studied by the Gentry. Every body studied it in hopes to avoid death; and the Women thro' natural Curiosity, as well as desire to prolong their life, applied themselves to it, wherein they exercise all sorts of Extravagancies, and give themselves up to all sorts of Impieties.
>
>   Those who have made this their professed business, are called *Tien fo,* that is, *Heavenly Doctors* . . . The Covenants which they make with the Devil, the Lots which they cast, their Magical wonders whether true or only seeming, make them dreaded and admired of the common Herd. (314–315)

The issue entailed not only charlatanism, but the religiously "false" pursuit of eternal life, which itself was taken to be evidence of the devil.

A longevity treatise in Du Halde presented an alternate religious approach. Describing his childhood illnesses, the anonymous physician-author pointed to his father's performance of meritorious deeds: "He set himself upon rebuilding Bridges, repairing publick Ways, giving Cloaths to the Poor, Tea to Travellers, and sending Victuals to the Prisoners, so that in one Years time he was at a considerable expence in these kind of charitable Works; nor was this done in vain, for it was visible that without using any Physick I by little and little regain'd an healthy Look, my Stomach and Strength return'd" (Du Halde 1736, 4:57–58). To petition for healing for oneself or one's family members was to emulate the Buddha's acts of compassion. Such measures included printing and distributing Buddhist texts, because one accrued merit by spreading the Buddha's teachings. Restored to health, the author returned to study, but he soon relapsed. Next he was given one hundred books on medicine and instructed to read them. Another decline followed. Finally he renounced all remedies and turned to practicing virtue. Ultimately the Confucian project of deepening oneself as a profound person provided the real healing, said the author, editorializing: "The Heart is in Man what the Roots are to the Tree . . . it presides over the whole Man, and as soon as the Art of governing that is known, the Faculties of the Soul and the five Senses are likewise under command; it ought therefore to be our first care to keep a guard over the Desires and Affections of the Heart" (4:59). Of course, the author suggested additional measures: regulating one's diet and drink (a measure also favored by the Kangxi emperor), chewing thoroughly, not sleeping after meals, and not engaging in excesses. It was the difference between the *daoshi* and the doctor, suggesting plural approaches to longevity.

Western observers commented on Chinese responses to death and their connections with health. Nieuhof (1669) was struck by funerals, during which "several images of Men, Women, Elephants, Tygers, Lyons, and such like Beasts, made all of Paper and Painted with several Colours, are carried before the Coffin, and at last burnt at the Grave" (205). The burning conveyed such things, along with paper figures representing life's comforts, to the *yin* world of the dead. (It is not clear why elephants, tigers, and lions.) The Jesuits belittled overt connections between grave alignment and a family's fortunes and health. Du Halde (1736) wrote, "If any Person . . . attains his Doctor's Degree early, or is raised to a Mandarinate, if he has several Children, or lives to a good old Age, or succeeds in Trade, it is neither his Wit, Skill, or Probity that is the Cause, it is his House happily situated, it is the Sepulchre of his Ancestors that has an admirable *Fong choui*" (3:63).

In a landscape alive with *qi, fengshui* presumed that the forces of dragons and mystical tigers permeated the ground. Rocks, trees, streams, and lakes were thick with ghosts, demons, and spirits. Martini had listed sacred hills and mountains, including an engraving of a mountain god (see Figure 12) that Kircher published—all of which le Comte (1698) dismissed. "The idlest Dream, and that to which they give most Faith is, That there is a Dragon of an extraordinary Strength and sovereign Power" (93–94). Still, he described mountains as widely visited pilgrimage sites. "The Women especially are very exact in the Performance of this piece of Devotion, for having no other Opportunity of going abroad, they are glad of that Pretence. But these Holy Travels being somewhat prejudiciall to their Vertue, their Husbands are not over-well pleased at it; therefore only your ordinary sort of Women undertake these Pilgrimages; but as for Persons of Quality, they force their Wives Zeal into a narrower Compass" (94–95). Women might visit shrines for Guanyin or other female deities who helped one get pregnant or healed one's children, much like the Virgin or certain Christian saints.

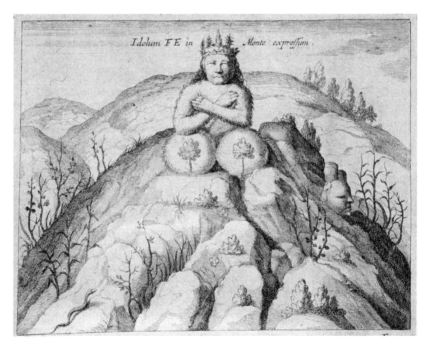

Figure 12. A mountain god. Athanasius Kircher, *China monumentis illustrata,* 1667. By permission of the Houghton Library, Harvard University.

The missionaries, schooled in the Church's history of healing, created their own pilgrimage sites. Eighteen years after Martini's death, Couplet described visiting his miraculously intact body: "No hair has fallen from his head nor whiskers from his face. There is no sign of putrefaction. There were people who cut his hair and nails, who washed his face and applied cosmetics to it . . . There are numerous visitors, including friends of the deceased, and all of them declare: the Jesuit is protected by the people and by the divinities because of his sublime virtues" (Liu 1996, 331). Martini had achieved a status analogous both to saint and local god, evidence not only of heaven-sent preservation but also of the implicit capacity to heal.

Le Comte admitted the temptation of religious wonderworking, describing a drought during which he and his fellow priests considered praying for rain, provided local Chinese discard their "idols." Prudence prevailed. Exorcism seemed less problematic—he hung a picture of Jesus in one afflicted house to expel afflicting demons. Du Halde (1736), while believing some possession stories probably false, still thought "there are in reality many Effects that ought to be attributed to the Power of Demons" (3:34). Possession, however, was not the only religious "affliction." Le Comte compared Buddhism to a plague: "This poison began at Court, but spread its infection thro' all the Provinces, and corrupted every Town: so that this great body of Men already spoiled by Magick and Impiety, was immediately infected with Idolatry, and became a monstrous receptacle for all sorts of Errors. Fables, Superstitions, Transmigration of Souls, Idolatry and Atheism divided them, and got so strong a Mastery over them, that even at this present, there is not so great impediment to the progress of Christianity as is this ridiculous and impious Doctrine" (le Comte 1698, 315[320, due to errata]). Note the language of poison and infection in relation to the social body of China. If Christ was the Physician, then the Church functioned as healer.

The missionaries, however, had no experience with another practice dating back at least to the Zhou dynasty. *Gu*—a deadly worm spirit—resulted from putting poisonous insects, worms, and snakes into a container for one hundred days. They devoured each other, leaving only one to inherit the others' poisons. The survivor was placed in water, with another of its species. They mated, producing deadly venom that could be put in an enemy's food or drink. Du Halde (1736) described the effects: "Those who are attacked with it have frequent Cardialgias, and something seems to gnaw them at the Heart, the Visage often becomes blueish; and the Eyes yellow, and several other extraordinary and irregular Accidents of the same nature happen: This Animal generally attacks the Midriff first, whence ensues spitting or vomiting of Blood; and if not prevented he'll devour the *Viscera* [*zangfu*] . . . and bring on Death" (3:457–458). No direct European correlate existed, but the practice resembled the lore of curses and occult afflictions. There were reported cases of witchcraft in Europe and the colonies— of objects being used as media through which to harm others (Butler 1990). Poisonous worms would have found a ready place among supernatural etiologies, malicious spells, and pacts with the Tempter—all condemned by the Church.

By the end of the period, the Chinese had been racialized as primarily white. Brownness carried class overtones, as it did in Europe, and yellowness lingered at the margins as a potential classifier. Chinese culture and intellectual traditions were considered superior on many counts. Where Europeans recognized analogies between the two worlds, they examined which practices to adopt and which to reject. The results ranged from pseudo-Chinese material culture to the fragmented exploration of Chinese approaches to healing, some of which—like astrology, divination, and ancestor practices—were no more seriously considered by a European intellectual elite than were their Western analogues. Pulse taking, herbal medicine, moxa, and acupuncture seemed more appealing.

Few physicians other than Abercromby and Floyer discussed actual attempts to adopt pulse taking. Its conceptual substrate and complexity, which few understood, together with the absence of teachers, figured as high barriers. Moreover, despite strong interest in Chinese herbal medicine, few Chinese herbs were available with which to prepare the formulas described in Du Halde. That "the very Names of the Roots and Simples, of which the *Chinese* Physicians compose their Medicines, are absolutely unknown" only complicated matters. Du Halde (1736) described his intent, therefore, as simply to illustrate how the Chinese used "a certain number of Remedies into the Composition of which their Roots, Plants, Simples, Trees, Animals, and even

Insects enter'd, and to give a Specimen of each Sort," facilitating an assessment of their skills (4:54). With few exceptions, such illustrations remained largely intellectual exercises.

A hint that *materia medica* could have been more widely imported to Europe appears in passing, under Du Halde's description of *Tang Couè* [*danggui*], which nourished the blood and helped its circulation. The drug could be obtained cheaply and shipped without spoiling, if one adopted precautions used by the Chinese: "This Root, like all others, is cut into very small Slices by those who retail it, for which reason if the *European* Merchants wanted to purchase Drugs of the *Chinese* at *Canton,* they ought to buy it out of the grand Magazines [stores] where the Roots are kept whole, and not from the Shops where they are cut into small Pieces before they are sold" (Du Halde 1736, 4:46–47). Yet apart from ginseng and drugs long part of Western medicine trade, like rhubarb and China root, it appears there was little demand for other *materia medica.* Only the tea trade flourished. That the leaves were successfully distributed throughout Europe and the American colonies attests to the feasibility of creating a market for Chinese medicines. Moxa was used by some, but acupuncture—apart from tapping—was primarily a matter of comparative curiosity.

Insofar as observers attempted to understand what they saw, heard, tasted, and felt, they did so with the assumption that China should be theirs to know, in tandem with a conviction that reality could be fully known and just as fully documented. The account, in its fidelity to the real, could be taken as authentic representation. In actuality, each web of reportage became another filter through which China entered the awareness of those who then went there, wrote more reports, and wove yet more layers of the web. As Edward Said (1979) has suggested, the fabricated Orient that resulted was not devoid of empirical substance. Many accounts provided considerable detail. But the substance had been so reworked that even when insider and outsider statements appeared to replicate each other, they often pointed in different directions, as in the condemnation of Daoist longevity practices. The observers—however intelligent and bent on rendering Chinese practices accessible—usually failed to notice the difference.

CHAPTER 4

Sinophiles, Sinophobes, and the Cult of Chinoiserie: 1737–1804

During the eighteenth century, a constructed European history rooted in ancient Hellenic thought erased historic connections between Greece and Africa, tracking a trajectory instead through Italy via the Renaissance, with "Europe" as the outcome. Eurocentric observers organized knowledge—including knowledge from other parts of the world—into "a systematic whole," applying their own intellectual structures to everyone else (Dirlik 2002). China became part of this project. Yet as the Enlightenment flourished, China also became a foil with which to assess the West. Writers like Voltaire (François Marie Arouet, 1694–1778), disillusioned by European institutions, generated a China imagined as the epitome of reason and good government. Other writers viewed it as despotic and corrupt. European and eventually American interest in Chinese healing arose as one facet of these perceptions of, and responses to, the Chinese and their practices.

Reports on China

The Jesuits continued to produce reports and translations. In 1743 the *Lettres édifiantes et curieuses* were translated as *Travels of the Jesuits, into Various Parts of the World*. Between 1776 and 1791, Henri-Léonard-Jean-Baptiste Bertin (1710–1792)—count of Bourdeilles and minister to Louis XV and Louis XVI—edited fifteen volumes of Jesuit letters and reports as *Mémoires concernant l'histoire, les sciences, les arts, les moeurs, les usages, &c. des Chinois* (Memoirs Concerning the History, Sciences, Arts, Customs, and Uses, etc., of the Chinese).[1] Bertin relied on missionaries like Fr. Jean-Joseph-Marie Amiot (1718–1793), whom he praised as unsurpassed in the sciences and the arts. Fr. Pierre-Martial Cibot (1727–1780) proved another important reporter.[2] From 1777 to 1785, Abbé Jean-Baptiste-Gabriel-Alexandre Grosier (1743–1823), librarian to "Monsieur, His Royal Highness," edited and published translations by Fr. Joseph-François-Marie-Anne de Moyriac de Mailla (1669–1748) of Chinese records as the *Histoire générale de la Chine*. The final volume—*De la Chine, ou description générale de cet empire* (A General Description of China, 1788)—was generally credited to Grosier. He expanded it to seven volumes between 1818 and 1820.

British reports remained few, reflecting England's ongoing difficulty in establishing a China trade. Lord George Anson (1697–1762), for example, was refused entry to Canton in the early 1740s. His vitriolic account, *A Voyage Round the World* (1748), became popular in England, setting a precedent for commentaries characterized by exaggerated faultfinding. The British East India Company, hoping to persuade the Qianlong emperor (1711–1799) to expand trade, dispatched the king's cousin, Lord George Macartney (1737–1806), in 1793. An Irish diplomat, Macartney had long believed it his destiny to go to China and had built a collection of China-related books (Peyrefitte 1993). The mission included Lord George Leonard Staunton (1737–1801), diplomat, physician, and friend of Macartney; Staunton's twelve-year-old son, George Thomas Staunton (1781–1858); John Barrow (1764–1848), originally young Staunton's tutor and now comptroller; physician Hugh Gillan (1745?–1798); Macartney's valet, Aeneas Anderson (dates unknown); painter William Alexander (1767–1816); and the Chinese translator Fr. Jacobus Li (b. 1750, called "Mr. Plumb" because *li* can mean "plum tree" in Chinese).[3] Macartney (Staunton 1797), Anderson (1795), Barrow (1804), and others wrote about their experiences. Barrow criticized the Jesuits for representing China as a paragon, to inflate their own successes.[4] He promised to "show this extraordinary people in their proper colours . . . as they really are" (Barrow 1804, 18), adding that it would be unfair to base one's opinion on Anson's account of his brief experience. That his own exposure to China was limited appeared not to trouble Barrow.

The *American Magazine* (Editor 1744) excerpted from Du Halde's *General History of China* (1736). When the American trade ship *Empress of China* reached New York in 1785, editors drew on le Comte's *Memoirs and Observations* (1698) and on Du Halde. By 1790, Harvard College's library included Du Halde, Hakluyt's anthology, Anson, and the *Lettres édifiantes* (Bond and Amory 1996). Americans also read accounts from the Macartney embassy and works by Voltaire, often borrowing them from "social libraries" like the Philadelphia Library Company founded by Benjamin Franklin. Such sources regularly included discussions of Chinese healing practices.

Jesuit access to China diminished with the order's suppression by Rome in 1773. Adversaries accused the Jesuits of distorting Christian teachings, and rites involving ancestor veneration remained a sticking point. Three members of the Vincentian order were sent to direct the Beijing mission, including the astronomer-geographer-botanist Fr. Nicolas-Joseph Raux (1754–1801). In 1811 the emperor expelled all but three Portuguese Vincentians from Beijing. Although the Jesuits were reinstated as an order in 1814, the hiatus proved disastrous to their role in China. Additionally, financial assistance from Spain and Portugal shrank, and the French Revolution ended French support. Catholic missionary narratives dwindled accordingly.

The Social Frame

The association of Chinese merchants in Canton known as the Co-Hong (*gonghong* or *gonghang*, "combined merchant companies") and its member "Hong" merchants were presided over by a "Hoppo," who reported to the local governor-general. By 1755 the Co-Hong's monopoly was well consolidated (Pritchard 1936; Gibson 1992; Downs 1997). In 1757 the Qianlong emperor restricted Western traders to a district in Canton through the trading season ending in the spring. Traders returned to Macao until early fall. Forbidden to learn Chinese from locals, they had to use the Hong merchants' "linguists," who generated a commercial *lingua franca*—pidgin (business) English. Western traders, who interacted primarily with Hong merchants, servants, sailors, and shopkeepers, rarely met the literati who had so impressed the Jesuits. It might not have helped; the literati considered merchants morally suspect, given their commitment to profits.

By the end of the century, conflicts between England and France—King William's War (1689–1697), Queen Anne's War (1701–1713), and King George's War (1744–1748)—brought French accounts of China under growing suspicion in England. The bias was compounded by a British and American tendency to identify the atrocities of the French Revolution with the influence of French *philosophes* like Voltaire, who had idealized Confucian thought and government. The emphasis on "progress" as the test of a culture's worth exacerbated a rereading of Jesuit accounts as unreliable.

China's own stability faced new challenges. The population increased from approximately 143 million in 1741 to approximately 200 million in 1762 and 286 million in 1784. Expansion, colonization, and emigration absorbed only some of the growth. The aging emperor became enmeshed with a handsome twenty-five-year-old bodyguard, Heshen (1750–1799), elevating him to chief minister. Through networks of corrupt officials and soldiers, Heshen plundered the empire for over twenty years, suppressing popular rebellions organized through the secret White Lotus Society led by Wang Lun, a martial arts master and herbalist.

Open rebellion broke out in 1796. The revolts—largely resulting from Heshen's corruptions—were protracted and costly because Heshen misled the government with falsified reports. When the emperor Jiaqing (1760–1820) came to power in 1799, he removed Heshen. Though the emperor eventually quelled the uprisings, they lasted until 1804, creating drastic deficits. At the time of Heshen's removal his private wealth approximated 800 million ounces of silver (Fairbank, Reischauer, and Craig 1978). The political system rewarded officials with government positions but paid low salaries, which the officials' friends and family expected them to supplement through tax increases and bribes. The poor bore the brunt. Nevertheless, China continued to view itself as "the central kingdom" and as economically and ideologically self-sufficient. It had little interest in expanding trade with European countries, or in new religious systems (Wright 1992).

Emerging intellectual trends in Europe reshaped discussions of China. Reason and nature, assumed to be universal, became the basis for knowledge, aesthetics, and judgment—also assumed to be universal—and the impetus underlying the movement known as the Enlightenment. Knowledge was classified according to categories of the day, predicated on the ostensible self-evidence of reason's constructs. This privileging of reason came in response to current political realities. French *philosophes,* for example, faced regular censorship and arbitrary imprisonment. Voltaire, educated by Jesuits, challenged the authority of the church as a source of disorder, ignorance, and barbarism.

Such men circulated between intellectual capitals, with Paris considered the central capital and French the international language. In the

British colonies, in Philadelphia, Benjamin Franklin and others organized the American Philosophical Society, some twenty members of
which actively promoted learning more about Chinese technology, agriculture, and trade. Authors from both continents corresponded and
exchanged publications. British colonies generally were better connected to London than to each other. Louisiana in particular maintained ties with France. European intellectual and fashion trends were
disseminated through American port cities. The wealthy sent their
sons, and sometimes their daughters, abroad for education, often to
England or to France, where they encountered the European representations of China discussed here.

French–British conflict spilled into the American colonies in the
Seven Years' War (the French and Indian War) in 1745. In 1759 the
British defeated the French, effectively ending France's colonial power.
To recover England's wartime financial losses, minister George
Grenville imposed import duties and, in 1765, a Stamp Tax—a reve-
nue-generating stamp affixed to all printed matter—which precipitated boycotts and public demonstrations. During this time, China
unwittingly intensified tensions by requiring silver in payment for tea,
creating a British trade deficit. To offset these losses, Parliament
passed the 1773 Tea Act, rebating duties on Chinese tea paid by the
British East India Company, but leaving in place those paid by American merchants who generally bought tea at auction in England. The
Company was authorized to sell directly to the colonies, often at lower
prices. In part, the act also came in response to decades of tea smuggling by American merchants, who purchased tea from Dutch free
traders in the Dutch West Indies (Goldstein 1978).

Colonists reacted by dumping a shipment of Chinese tea into
Boston Harbor, in what became known as the Boston Tea Party. By
September 1774, fifty-five delegates from twelve colonies met in Philadelphia for the first General Continental Congress, leading to the
American Revolution and the founding of the United States. France's
financial assistance to the colonists exacerbated French fiscal woes,
which in turn contributed to the French Revolution in 1789—the year
of the signing of the United States Constitution. By 1793 France was at
war with most of Europe. Fighting continued until 1815. The repercussions of China's policies thus had farther-reaching implications than
her ministers anticipated (or than would have concerned them).

American expansion was modeled on the American colonies' own origin—British imperialism, particularly in relation to non-European groups. Ongoing economic and cultural relationships with England reinforced dispositions to emulate British treatment of other peoples. Prior to the American Revolution, British laws had prevented American ships from trading directly with China. Such laws did not prevent Benjamin Franklin and wealthy Philadelphia merchant William Allen from sending expeditions in 1751, 1753, and 1754 to try to locate a northwest passage to China. The attempts failed, and antagonized London-based merchants, who viewed them as violations of the Navigation Act and other British trade laws (Goldstein 1978). In 1783, however, a privateer built for the Revolution was converted into a trade ship, the *Empress of China*. She sailed in February 1784, by way of the Cape of Good Hope, landing at Canton in August. Her cargo included a shipment of American ginseng destined for the Chinese medicine trade. The ship returned to the United States in 1785 with tea, porcelain, spices, silk, and nankeen (a sturdy cotton cloth), earning her investors a 26 percent profit of $30,727. By 1789, according to British captain John Meares (1791), fifteen American vessels were trading with China, sailing from ports like Salem, Boston, and New York. The sailors and merchants on these vessels were among the early American observers of China. Few, however, recorded their observations in forms that reached a broader public. One exception was Amasa Delano, whose *Narrative of Voyages and Travels* ([1817]1994) included his observations of Canton.

The Macartney embassy failed to expand trade between Britain and China. Macartney brought six hundred crates of gifts, including scientific instruments and British manufactures, not understanding that the Jesuits had already introduced more sophisticated mechanisms. Worse yet, visiting dignitaries were expected to *ketou* (kowtow) to the emperor. Macartney refused. Finally he proposed going on one knee and inclining his head, as he did for his own king.[5] Qianlong was insulted. Beyond a courtesy audience, he entertained none of Macartney's proposals. Even Macartney's efforts to express interest in Chinese culture and history met with apprehension. He returned disappointed. Subsequent representations of the mission produced some of the first scurrilous caricatures of the Chinese, as in one carton by James Gillray (see Figure 13).

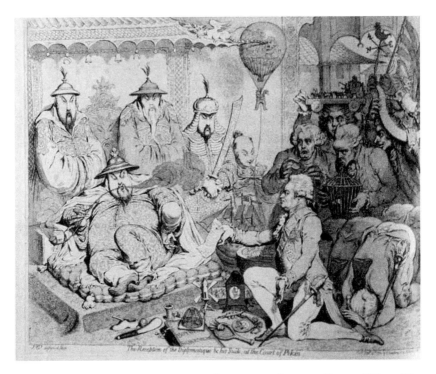

Figure 13. Macartney embassy visit to the emperor's court. James Gillray, *The Genuine Works of James Gillray*, 1830. By permission of the Houghton Library, Harvard University.

Of Time, Space, and Humankinds

As in earlier periods, Westerners continued to interpret Chineseness in temporal and spatial frameworks, and within constructs of human types. These endeavors merged imagination, fascination, and suspicion with aesthetic and moral assessment. Some of the very authors who generated discussions of Chinese healing practices also commented on these other factors. The resulting images and accounts illustrate the complexity of converging and sometimes conflicting representations.

Assessing Antiquity

Revisiting Noachide time frames, some Jesuits proposed that Noah's ark had landed in China, that early Chinese law had been Hebraic, and that China's classics foretold Christianity. John Bell (1691–1780), a Scotch physician who accompanied a Russian embassy (1719–1722), wrote that the Kangxi emperor acknowledged "a great deluge in China [had] destroyed all the inhabitants of the plains; but such as escaped to the mountains were saved" (Bell [1763]1965, 154). Barrow cited a confirmation of the flood by Carl von Linné (Linnaeus). The Jesuits might therefore be right that Noah had gone east, "and that he is the same person as the Foo-shee of their history" (Barrow 1804, 291).[6]

European understandings of "antiquity" underwent reassessment. Herculaneum was excavated in 1738; Pompeii, beginning in 1760. China provided some with further inspiration. For others, classicism was folded into an emerging construction of time and change, understood as history and progress. For them, although one could admire ancient China, the country was read as having stagnated—a trope that resurfaced in Barrow (1804): China was "among the first nations . . . to arrive at a certain pitch of perfection, where, from the policy of the government, or some other cause, they have remained stationary: that they were civilized, fully to the same extent they now are, more than two thousand years ago, at the period when all Europe might be considered, comparatively, as barbarous; but that they have since made little progress in any thing, and been retrograde in many things" (238). Barrow proposed to enable the reader to rank China's current place "in the scale of civilized nations" (4). This ranking almost invariably positioned Europe as the rising exemplar of progress.

In the Space of Fashion and Art

Space and the Chinese ceased to be primarily a matter of maps. Rather, a constructed China reoriented Western material and metaphoric experiences of space, through style and fashion. Architectural innovation, for example, followed an imagined Chinese aesthetic. William and John Halfpenny published *Rural Architecture in the Chinese Taste* (1750–1752), and Eva Dean Edwards and Matthew Darly, *A New Book of Chinese Designs* (1754). The wealthy built "Chinese" rooms and pavilions. In Paris a Chinese café boasted an actual Chinese porter; the waitresses dressed *à la chinoise*. Landscaping also underwent sinification. The most famous example was the Duke of Kent's Kew Gardens, near London, designed by former supercargo Sir William Chambers (1726–1796) according to a "Chinese" model—including a nine-story pagoda. In his *Designs of Chinese Buildings* ([1757]1969), Chambers cited Du Halde as saying that Chinese cities looked alike, justifying Chambers's Canton-based drawings as typical. A concurrent fascination with the Gothic led to novels set in ruined castles, tombs, and dungeons (the wealthy built fake ones). Both fashions appeared in William Halfpenny's *Chinese and Gothic Architecture Properly Ornamented* (1753).

Individual bodies were wrapped in chinoiserie. Italian artist Antonio Canal ("Canaletto," 1679–1768) included women in Chinese gowns in his *English Landscape Capriccio with a Palace* (ca. 1754). Locals witnessed John Bell riding the moors in Chinese robes. These influences crossed the Atlantic, where in Salem, Massachusetts, men wore such robes at public assemblies. Residents of American ports encountered Chinese goods: "In the shops where one might purchase Bohea and Souchong teas, nankeens, India muslins, Chinaware, Bengal ginghams, lacquer boxes, camphor wood sea chests; while reading the newspaper where notices of new arrivals of vessels from Canton and Calcutta regularly appeared; or perhaps while sauntering along the wharves where one might encounter Chinese and Indian servant boys brought home by the sea captains" (Jackson 1981, 7). Boston merchants sold reproductions of Chinese wallpaper, and the furniture of Thomas Chippendale, with design elements like the ball-and-claw foot, modeled after the Chinese dragon-foot. In 1755 George Washington paid three hogsheads of tobacco for Chinese porcelains. Thomas Jefferson possessed an edition of Du Halde. He considered imitating the pavilion at Kew and erecting a Chinese temple at Monticello (Tchen 1999).

A fictitious China entered the space of popular media and literature. Some authors imitated Chinese poetry. A Mme du Boccage (1786, xi) described inheriting her penchant for things Chinese from her parents, noting her "wish to put into French verse several from the Chinese poems." In England, Bishop Thomas Percy translated a Chinese romance, proverbs, and fragments of poetry as the *Hao Kiou Choaan: or the Pleasing History* (1761). Readers continued to read pseudo-Chinese fiction, like *Chinese Tales* and *Tartarian Tales,* which Samuel Taylor Coleridge loved as a child. Even Benjamin Franklin concocted a story involving two Western sailors in China. Robert Dodsley's *Economy of Human Life* ([1750]1817), purportedly authored by a Chinese imperial scholar, grouped platitudes under headings like

"Benevolence" and "Charity." Letters supposedly written by Chinese travelers (Chinese Traveler 1745) lampooned European cultures, as in Oliver Goldsmith's 1762 "The Citizen of the World" (Goldsmith [1762]1901). Chinese elements also appeared in theatrical space. In 1754 the ballet *Les fêtes chinoises* triumphed in Paris. In 1755 David Garrick brought it to England. Anti-French sentiment, however, prompted riots, closing the theater. He had better luck with Voltaire's rendering of a tale of revenge from Du Halde. The *Orphelin de la Chine* (Orphan of China) played in France, England, Italy, and the United States.

As Theodore Foss and Donald Lach (1991) note, "Europeans manufactured chinoiseries, composed unreal images, imported objects for which they misunderstood the usages, called these things Chinese, and then applauded the Chinese for having good taste!" (181). Nevertheless, these products of Western imagination were circulated and advertised, the advertisements themselves contributing to a fabricated China. Tradesmen's business cards utilized racialized images to sell products like tea, representing the Chinese as trading partners at once exotic and familiar (Kim 2002)—the very contradiction implicit in the broader process of imagination.

The Space of Social Vision

On more intangible levels, representations of China provided lenses through which Europeans and Americans rethought the inner space of the mind. Intellectual chinoiserie selectively appropriated Chinese thought, French *philosophes* admiring a system whose philosophers appeared to run the state. They saw in Confucius an agnostic rationalist because translations either omitted his cosmological commitments or transposed them into Deist keys, registering a moral civilization independent of Christianity. An advocate of agrarian economy, Louis XV's physician François Quesnay (1694–1774) saw in China a model state; this earned him the sobriquet "Confucius of Europe." Franklin knew and visited Quesnay, and Jefferson translated Count Destutt de Tracy's *Treatise on Political Economy,* a work informed by Quesnay's version of Confucian economics (Tchen 1999). British intelligentsia construed the literati as landed gentry, committed to public service—much like themselves. Samuel Johnson described China as "a country where Nobility and Knowledge are the same, where Men advance in rank as they advance in Learning, and Promotion is the Effect of virtuous Industry" (Eubulus 1738, 365).

American Magazine printed excerpts from Du Halde and described the *Analects* as containing "a great Number of Reflections and Precepts very affecting and important" (Editor 1744, 632). In a 1749 letter, Franklin advised evangelist George Whitefield to win over political leaders, setting examples for other social classes. "On this principle," Franklin added, "Confucius, the famous eastern reformer, proceeded. When he saw his country sunk in vice, and wickedness of all kinds triumphant, he applied himself first to the grandees; and having by his doctrine won them to the cause of virtue, the commons followed in multitudes" (Franklin 1987, 439). The model of Confucius thus informed political thought and behavior throughout the eighteenth century.

Chinoiserie did not attract everyone. Goldsmith (1901) mocked fashionable women's "sprawling dragons, squatting pagods, and clumsy mandarines . . . stuck upon every shelf: in turning round, one must have used caution not to demolish a part of the precarious furniture" (306). Such excesses generated a reactive defense of Europe's Greek and Roman roots. Two counter-trends emerged. The first depicted the literati as atheists; the rules of morality central to Confucian thought, one author asserted, were nothing more than "the Dictates of your own Heart" (Anonymous 1740, 30). The second viewed Chinese religious pluralism with growing suspicion, suggesting that Buddhist and Daoist superstition riddled the country. Because the Jesuits had represented Buddhism and Daoism as minority traditions, some European journals charged the order with distorting the truth to serve its own interests. One correspondent to the *Gentleman's Magazine* equated China with the anti-Christ (Appleton 1951, 151).

Taxonomies of Human Variety

Discussions of the Chinese became part of ongoing efforts to refine human typologies. Taxonomies based on color and phenotypes assumed increasing importance, although they were still distributed along a black–white polarity. The Chinese routinely either were said to constitute distinct types or were included in clusters of subtypes.

Physician John Hunter (1728–1793), for example, posited a gamut ranging from black and swarthy (northern Africans) to copper-colored (East Indians), red-colored (American Indians), brown-colored (among whom he included the Chinese), brownish (Turks, Laplanders, and southern Europeans like Sicilians and Spaniards), and white (northern and eastern Europeans) (Editor 1775b, 368). In his *Natural History* (1749–1788), George-Louis LeClerc, the Comte de Buffon, applied the term *race* to categorize different complexions. His typology consisted of copper, purple, tawny, olive, yellow, and brown, positioned between whiteness and blackness. It acknowledged varieties within national groups, such as sun-darkened French peasants and lighter-skinned urbanites, whose differences corresponded to earlier distinctions related to color variations among the Chinese due to sun exposure.

The term *Caucasian* entered the racial lexicon through a taxonomy developed by German anatomist and naturalist Johann Friedrich Blumenbach (1752–1840) in *De generis humani varietate nativa* (On the Natural Variety of Mankind, 1795). Building on the work of his teacher, Linnaeus, Blumenbach proposed five groups: Caucasian (his own addition), Mongolian, Ethiopian, American, and Malay. "Caucasians" inhabited the Caucasus Mountains, as the original humans. Over time, Blumenbach argued, part of the group had degenerated in two directions, yielding the other four types. On one side were Americans, from whom emerged Mongolians; on the other, Malays, yielding Ethiopians. "Caucasian" was white, with red cheeks, while "Mongolian" was "yellow, olive-tinge, a sort of colour half-way between grains of wheat and cooked oranges, or the dry and exsiccated rind of lemons" (Blumenbach [1795]1865, 209–210). Aesthetics intruded as Blumenbach ranked the groups according to notions of relative beauty: At the zenith he placed Caucasians—light-skinned Europeans, northern Africans, and peoples of western Asian countries. Black Africans and East Asians stood farthest from this ideal, both represented accordingly as the ugliest (see Gould 1997). Blumenbach's system was soon equated with "Anglo-Saxon" ancestry—a construct including those of Teutonic descent. Over time, Anglo-Saxon identity assigned itself the mystique of a peculiar purity, presumed superiority, and racialized whiteness.

Eighteenth-century writers also attempted to locate causes for color

differences. One camp defined them as variations within a single species; the other, as evidence of multiple species. The first resorted to
humoral theory, associated with different "complexions" and geography. Voltaire, for example, believed that Europeans, Africans, and
Native Americans represented distinct species (Smedley 1993).
Polygenesis theories drew on biblical narratives involving the flood or
the Tower of Babel. Blumenbach (1865), for whom "degeneration" explained difference, attributed some of it to climate (197). Another approach drew on the Great Chain of Being, which organized all living
things hierarchically, and into which newly discovered forms could be
inserted. Gradually a temporal dimension was inserted, such that organisms might "climb" the chain as if it were a sort of ladder (Rolfe
1985, 302).

Reality routinely undermined efforts to delineate absolute racial
types. Medical journals reported cases of blacks who turned white
(and, occasionally, vice versa), as did Henry Moss, who became something of a celebrity in 1796. Children from intermarriages were viewed
differently in different contexts. Thomas Jefferson and Patrick Henry,
for example, promoted white–Indian intermarriage. Marriages between Indians and blacks were not uncommon, particularly because
escaping slaves often sought refuge with the tribes. The period thus
witnessed the irony of efforts to type difference concurrent with realities that persistently confounded the types.

Racializing Chineseness

Jesuit Fr. de Tartre wrote in 1701, "The Usages and Customs of this
Empire are so different from ours, that an *European* must quite new
mould himself . . . to become a perfect *Chineze*" (de Tartre [1701]1762,
145). The policy presumed that newly arrived priests knew what a "perfect Chineze" *was.* Descriptions abounded, some providing phenotypical details. Blumenbach colored "Mongolians" "yellow," departing
from earlier Jesuit reports of whiteness. Rejecting *Tartar* (a term he
blamed on Matthew Paris), he applied the term *Mongolian* to all East
Asians. Barrow distinguished Tartars (Manchus) from the Chinese,
while Macartney critiqued tendencies to confuse them, given their mutual contempt. Barrow rejected a China–Egypt connection, believing
the Chinese were a distinct race.

Some discussions of color were more nuanced. Macartney thought Chinese peasants were "copper-colored" from the sun but "naturally fair" (Barrow 1807). Barrow (1804) found the Chinese and Manchus ranging from fair to dark, while "women of the lower class, who labour in the fields . . . are almost invariably coarse, ill-featured, and of a deep brown complexion, like that of the Hottentot. But this we find to be the case among the poor of almost every nation" (124). He drew further comparisons with "Hottentots," including an illustration of the heads of a Chinese man and a Hottentot (see Figure 14): "I am the more convinced of their near resemblance in mental as well as physical qualities. The aptitude of a Hottentot in acquiring and combining ideas is not less than of a Chinese, and their powers of imitation are equally great, allowance being made for the difference of education" (49–50). Hottentots, Barrow suggested, lacked only education to equal

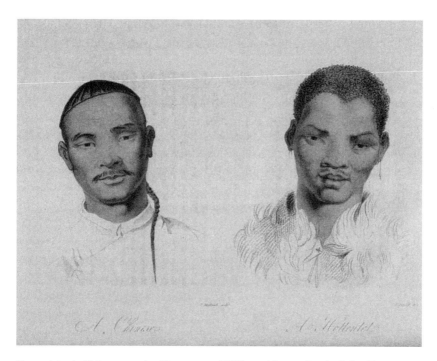

Figure 14. A Chinese and a Hottentot. William Alexander, in John Barrow, *Travels in China,* 1804. By permission of the Houghton Library, Harvard University.

Chinese cultivation. Yet opinion at the time viewed them as barely human (Gould 1985), rendering Barrow's assessment ambiguous.

The racializing process also assessed behavior and purported moral
disposition. Europeans continued to express mixed perceptions of
Chinese manners, for example. Bell (1965) wrote, "Above all, their regard for their parents, and decent treatment of their women of all
ranks, ought to be imitated and deserves great praise" (182). He described sightseeing, shopping, and dining with "one of my Chinese
friends" (166). Macartney described a Manchu viceroy who "behaved
with refined and attentive politeness; but without the constraints of
those distant forms, or particular ceremonies, which are sometimes thought proper . . . in China between persons of unequal rank"
(Staunton 1797, 1:261). Mandarins who visited the party proved "in-
quisitive, lively, and talkative, and totally void of that composure, gravity, and seriousness, which we had been taught to believe constituted a
part of the Chinese character" (Barrow 1804, 193).

Yet surgeon François Dujardin (1738–1775) cited Du Halde, describing the Chinese as "cold and tranquil," accustomed from childhood to order, reason, and custom, their behavior prescribed by rites
that "chilled the soul" and "extinguished feeling" (Dujardin 1774, 75).
The term *jealousy* increasingly entered British descriptions, implying unjustified suspicion—ignoring that such suspicion was sometimes
provoked, as when Anson (1748) demanded that local officials "give
him no further trouble, for he would go when he thought proper and
not before" (369). Offended, they prohibited anyone from selling him
provisions. Anson retaliated in print: "We are told by some of the Missionaries, that . . . the morality and justice taught and practiced by [the
Chinese] are most exemplary . . . But our preceding relation of the behaviour of the Magistrates, Merchants and Tradesmen at *Canton*,
sufficiently refutes these jesuitical fictions . . . For we have seen that
their Magistrates are corrupt, their people thievish, and their tribunals
crafty and venal" (413–414). Macartney found some high-ranking men
"ceremonious without sincerity, studious of the forms only of politeness" (Barrow 1807, 119). He voiced frustration at "that same strange
jealousy . . . which the Chinese government has always shewn to other
foreigners, although we have taken such pains . . . to conciliate their
friendship and confidence" (269). Some observers criticized what
they viewed as elegance masking dirt. Barrow commented that neither

sovereigns nor peasants changed their undergarments or bathed frequently. Even officials, he wrote with distaste, summoned attendants to remove lice from their necks. He also disliked that they "spit about the rooms, or against the walls, like the French" (Barrow 1804, 52).

European writers, who adopted Chinese pseudonyms to criticize their own cultures, perpetuated challenges to Chinese honesty. Jean-Baptiste de Boyer, the Marquis d'Argens (1704–1771), author of *Chinese Letters* (Argens 1741), feigned Chinese identity to write:

> One Day when I was in the Province of *Canton,* I could not help being angry at what a Countryman of ours said to an *English* Merchant, to whom he had sold a great many Bales of Silk. The *European,* before he put them on board his Ship, was resolved to examine them. The first that he opened, he found in a very good Condition; but when he came to inspect the others, he perceived that every Piece of the Silk was rotten. He smartly reproached the *Chinese* for his Knavery; but the latter, with a Gravity as surprizing as it was unfathomable, made him Answer, *I should have served you better, if your Rogue of an Interpreter had not assured me positively that you would not look into your Bales.* (Argens 1741, 15)

Years later, in his autobiography, Barrow (1847) remembered "Vantagin" (Wang Wenxiong, 1740?–1800), a soldier who accompanied the party, and "Chou-ta-jin," a provincial governor, as "two most amiable, well-conditioned, and cheerful men . . . who gained the esteem and affectionate regard of everyone in the embassy, having been ever ready to please and make us all comfortable" (65). Yet his embassy narrative also characterized many Chinese as "well skilled in the arts of cheating. They have, indeed, found many Europeans as great proficients in that art as themselves. And if you cheat them once, they are sure to retaliate on the first opportunity" (Barrow 1804, 184). Anderson (1795) blamed interactions with foreigners for the "knavish" character of Cantonese traders (278). Barrow again differentiated along class lines, pointing to the care with which the embassy's crates were transported, likening Hong merchants to eminent English traders. This class-divided perception allowed him to speak with equal sincerity in praising his Chinese friends and criticizing street merchants.

Chinese treatments of bodies were selectively emphasized. George Henry Mason's *Punishments of China* (1801) praised Chinese decency, modesty, and self-control but slid into an illustrated folio of punishments. The collection not only joined the lurid genre of William Jackson's *Newgate Calendar,* whose extended title promised "notorious criminals . . . who have suffered death, and other exemplary punishments," but also contributed to a trope focused on "Chinese torture." Such works represented the Chinese as having been made "indifferent, unfeeling, and even cruel" by "the state of society, and the abuse of the laws by which they are governed" (Barrow 1804, 107). The exposure of infants was cited as evidence, Barrow claiming to have seen an infant's body in the river. Such descriptions generated more persisting impressions than Bell's (1965, 183) description of public hospitals that recovered abandoned babies or Delano's (1994) speculation that exposure represented the desperation of poor women. No one drew comparisons with infants exposed in Europe, although in 1771 alone Paris's Enfants-Trouvés hospital retrieved 7,600 cast-off babies, many of whom died. In 1778 the city's register of grievances included the complaint that abandoned newborns fell prey "to the voracity of animals" (Peyrefitte 1993, 159).

Foot binding was still equated with fashionable corseting. Barrow (1804) added, "We had certainly no great reason to despise and ridicule the Chinese . . . seeing how very nearly we can match them with similar follies and absurdities of our own" (50). More problematic for him was homosexuality, which even "the first officers of the state make no hesitation in publicly avowing" (101). Staunton singled out court eunuchs. Both practices appeared to render Chinese manhood suspect—reactions situated within a larger, gendered rationale for British imperialism, as when one author (Anonymous 1773) suggested that Providence had given India to England partly because of the "effeminacy" of its inhabitants. These representations of body-related practices contributed to a racialized Chinese identity, in which color and purported unnatural cruelty became intertwined, alongside representations that idealized Chineseness. Two opposites emerged—one unfeeling and suspect, the other a paragon.

Chinese Abroad

The Qing government prohibited emigration, fearing that overseas Chinese might organize to challenge its authority. The policy limited direct encounters in Europe and America. Many Chinese seminarians were orphans or from poor families, and merchants were not schol-ars.[7] Neither exposed the West to Chinese elite culture. Around 1751, Chinese Jesuits Louis Guo (Gao Leisi, 1732–1790) and Etienne Yang (Yang Dewang, 1733–1798) reached France, staying for thirteen years as Bertin's protégés, known as "Bertin's Chinese." Prior to their re-turn, Anne-Robert-Jacques Turgot (1727–1781) invited them to re-main an additional year to study science, agriculture, and industry, and conduct a comparative inquiry into Chinese practices. Reaching Beijing in 1766, the two encountered unanticipated difficulties. Hav-ing left China illegally, they dared not attract the attention of govern-ment officials. Instead, their Western superiors posed Turgot's ques-tions and sent the responses back to France, providing the *Mémoires* with discussions of China's history, sciences, and letters (see Cordier 1909; Silvestre de Sacy 1970; Lottes 1991). Guo and Yang also received some medical training in France, practicing it after returning to China.

In 1756, Portuguese-speaking merchant Loum Kiqua visited Eng-land and was received by the royal family, although disappointed British intellectuals could not communicate with him. Daniel Serres painted his portrait. He returned to China in 1757. Merchant Tan Chitqua, who made clay busts, came to England in 1769, conversant in pidgin English. He, too, met royalty, and he received commissions to craft busts of the Royal Infantry. Invited to the first official dinner of the Royal Academy, he was included in Johann Zoffany's portrait of the group. He returned home in 1772.

It became fashionable to have Chinese pages, as did Giovanna (Janette) Bacelli—the Duke of Dorset's Italian mistress—in "Hwang-a-tung": "a young man of twenty-two, and an inhabitant of Canton, where having received from Chitqua, the Chinese figure-maker, a fa-vourable account of his reception in England . . . he determined to make the voyage likewise, partly from curiosity, and a desire of improv-ing himself in science, and partly with a view of procuring some advan-tage in trade, in which he and his older brother are engaged" (Gentle-man 1775).[8] John Bradley Blake (1745–1773), an East India Company supercargo, may have sponsored Hwang's trip. Hwang was mentioned in letters and diaries of literary men he met, appeared in sketches for Gainsborough's portrait of Bacelli, was painted twice by Sir Joshua Reynolds (see Figure 15), and received education at the Grammar School in Sevenoaks at the duke's expense. The servants called him

"Warnoton." Following his return to Canton, he corresponded with Sir William Jones, with whom he briefly considered translating the *Shijing* (Classic of Poetry) (Sackville-West 1991).

In the United States, three Chinese sailors were reported stranded in Baltimore, Maryland, during 1785. In 1788 John Meares hired craftsmen and sailors out of Canton, speculating that such men would be invaluable to a potential Pacific Northwest trading post. Unfortunately, Spaniards captured Meares's men, detaining the Chinese to dig in the mines. As of 1796, eight Chinese were working as servants in the New York household of André Everard Van Braam Houckgeest (1739–

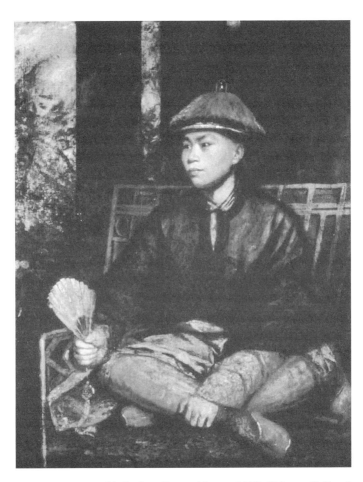

Figure 15. Wang-y-tong. Sir Joshua Reynolds, ca. 1776. Private Collection.

1801), who was a member of a Dutch East India Company embassy to China in 1794–1795 (Chen 1980, 4). In 1798 a Chinese sailor died in Boston Harbor. His captain arranged for his burial in the Central Burying Ground on the Boston Common. The weathered stone reads:

> Here lies interr'd the Body
> of CHOW MANDERIEN
> a Native of China
> Aged 19 Years; whose death
> was occasioned on the 11th Sept
> 1798, by a fall from the Masthead
> of the Ship Mac of Boston.
> This Stone is erected to his Memory
> by his affectionate Master
> JOHN BOIT Junr

Chinese continued to enter Spanish territories. Two were baptized in Monterey—one in 1774, the other in 1793. German author Ludwig Louis Salvator mentioned a Chinese man living in Los Angeles in 1781 (Chen 1980, 4).

The temporal, spatial, and phenotypical constructions of the Chinese converged in what amounted to a kind of proof-texting (randomly taking passages out of context to "prove" an argument). Resulting reports about China were used to support a broad spectrum of European interests and undertakings, ranging from interior decorating to political theory. The various self-interested readings yielded multiple Chinas. Whether debates over how to interpret China and the Chinese were cast in terms of faith versus reason, or science versus superstition, deeper issues involved the authority of chosen forms of knowledge, and related versions of personhood and social order.

The State of Physic

Amid these complex perceptions of China, we find Europeans exploring Chinese healing. Some were Jesuits, some traders, some diplomats. Some represented a new category, the naturalist, engaged in studying the world's plants and *materia medica*. Some were physicians and surgeons. It is not difficult to imagine them wearing Chinese robes, strolling through pseudo-Chinese gardens, crossing a brook with arching

Chinese bridges, and returning to studies decorated with wallpaper, curtains, and furniture inspired by Chinese motifs. There, over cups of Chinese tea, they might read Du Halde or perhaps one of the thirty-five topics in the *Mémoires* indexed under "Medicine of the Chinese."[9]

Medical Training

Some discussions of Chinese physicians involved their training. China continued the lineage system, although physician Xu Daqun (1693–1771) challenged his contemporaries' failure to follow the ancient sages and "forgotten traditions." He disliked innovations from the Song period, as did Dai Zhen (1724–1777), who targeted various Song teachings as falsifications of older Confucian texts (Unschuld 1986a). Comments attributed to emperor "Cheng-Tzu-Quogen" offered additional critiques: "If the doctors of today, instead of wasting their time in conversation, joking with their friends, would employ it in reading, learning, examining, seeking, digesting, and deepening the marvelous secrets of their art . . . if they would apply themselves to knowing the pulse, and to drawing accurate inferences . . . they would not be subject to making mistakes" (Cheng-Tzu-Quogen-Hoang-Ti 1783, 242–243). Physician Hugh Gillan (1962) wrote, "There are no public schools or teachers of medicine, no professors of the sciences connected with it, no regular united body or college of physicians throughout the whole Empire" (279). He viewed apprenticeship as a poor alternative, dependent on a single master, and noted that Chinese physicians generally earned low fees, although the imperial family and court officials had doctors in their households (280).

The Western frame of reference still included apprenticeship but also saw growing formalization of medical education for an elite few. London teaching hospitals grew. After 1778 the Royal College of Surgeons in Edinburgh became another leader. Paris remained a medical center, as faculties in Montpellier, Toulouse, Strasbourg, and Rheims also flourished. In 1776, Drs. François de Lassone (1717–1788) and Félix Vicq d'Azyr (1748–1794) founded what would two years later become the Société Royale de Médecine. American medical students usually went to London for one to three years, and then to Scotland, sometimes including a stint in Paris. Formal training in the United States began in 1750, with anatomy courses taught by John Bard and

Peter Middleton in New York. The first U.S. medical school, established in Philadelphia in 1765, became the University of Pennsylvania. Harvard Medical School was founded in 1783. Philadelphia opened a general hospital in 1751 and a dispensary, or clinic, in 1786. Such developments did not necessarily increase trust in medical men. Novelists assigned them names like "Dr. Slop" and "Dr. Smelfungus" (Duffy 1993). Still, these practitioners presented themselves as superior to those trained in apprenticeships.

Gillan assumed that Chinese practitioners acted simultaneously "as physician, surgeon and apothecary," equating the overlap with quackery—a judgment deriving from European characterizations of quacks as those who exaggerated their abilities. He added: "And as it frequently happens in other countries, many of them take advantage of the obscurity in which their own art is involved and of the ignorance and credulity of the people to gain money by the sale of nostrums and secrets of their own, which they pretend to be of wonderful efficacy in the cure of the greatest number of diseases incident to the human body. They have hand-bills printed for this purpose, setting forth their medicines, and attested cures annexed to them, which they take all possible means to circulate among the people" (Gillan 1962, 279–280). Other members of Macartney's party issued similar criticisms, especially of street vendors. The methods of such peddler-doctors had been recorded by scholar-herbalist Zhao Xuemin (1730?–1805) in his *Chuanya* (Collection of Proper Methods, 1759), based on interviews with a country doctor. These methods—including acupuncture and purging through induced vomiting or diarrhea—were considered violent by the literati, who identified them with the lower classes (Leung 1993). Barrow described one man who displayed a poisonous snake, prompting it to bite his tongue, which swelled up. In apparent agony, he applied a powder. The swelling subsided. Barrow added, "Though the probability, in the city, of any one person being bit with a snake, was not less, perhaps, than a hundred thousand to one, yet every person present bought of the miraculous powder; till a sly fellow maliciously suggested that the whole of this scene might, probably, have been performed by means of a bladder concealed in the mouth" (Barrow 1804, 232–233). Literati physicians would have been equally critical.

Such descriptions may have inspired an anonymous mock advertisement in *Boston Weekly Magazine* for "Dr. Ching-Ching-Ti-Ching, from *Pekin,* Fellow of the Imperial Medical Academy of China, Second Grand Physician to the Imperial Seraglio," lately arrived. The "doctor" was selling "Magnum Imperiandum Braniorum Restorandum," or "Grand Imperial Brain Restorative," citing testimonials for his nostrum from Miss Fanny Flutter, Master William Muslin, and Mr. Walkbackward (Anonymous 1803, 185–186). The details suggest a rudimentary familiarity with sources on China; none indicates whether the Grand Physician grew from the same antimedical imagination as Drs. Slop and Smelfungus, or whether Chinese physicians were being targeted as quacks.

Medical Sources

Physicians in Europe and the colonies formed learned societies to control quackery, publishing "transactions" and journals and exchanging them internationally. Whereas medical books from early in the century had usually been in Latin, by the mid-eighteenth century many appeared in European vernaculars. Successful works were quickly translated. The interest in cataloging knowledge—it was, after all, an age of encyclopedias—contributed to interest in Chinese medical sources. Physician Jacques François Vandermonde (d. 1746) served in Macao from 1720 to 1731, marrying a local woman in 1724 and returning to France with his son Charles Augustin in 1732.[10] He sent twenty-four mineralogical samples from Chinese *materia medica* to Bernard de Jussieu, along with Chinese characters and a phonetic summary from the *Bencao gangmu,* which he included in his medical thesis (1736; see Boxer 1974, 21–26.). The samples were identified by Alexandre Brongniart (1770–1847) and later chemically analyzed by Edouard Constant Biot (1803–1850) (Huard and Wong 1968, 127).

Many Jesuit observers commented on Chinese sources. Fr. Cibot (1782) wrote: "First, most of the great compilations have been made with much order and method. After having established general principles and the fundamental rules that must direct medicine in particular cases, one deals with the illnesses of all parts of the human body, occasioned by the alteration in their organization or by exterior causes. Let one imagine the practice of Ethmuller, but even more detailed, better analyzed, and more precise in particularizing each illness, articulating the diagnostics, distinguishing the attacks" (260).[11] In 1786, Fr. Amiot sent Bertin "a complete collection of all the best that has been written about medicine since the most remote times up to our day. It is titled *Kou-Kin-yi-toung*, it is in 48 volumes, contained in 6 *tao* or envelopes" (Huard and Wong 1966, 166). Bertin thanked him for the manuscripts, "as well as for what will accompany it next year in figures of men and instruments for surgery." He meant *jingluo* diagrams for acupuncture, Amiot having already sent him "tempered needles, a remedy to quell rhumatismal pain," and "drugs that entered into the composition of the aforesaid needles" (Huard and Wong 1966, 166).

Many such works remained untranslated. Amiot (1791b, xiii) explained: "It is not enough to understand a language and to be simply a man of letters, to translate well what is written in this language about the sciences and the arts; it is necessary for the translator to possess the art or the science about which he writes, from what he has read in a foreign language, without which the translation will swarm with errors, will yield nothing from the original that he wishes to make known but a false idea. And, unfortunately, almost all the translations I have seen are of this kind." Blaming his advanced age, Amiot declined his Chinese doctor's offer to teach him enough medicine to translate medical works, "for want of understanding them, to make them say what they haven't said, to set them in contradiction with each other, even though they are perfectly in agreement, insofar as they express themselves in slightly different ways, etc." Instead, he periodically included discussions of medicine in his letters, and sent Bertin related resources (Huard and Wong 1966, 142–143).

Amiot meant the *Yizuan yizong jinjian* (the Imperially Commissioned Golden Mirror of the Orthodox Lineage of Medicine, 1742), commissioned by the Qianlong emperor as part of his effort to define orthodox practice in different domains of Chinese knowledge and to establish himself within the Chinese classical lineage. The *Golden Mirror's editors foregrounded the cold-damage (shanghan)* treatise of Zhang Zhongjing (150–219). Influenced by the Han learning movement and its reconstruction of Han dynasty texts through philological, historical, and textual analysis, they did so to privilege south China's medical lineage and elevate their own status. The work comprised ninety *juan,* or volumes, divided into fifteen headings, corresponding to the administrative divisions of the Imperial Academy of Medicine (Hanson 2003).[12]

Bodies, Diagnoses, and Diseases

Westerners continued to interrogate Chinese theories of the body, while guardedly acknowledging Chinese diagnostic and therapeutic skills. Abbé Lambert, who authored a history "of all peoples of the world," conceded that "one sees that their remedies almost always have a salutary effect" (Lambert 1750, 10:122–123). Ancient theory, he thought, must have been more intelligible; what remained were the mechanics. Voltaire wrote, "The theory of medicine is still, among them, only ignorance and error." Nevertheless, the Greeks had bled patients without understanding the circulatory system. "The experience of remedies and good sense have established practical medicine throughout the world: it is everywhere a conjectural art, which sometimes aids nature, and sometimes destroys it" (Voltaire 1878, 12:433). A Chinese doctor responding to questions about Chinese practice cautioned against quick judgments: "Our medicine has a language suited to the systematic teachings of the doctors from the Song dynasty, on the mechanism, the equilibrium, and the reaction of the humors in the human body. The general system that is its basis may be ridiculous and absurd, if you will; but it is integrated to such an extent into the general and particular theory of medicine, that all the reasoning is unintelligible if one does not have the key" (in Cibot 1779a, 394).

Anatomical Bodies

Such advice generally went unheeded, because the anatomical paradigm became more influential even as anatomists remained suspect. Medical students at Paris hospitals dissected the corpses of the poor. In 1752, England's Parliament passed an act authorizing public dissections of executed criminals, further linking the practice with grisly punishment. Connections between surgeons and grave robbers—"Resurrection Men"—exacerbated matters. Although humoral models persisted, Western physicians increasingly *saw* the body anatomically. Occasional Western writers recognized that the Chinese saw something

different. Cibot (1782) commented, "They have made many observations that have perhaps escaped our most famous anatomists" (261).
Grosier (1788) wrote, "It is true, they never use dissection, and that
they do not even open the bodies of the dead; but if they neglect to
study nature in dead subjects, which always leaves much to be guessed,
it appears that they have long studied living nature with profound attention and with advantage" (2:483). This attention to living nature remained outside the purview of anatomists.

Grosier praised Chinese forensics, which necessarily focused on corpses.
Cibot translated part of the *Si-Yuen* (Song Ci's *Siyuanlou*, Washing
Away of Wrongs, 1247). According to Cibot (1779b), *si* meant "to
wash" (it could also mean "to clear") and *Yuen*, "grave" (421). The text
explained practices related to detecting varieties of wrongful death.
"Lien-yen," for example, was used in cases of homicide or suicide: "The
sight of a cadaver, they say, is a lugubrious and distressing spectacle
that one must spare magistrates and the people. Zeal for the public
good cannot hold against the horror that the sight inspires, against the
infection it exhales and against the danger of breathing the air it cor-
rupts" (424). Nevertheless, viewing a corpse could deter criminals; this
was the intent of *Lien-yen,* which provided methods for determining
whether the deceased had been strangled, drowned, or murdered.
Still, Cibot concluded that Chinese forensics had little to offer Western
anatomists. Other authors, unaware of the forensic tradition, were
harsher still. Gillan (1962) wrote: "[The Chinese] are totally ignorant
of the anatomy and physiology of the human body . . . nor do they
seem to have any idea that such knowledge could be of any use to
them in the treatment and cure of diseases. Their pathology and therapeutics must of course be extremely deficient and are for the most
part erroneous" (279). Staunton (1797, 2:229) added that, even in
books showing internal structures, it was "perhaps oftener to find out
the name of the spirit under whose protection each particular part is
placed" than its form or location. The description suggested a suspect
animism.

French surgeon Pierre Sue (1739–1816)—librarian and professor of
anatomy and surgery at Paris's École de Médecine, and commissioner
of the Académie Royale de Chirurgie—proved a careful reader of the
Lettres édifiantes and the *Mémoires.* Citing Chinese forensics, he hypothesized that the ancients had studied anatomy and surgery. Yet he also

recalled the translation ordered by the Kangxi emperor of the anatomy text provided by the Jesuits. "Why then," he complained, "have the Chinese not profited from these examples . . . Why have they not used them to make some progress in anatomy and in surgery?" (Sue 1796–1797a, 139–140). Moreover, how could a nation that abhorred mutilation, while castrating males to produce eunuchs, progress? Western observers did not know that in 1797 physician Wang Qingren (1768–1831) was in Luanzhou during an epidemic that killed hundreds of children. Wang observed the interior cavities of bodies dug from shallow graves by dogs. He began to question Chinese body diagrams and to introduce revisions into Chinese medical knowledge, although not from a Western anatomical foundation (Unschuld 1985; see also Andrews forthcoming).

Circulatory Systems

Chinese theory also faced ostensibly irrefutable evidence concerning blood, air, and circulation, in tension with a lingering Galenism. *Icones anatomicae* (Anatomical Images, 1743), by Albrecht von Haller (1708–1777), detailed blood vessels. In 1775 Antoine-Laurent Lavoisier (1743–1794) named a gas isolated by Joseph Priestley and Karl Scheele "oxygen" and compared the exchange of gases in the lungs with combustion. Commentators on Chinese practice did their best to translate Chinese analogues: "The Chinese doctors of today assure one that their ancient masters knew that the blood circulated through the body, and that this circulation happened by means of vessels called *Kinglo:* these are the arteries and the veins . . . They have, they say, an old book . . . which gives an explanation, but it is difficult to understand . . . They add that this knowledge not being absolutely necessary to cure illnesses, they do not wish to waste their time in acquiring it" (Lambert 1750, 10:121–122).

Dujardin's *Histoire de la chirurgie* (History of Surgery, 1774) cited Martini, Cleyer, ten Rhijne, and Du Halde on Chinese systems, and reprinted ten Rhijne's meridian diagrams (see Figure 16). (He found Cleyer nearly unintelligible, and wished ten Rhijne had elaborated more.) Dujardin reviewed relationships between blood ("the captain") and "spirits" ("his escort"). Blood flowed *in* the vessels, and the spirits outside them, in a circuit related to breath and pulse (77). Dujardin, too, translated *yin* and *yang* as vital heat and radical moisture, identifying "spirits" as the vehicles for the first, and blood for the second. Like other authors, he alternately referred to the *jingluo* as veins, vessels, pathways, channels, and arteries, through which *"yam"* and *"yn"* passed. He acknowledged, "The name *artery,* among the Chinese . . . does not have the precise meaning that we attach to it: it is used indis-

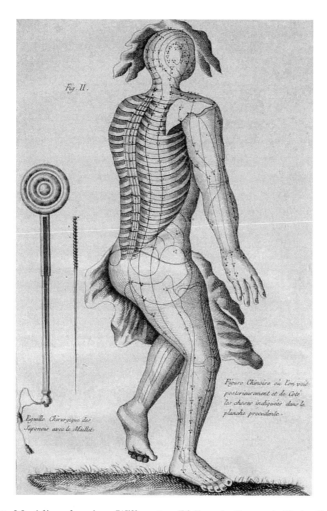

Figure 16. Meridian drawing. Willem ten Rhijne, in François Dujardin, *Histoire de la chirurgie,* 1774. Courtesy of the Boston Medical Library in the Francis A. Countway Library of Medicine.

criminately for the veins, the arteries, and the nerves" (80). Ultimately, he judged Chinese theories "no more than a shapeless mass of systems, of tentative efforts, of conjectures" (77) because the Chinese rejected dissection.

Grosier, too, wrote that blood and spirits served as vehicles for vital heat and radical moisture, with the latter seated in specific organs— radical moisture in the heart, lungs, liver, and kidneys, and "vital heat [in] the intestines, the number of which they make amount to six" (Grosier 1788, 2:481). He committed the fatal error, however, of claiming that "the Chinese were acquainted with the circulation of the blood long before any of the nations of Europe" (2:482). Sue quoted him, adding that if one defined "circulation" as a movement of blood and humors, then pre-Harveyan physicians had known the same thing, and protesting:

> What! Because . . . because the Chinese have acknowledged twelve ordinary pathways for the circulation of blood and humors, and eight other extraordinary pathways, for which Cleyer has given . . . an extremely obscure description; because the Chinese have imagined that radical moisture and natural heat spread themselves throughout the body, by virtue of a so-called circulation of the blood and the spirits, that is accomplished by means of the veins and other vessels of the twelve members . . . because, finally, the Chinese have established, based on this crazy and ridiculous theory, the revolution of the fluids in the human body, one will give the honor of a discovery as beautiful as that of the circulation of the blood, to a people who do not even have the first knowledge of anatomy! (Sue 1796–1797a, 22–23)

Later British observers would flag Grosier's unfortunate assertion to demonstrate Jesuit fallibility and dismiss Chinese theory. Barrow (1804), for example, described Chinese doctors as ignorant of the circulatory system, "notwithstanding the Jesuits have made no scruple in asserting it was well known to [them] long before Europeans had any idea of it" (345).

In 1799 Dr. William Scott, who accompanied Macartney to Beijing, informed leading American physician Benjamin Rush that Chinese physicians "believed the arteries carried air, and that when the pulse was slow air stagnated in the vessels" (Rush 1948, 245). As a promoter of bloodletting, Rush could hardly have found this detail appealing. His writings say nothing further about Chinese medicine.

Pulse Diagnostics

Pulse reading continued to figure in Western practice, as did observing a patient's coloring, tasting urine, smelling for decay, and listening for respiratory irregularities. In 1741 Irish doctor James Nihell translated a work on pulse theory originally published in 1731 by Spanish physician Francisco Solano de Luque (1685–1736?). In reviewing earlier sources, Nihell (1741) grudgingly acknowledged that Floyer had produced "the nearest Hint to this Proposition . . . Some Readers may expect I should . . . take Notice of the so much vaunted *Art of Pulse-feeling* among the *Chinese:* But, notwithstanding the wonderful Tales that are written and told of these famed *Asiatics,* and the painful Efforts of a Modern Author to explain and support them, whoever is pleased to peruse what is published on this Subject from the best original Writings of the *Chinese* Physicians, in *Père Du Halde's* late History of *China,* will readily forgive the Omission of such impertinent Trifles, and gross Absurdities, as are there related" (xxvi–xxvii). A note identifies Floyer as the "Modern Author." Far from seeking rapprochement, Nihell rejected Floyer's efforts and ridiculed Chinese practice.

Physician Richard Brookes (fl. 1721–1763) explained that the four pulse "motions" were "*great* and *little, quick* and *slow*" (Brookes 1751, lxxvi). Pulses could be tense, remittent, and hard, or flaccid, soft, and lax. Different combinations corresponded to different conditions. Diagnosis included examining the patient's state of mind, "because there is a wonderful Connexion between the Mind and the Body" (iii). Théophile de Bordeu (1722–1776) cited Nihell as having made "a happy application" of Solano de Luque. Acknowledging Galen's contributions, he quickly added, "there are few who do not look upon this system as entirely destroyed by the doctrine of the moderns: it is in fact fallen into oblivion" (de Bordeu [1756]1764, x).

Galen had used natural phenomena to characterize different pulses. Here, de Bordeu suggested, lay the core resemblance between Galenic and Chinese pulse vocabulary. He posited a common origin between China and Egypt, resulting in Chinese pulse descriptions like "a *rolling* pulse, that which moves like a *frog,* another which resembles the *glanc-*

ing of a fish, another that is like the *boiling of a pot,* and a fourth that resembles the *bill of a Hen*" (xii). Subsequently, however, the moderns had been abandoning Galen's terminology for "*strong* and *weak, frequent* and *slow, great* and *small, hard* and *soft,* &c."—terms that had also been used by Galen (xii–xiii) and appeared in Brookes's lexicon. In contrast, de Bordeu proposed his own system as a true departure from Galen, the Chinese, *and* the moderns. Regardless of actual differences, the Chinese were being marginalized from discussions of pulse theory.

In 1758 an anonymous physician reviewed Boym's pulse treatise in *Le Conservateur,* a journal dedicated to "rare pieces, and ancient works." The author associated Boym's discussion with European efforts to refine pulse analyses, and supported the undertaking: "If the knowledge of pulses is so important, why would we hesitate to share the riches that foreigners have amassed with so much care, & that have as their object the certainty of a science whose practice, for the great part, has been given over, up to the present, to conjectures and to systems?" (Anonymous 1758, 135). The author identified European physicians, including Solano de Luque and Nihell, who linked specific pulses to the onset of particular health crises. He emphasized being able to discern "the natural pulse for each individual, each age, each temperament, &c., since if one did not know the measure of the natural pulse of each being, how could one know that it diverged more or less from its perfect state?" Boym's work was little known, he thought, "because of its obscurity, the continual language of the Paripatetic school, & the Chinese terms that are frequently scattered through it" (142).[13] Yet it connected Chinese pulses with specific conditions, particularly those heralding impending death. The author recommended experimenting, where the Chinese reported "all the different modalities of the circulation of innate heat and radical moisture" (147). He selected pulses called "monstrous or mortal."

> The first monstrous pulse is called leap of a frog, because it seems to imitate the leap of this animal. It only beats one time in the space of a breath. It denotes a malignant fever, and that death will arrive on the third day.
>
> The movement of the second type of pulse bears a resemblance to the immobility of the tail of a fish that is swimming. The pulsations appear and disappear. This is a sign of malignity in fevers, and that the

bladder and kidneys are affected. Death must follow at the end of two days, & if it is an old man, it will not delay in arriving. (147–148)

The author explained that reviewing Boym did not mean uncritical endorsement of Chinese practices. Rather, "we claim to give a place to new experiments, & to furnish ideas to those who are devoted to an art whose most certain principles consist in observation" (154).

Dujardin (1774) understood that Chinese theory connected pulses to planetary, environmental, and seasonal influences. "Just as the springtime exercises its control over plants, so it exercises the same over the liver; the summer dominates the heart, the autumn the lungs, the winter the kidneys, and the stomach is subject to each of the four seasons of the year" (82). The Chinese diagnosed from the color of "the face, eyes, [and] nails, from the state of the nostrils and ears," the voice, the tastes one experienced or craved, and the disposition of one's temperament (84). The head functioned here not as the seat of reason, but as the locus of the senses.

Grosier (1787), borrowing Du Halde's metaphor, compared pulse diagnosis with playing a lute. He encouraged European doctors to study Chinese methods, alluding as well to Solano de Luque. In contrast, Staunton described a Chinese doctor playing "foolishly" upon the pulses. Barrow (1804) was equally disparaging: "Thus, they suppose one pulse to be situated in the heart, another in the lungs, a third in the kidneys, and so forth; and the skill of the doctor consists in discovering the prevailing pulse in the body, by its sympathetic pulsations in the arm; and the mummery made use of on such occasions is highly ludicrous" (345). He claimed that taking a woman's pulse involved tying a cord to her wrist and passing it through a hole in the wall, where a doctor in the adjoining room felt the pulse through the cord—"a due observance of solemn mockery" (233).

Cibot (1782) referred to the Latin translation of a pulse treatise, suggesting that readers would appreciate the illustrations. He had relied on "a bad edition from Province" (261). (Cibot may have meant *Les secrets de la médecine des Chinois* [1671]—Grenoble, although not in Provence, was in the same quadrant of France.) Sue reviewed both Cleyer's *Specimen medicinae sinicae* (1682) and Boym's *Clavis medica* (1686), linking Cleyer's text with Chinese physician "Vàm Xo Ho" (Wang Shuhe, 210–285 CE). Summarizing Cleyer, Sue (1796–1797b) offered illustrative details: "If the pulse is falling, *cadens,* it is a sign of bad digestion: the small pulse indicates abdominal pain without respite" (145). He suggested that Cleyer's plates detailing the circulatory system were the book's key failing, tracing that failing to "the doctrine as well as to the physical and anatomical system spread throughout the work" (152). Sue's review of Boym included descriptions of the twelve "ways," their relationship to pulse taking, and a discussion of the related diagrams. This, Sue wrote, was the extent of Chinese anatomy, "because they are persuaded, and claim, that almost everything is destroyed [in death] and changes form in the body, in such a way that the most clairvoyant anatomist can discover only very little, relative to life" (154–155). From these explanations and diagrams, he concluded, one had to be Chinese to understand that system of pulse reading.

This was not necessarily the case, of course. Charles Jacques Saillant (1747–1814), son of a Paris bookseller, was a member of the Faculté de Médecine de Paris and of the Société Royale de Médecine, moving in the elite circles of French medicine. In 1784 he wrote to the Beijing mission, "I have tried for almost twenty years to take pulses in the manner of the Chinese . . . In examining the pulse in this way, it has often happened that I have intuited the cause and seat of the illness and diagnosed diseases for patients of which they were not aware" (Grmek 1962, iv). Like Sue, he sent questions. In 1786 Amiot relayed the responses of a Chinese doctor, who acknowledged that pulse taking had "always been the principal object of our studies . . . since there have been physicians in China, that is to say, for more than four thousand years." In response to whether modern or ancient Chinese knew more about reading pulses, the doctor replied, "The ancients had the advantage of genius over us, and we have a longer experience over them" (Grmek 1962, vii). It was change, in particular, that physicians sought to detect, through changes observed in the pulses. Amiot referred Saillant, as well, to Boym's *Clavis medica.*

The letter arrived in 1787. Within months Saillant replied, comparing the doctor's responses to Galen and de Bordeu. It was here that Saillant, unlike his contemporaries, demonstrated his grasp of the essence of Chinese pulse taking. "The pulse seems to be like a clock," he wrote:

> like the indicator of the vital principle and its diverse states, whether in the entire mechanism or in some particular organs. All the modifica-

tions that it can undergo can be related to the two great principles of Hippocrates who is later made the basis of all the doctrines of the different sects on the temperaments, fire, and water.

Too much or too little heat, or to use the expression of our modern chemists, too much or too little caloric; too much moisture, too many humors and of such and such a humor, or too much dryness. Here is what has been recognized for all time as affecting the vital principle, as altering or modifying the principles of life. (in Grmek 1962, xiv)

Although not referring to *qi, yin,* or *yang,* Saillant recognized the link to vitalism. For reasons that are not clear, he seems not to have published these insights. Amiot later published only the questions and the Chinese physician's replies (Amiot 1791b). One is left wondering what might have happened had Saillant more actively and publicly linked Chinese pulse taking with vitalism.

Some Europeans reported direct experiences of pulse taking in China. Barrow, having developed stomach pains after eating unripe fruit, asked the local governor for opium and rhubarb. He was referred to a doctor whose style of pulse taking struck him as being virtually identical to that of a London or Edinburgh physician: "[He] fixed his eyes upon the ceiling, while he held my hand, beginning at the wrist, and proceeding towards the bending of the elbow, pressing sometimes hard with one finger, and then light with another, as if he was running over the keys of a harpsichord. This performance was continued about ten minutes in solemn silence, after which he let go my hand and pronounced my complaint to have arisen from eating something that had disagreed with the stomach" (Barrow 1804, 345–346). Barrow wondered whether the diagnosis derived from pulse reading or from knowing about the medicines he had requested. He maintained his previous pejorative assessment.[14]

A second episode involved the corrupt minister Heshen, who consulted with Gillan in Beijing. Heshen had experienced chronic seasonal inflammation for ten years, and, for eight, swelling and pain near his abdomen from horseback riding. Gillan (1962) reported, he "presented me first his right arm, and next his left, rested upon a small pillow covered with yellow silk and embroidered with gold" (282). To avoid offending, Gillan enacted the expected pulse reading. He then explained that European doctors did not take different pulses, because all were connected to the heart and to each other through the

circulatory system. Requesting the minister to place his right forefinger on his left artery, and his left forefinger to his right ankle,
Gillan demonstrated that the pulses were identical—after which he
took the history of Heshen's complaints, diagnosing rheumatism and
a hernia. He warned the minister that if he allowed the Chinese doctors to needle the hernia as planned, "the worst consequences" would
likely ensue. He prescribed, instead, another, unspecified medicine.
Following discussion between Heshen and his physicians, an interpreter was instructed to tell Gillan that his "ideas and all [he] had said
were so extraordinary that it appeared to them as if it had come from
an inhabitant of another planet" (282–283).[15] Sue (1796–1797a) repeated the story to show that Chinese pulse reading was overrated, the
object lesson being the superiority of Western medicine.

Theories and Illnesses

In 1737 physician Jean Astruc (1684–1766) also sent a questionnaire
to Beijing, regarding venereal diseases. In 1739 he received a first response, which he included in the 1775 edition of his *Dissertation sur
l'origine, la dénomination et la curation des maladies vénériennes à la Chine*
(Dissertation on the Origin, Denomination, and Cure of Venereal Diseases in China) and the fourth edition of his book on venereal diseases. The Chinese, he wrote, employed two cures—one attacking the
illness forcefully, the other expelling it through induced sweating. "In
the first case, these are pills composed of different powders and wheat
flour, which one gives the patient twice a day, morning and evening,
for more or less time according to whether the illness is lighter or
more serious . . . The use of these pills ordinarily causes toothaches,
and procures abundant very fetid salivation; which is the sign of a
prompt cure; but the Pox thus cured is subject to recur" (Astruc 1777,
343). Astruc incorporated into his bibliography the Chinese references provided him by Frs. Pierre Foureau (1700–1749), Dominique
Parennin (1665–1741), and Étienne Rousset (1689–1758), and by Dr.
Vandermonde. He also reproduced the Chinese characters for syphilis
(Huard 1968).[16] Astruc concluded that the Chinese and Europeans
did not have equivalent success in curing venereal disease, because it
was less severe among the Chinese. "One cannot count on the efficacy
of a decoction of toads: as what effect could this decoction produce,

since vipers which have greater virtue, cooked several times in broth have never done anything very useful in Europe?" (Astruc 1777, 382). Only because Chinese pox was less serious, he argued, did their remedies appear so successful.

Portuguese physician Antonio Ribeiro Sanches (1699–1783)—a student of Boerhaave—wrote his own dissertation on venereal disease, arguing that it had originated not in the Americas, but in Europe, as the result of an epidemic. To test his theory, he wrote to the Portuguese Jesuits in Beijing to learn whether Chinese records of the disease predated Columbus's voyages. From what Bishop Polycarp de Sousa could learn, no one seemed to know its origins, nor did anyone blame the Portuguese. "And certainly, if the Portuguese had brought it, I believe that they would have indicated as much in the wording thereof, as they have done with various other things which have come from Europe" (Boxer 1974, 10).

China, like Europe and United States, routinely faced epidemics. According to Gillan (1962), diseases arose from fluctuating seasons and, among the poor, "debility and inanation. In the hot seasons inflammatory fevers, sunstroke, phrenitis, hepatitis and cholera morbus prevail. In the cold seasons catarrhs and peripheumonias, and among the poor people fluxes, dropsies, and typhus fever are the reigning diseases" (285). Barrow (1804) added crowded urban conditions and "the want of cleanliness" to the causes in Beijing. He noted, however, that in the south, people wore "vegetable substances" more than clothing made from "animal matter." Windows were left open, resulting in greater ventilation (233–234). Still, the observers did not see epidemics particular to China.

In reviewing Chinese illness theories, Dujardin followed ten Rhijne, discussing winds and *yin-yang* imbalances. Review, however, did not ensure acceptance, as Sue's subsequent critique of the Chinese doctors in Gillan's narrative indicated—particularly of what they called a "malign vapor." In Europe, *vapor* meant harmful exhalations from different organs, particularly the stomach. Other common association involved "miasmas"—vapors from rot in sewers and drains, wet and decomposing matter, and diseased bodies. Miasmas were thought to taint the air, causing sickness and epidemics (Halliday 2001). None of these meanings was the same as harmful *qi*.

In contrast, Amiot described experiencing "a serious illness, of the

genera of those called *shanghan*." He went to the Chinese doctor who
had treated him for forty years, and described his symptoms—"such
sharp pains under the left breast that they prevented me from drinking, eating, sleeping, and the free exercise of all animal functions."
The doctor took his pulse, assigning the problem to Amiot's liver function—"it came from elevated *yang*, which would soon inflame the
whole machinery, if one did not promptly set an obstacle, by temper-
ing it with *yin*" (Amiot 1791a, vi). The Chinese doctor, when asked to
explain "malign fever"—replied that he could not do so without translating voluminous works on the subject. Moreover, he wrote, it referred "to one of the three hundred and ninety-seven branches of the
illness that we call by the general name, 'cold-damage disorder'" (x).
He invited his questioner to judge how difficult it would be to provide
detailed explanations.

On *Materia Medica*

Interest, ambivalence, or indifference toward reports about Chinese
materia medica were shaped by trade possibilities, the conceptual systems within which Western researchers classified their own medicines,
and issues of access. As trade introduced a growing *materia medica* to
Europe, wholesale companies formed to distribute them. Medical authors and societies produced new pharmacopoeias, including more
recently available drugs. Linnaeus's taxonomy gained influence, but
plants were still read as having "signatures," their physical forms suggesting body parts to which they were therapeutically related. Prayers
and charms accompanied certain remedies. Nicholas Culpeper's astro-
logical-medical work stayed in print, even though a revised Culpeper
also praised the "Linnaean System."

  Family medicine books—like George Cheyne's *Essay on Health and
Long Life*, in its tenth edition by 1745, and Methodist minister John
Wesley's *Primitive Physick* (1747)—democratized care. One of the most
popular was William Buchan's *Domestic Medicine* (1769). Such sources
frequently retained ingredients dropped by more elite publications.
Evangelist John Tennent's *Every Man His Own Doctor, or The Poor
Planter's Physician* (1734), for example, included the dung of asses,
cows, deer, and humans; human breast milk, deer's horn, bear's oil,
brimstone, and peach blossoms. In the United States, a growing

nationalism focused on indigenous *materia medica.* Samuel Stearns's *American Herbal* (1801) dealt with "our American productions only, and [giving] no general account of those found in other parts of the world, unless some of the same kind are produced here" (17).

Western naturalists were more interested in Chinese plants, including medicinal ones. Linnaeus's collection included *Astragalus chinensis* and *sinicus;* the version of China root (*Smilax China*) often used in Europe; and *Artemesia chinensis,* identified with *Artemesia vulgaris,* used in moxibustion. Magnus von Lagerstroem (1696–1759), director of the Swedish East India Company, solicited specimens from employees in Canton, amassing some thousand Chinese drugs. He also owned a copy of the *Bencao gangmu.* For close to forty years, Portuguese Jesuit Ioannis de Loureiro collected plants in Vietnam and Canton, returning to Lisbon in 1782 and writing *Flora cochinchinensis* (Vietnamese Flora, 1790).

Naturalist-physicians like Sir Hans Sloane (1660–1753), John Fothergill (1712–1780), and Sir James Edward Smith (1759–1828) built collections including Chinese plants. Sloane, president of the Royal Society, leased a manor in Chelsea to the Society of Apothecaries to establish the Physic Garden, a teaching collection. Upon his death, he left natural history specimens, his books and manuscripts, and his herbarium, which included Kaempfer's dried specimens and drawings, laying the foundation for the British Museum. Fothergill, a well-known botanist and fellow of the Royal Society, cultivated a large botanical garden from 1752 on. It contained Chinese specimens, some of which he was the first to plant in England. Smith purchased the Linnaean collections and herbarium in 1784. In 1788 he founded the Linnaean Society of London, eventually bequeathing it the entire collection. Kew Gardens—site of the chinoiserie described above—became a repository for the fruits of botanical research throughout the world. Supercargo John Blake (possibly the sponsor of "Hwang-a-tung") sent seeds and plants.

Pierre-Joseph Buc'hoz produced the *Herbier, ou, Collection des plantes medicinales de la Chine* (Herbarium, or, Collection of Medicinal Plants of China, 1781), supposedly based on a manuscript in the Chinese emperor's library. It may also have derived from hand-painted albums of Chinese plants in the Institut de France and the Bibliothèque Nationale (Huard 1968). Buc'hoz's *Herbier* contained a romanized list of the Chinese names, but no other explanations. In 1787 William Curtis founded the more highly regarded *Botanical Magazine,* with descriptions and drawings. European naturalists could, therefore, observe a limited sample of Chinese medicinal plants in a variety of visible forms (Bretschneider [1898]1981).

Chinese *Materia Medica*

Ribeiro Sanches asked not only about venereal disease, but also about Chinese *materia medica*—questions the Jesuits referred to Chinese physician acquaintances. The answers did not always impress the Portuguese fathers: Fr. André Pereira judged Chinese medicinals inferior to those of Europe, particularly because the Chinese did not bleed or purge. More detailed information was provided by three French missionaries, Frs. Parennin, Cibot, and Pierre Nöel Chéron d'Incarville (1706–1757). After Parennin's death, d'Incarville continued sending information, such as lists of "Plants and Simple Drugs, which I have seen in China, with several observations I have made over 15 years that I have been in the country."[17] Cibot (1782) commented, "The medicines of China are scarcely more than strong infusions, of which one always takes two doses; but rigorous diet and regime facilitate their effects" (261).

Grosier, while characterizing them as "almost all quackery," praised herbal texts: "What would afford matter of surprise, even in Europe," he added, "is, that much order, precision, and perspicuity, appear in all these collections" (Grosier 1788, 2:487). Another Jesuit described how physicians tailored formulas to the patient. Some remedies were administered to elderly patients "because of their temperament and the state in which they find themselves in certain seasons and circumstances, so it would be dangerous to advise, to all, the use or even the habit to those to whom they might seem the most profitable" (Anonymous 1779b, 241). Ironically, Gillan (1962) criticized this very aspect, complaining of the absence of uniform practice: "The composition, the doses, and the method of administering them of course are arbitrary and capricious, and vary not only in different provinces and towns but in the hands of every physician and dabbler in physic" (279).

Observers appear not to have encountered alternative formulations, such as Zhao Xuemin's *Chuanya* (Collection of Proper Methods). This work did not refer to *yin-yang* or the Five Phases. Instead it described how some drugs had ascending effects, others descending, and still others that of interrupting an illness. Zhao's work is evidence that the Chinese theories represented in European sources failed to reflect the full spectrum of actual practice (Unschuld 1985).

Frs. Guo (Gao) and Yang included discussions of medicine in their correspondence with Bertin. In 1774 Bertin wrote to request not only discussions of illnesses, but also samples of drugs and discussions of cures, "since I am determined to have printed each year everything that you send so that the public may enjoy at once the literary and scientific riches . . . Secondly, I have formed a cabinet where everything that I receive from China is preserved to provide communication about them to all those who are interested" (Huard and Wong 1966, 167). In 1776 he wrote that he had not dared touch the medicines they had sent, without a catalog detailing their origins, properties, and applications. Still, a Monsieur Lefebvre had informed him— after curing himself of a violent illness—that Chinese medicine was notable not only for pulse reading, but also for its simples (herbal formulas): "It is thus a capital—and I dare say an inappreciable—service to make known to Europe this method of curing the most serious illnesses without bleeding and without purging. I agree that the Chinese can contribute to it infinitely, but always it is a constant that Chinese medicine seems as rich in remedies as that of Europe is poor in this genre, while [the latter] has been raised to the highest level in anatomy and surgical illnesses or that require operations by hand" (Huard and Wong 1966, 167).

Yang wrote from Canton in 1775 that he agreed about the value of Chinese drugs. The *Bencao gangmu* discussed everything contributing to healing illness: "I have wished to attempt to translate it, but I have found it very difficult due to my lack of knowledge about appearances and plants, to medical terms I don't know, and to the difficulty of finding examples of plants in nature, since ordinarily in the shops they only sell them when they have been prepared in the same place where they are found, and which sometimes is a foreign place, at least they are always dried" (Huard and Wong 1966, 167). Nevertheless, a delay in the departure of the ship *Dauphin* allowed Yang to gather seventy-four drug samples that were not likely to rot or become worm infested, each of which he numbered. If there were questions, Bertin only had to cite the number and he could check it against his list. Years later, surgeon François-Albin Lepage (1813) cited the notices and memoirs sent by the two priests, "these two interesting men" (43).

One anonymous Chinese physician observed: "Beyond its using many plants that are particular to China . . . [Chinese medicine] reasons about their virtues and qualities according to a manner that is very different from the medicine of Europe. That given, how to find a way to make it understood to the latter?" (Cibot 1779a, 395). Western authors generally ignored this issue, focusing instead on four broad topics: (1) drugs imported *from* China, whose Chinese uses were sometimes described, without expectation that Western practitioners would adopt those uses; (2) comparative discussions of Chinese drugs used in both China and the West; (3) some substances unknown in Europe, discussed to illustrate Chinese practice; and (4) drugs exported from the West *to* China and used in both settings, although not necessarily in the same ways.

The Composition of Their Medicines

The list of drugs imported from China continued almost unchanged from the earliest trade—rhubarb, ginger, camphor, cassia, and China root. Some European writers assumed that these were also the drugs most widely used in China. Gillan (1962, 284) defined the "chief remedies" as "rhubarb, ginseng, ginger, pepper, camphor, tea, opium and oil." Fr. Lambert (1750) relayed Chinese representations of camphor as bitter and hot: "It serves to dissolve, to carry away phlegm and excess saliva from the bowels; it dissipates impurities of the blood, and remedies discomforts caused by cold and humidity: it calms violent stomach-aches and *cholera morbus,* ailments of the heart and the stomach. It cures scurf, gall, and inopportune itching: it is used advantageously to harden damaged teeth" (10:208–209). Grosier (1788) differentiated between China root *(Smilax China)* and *fou-lin* [*fuling*], which Chinese doctors recommended for "asthma, dropsy, suppression of urine, flatulencies, and dissolving phlegm. They assert that it stops vomiting, prevents convulsions in children, and that, by strengthening the reins [kidneys] it procures females a safe and easy delivery" (1:554). In America, Stearns (1801) wrote that China root *(Smilax china)* was compared or identified with sarsaparilla, although it was then called pseudo-China.

Lambert (1750) commented that the Chinese rarely used rhubarb raw or alone. "It tears out the guts, they say . . . they more voluntarily take rhubarb in a decoction, with many other simples" (10:8). Citing the case of a severely constipated mandarin: "A Chinese doctor had him swallow the decoction of a double dose of this rhubarb, prepared with a little white honey" (10:10). The patient recovered. Culpeper's herbal, reissued in 1792, identified rhubarb as coming from "Great Tartary" and northern China. His editor, Joshua Hamilton, boasted, "But we have now as good rhubarb plants growing in our physic gardens as any that come from abroad" (Culpeper 1792, 2:92). Stearns, too, had observed rhubarb in American gardens.

The editor of the *Foreign Medical Review* noted the debate over species (Editor 1780). Were *Rhabarbarum sibericum* and *Rhabarbarum chinense* different? Physician Simon Morelot identified *rheum undulatum* and *rheum compactum* as Chinese, but proposed growing *rheum palmatum* in France. Almost a century earlier, wrote Morelot (1797–1798), "the Chinese, not foreseeing the consequences that might result to the prejudice of the business they conducted in this root . . . gave several plants to French travelers, to satisfy what they called their curiosity" (305–306). Much as Europeans had appropriated lacquer and porcelain technology, why not do so with drugs?

Musk was "taken from the Musk-animal of the Goat-kind" known as *Che-hiang* (Brookes 1754, 286). Chinese hunters applied it to wounds, among other uses (Anonymous 1779a). William Black (1782) wrote, "By experiments of Dr. Wall, published in the *Philosophical Transactions,* musk taken internally is represented as of considerable utility in some convulsive and hysterical diseases, and in dangerous cases of malignant fevers, accompanied with twitchings of the tendons and convulsive starting" (214).

French Citizen Delunel (1798–1799, 50) speculated that tea might "be a great cause for the manifest effeminacy and diminutiveness of [the Chinese]." Acknowledging, however, that if it *were* poisonous, such constitutions would have quickly felt the effects, he left the slur unresolved. The *American Magazine* credited tea with Chinese freedom from gout and kidney stones, and described it as an astringent and diuretic that strengthened the stomach and bowels. It was also, the editor added, an aphrodisiac, "and Dr. Percival imputes the amazing population of China among other causes, to the general use of it" (Editor 1788, 411).

Comparisons of plants used in both China and the West led Cibot (1782) to recommend the *Shennong bencaojing*, "filled with details and observations . . . which merit the attention of naturalists, and above all of physicians and doctors" (232). Lambert commented on plants familiar to both: angelica, dittany, asparagus, wild fennel, cinquefoil, pimpernel, and others. Describing bellevedere, he wrote: "It is cold by nature, with a sweet taste, full of a benign juice; it relieves excessive internal heat: it is a diuretic . . . it procures sleep. Being roasted, reduced to a powder, and taken at a weight of about two drams in a drink, it releases the lower intestine of its flatulence. It is a salutary remedy against all illness caused by the hot season. Finally, the root of this plant, reduced to ashes, dissolved in a little oil, and applied to the bites of snakes and other poisonous insects, absorbs the poison, draws it out, and heals the wound" (Lambert 1750, 10:198–199). Another Jesuit described both medicine systems as agreeing about oak bark, leaves, and acorns, detailing Chinese practice: "to reduce the acorns with their caps to ashes; then to infuse the ashes in boiling water, to extract the salt that they have deposited in them, and to give it in an appropriate manner in diarrhea [and] dysentery; and . . . to wash and clean wounds and ulcers often . . . with the water in which one has boiled the bark" (Anonymous 1778, 489). The Chinese also used raisins (as did the French) in infusions to promote smallpox eruptions, or to induce sweating in pleurisy and fever (Anonymous 1780b). One herb known to the Chinese, *kaolin,* was discovered in western Europe in 1771 by PierreJoseph Odolant-Desnos (1722–1801) and Jacques Etienne Guettard (1715–1786) (Huard 1968).

Lady Mary Wortley Montagu (1689–1762), wife of the British consul in Constantinople, had observed smallpox inoculation among Turkish women, who inserted lymph or scab matter into a healthy person's skin. Lady Mary had her own children inoculated, after which the procedure was tested on condemned felons. Surgeon Robert Sutton (1707–1788) and his sons applied the material to small scratches. Edward Jenner (1749–1823) later substituted cowpox matter, resulting in "vaccination" (*vacca,* "cow"). Western observers agreed that the Chinese had developed related methods early on. Dried matter from pustules was sprinkled on cotton, inserted in the patient's nose and plugged with wax for three days, after which it was determined whether the patient had contracted a mild case. If not, the process was repeated (Cibot 1779a). The French Bibliothèque Nationale acquired a hand-painted album showing sixty-two drawings of children with smallpox, the pox patterns indicating relative likelihood of survival, and referencing medical texts with appropriate treatments. Despite such sophistication, Gillan (1962) characterized the Chinese method as both different and "undoubtedly much inferior" (290).

Nao-cha, or sal-ammoniac, was used in both China and Europe. Jesuit Fr. Collas (1786), after requesting some from a Chinese pharmacy, was surprised to receive three different kinds, all under the same name and all equally unfamiliar to him. Another pharmacist provided the same three, plus a fourth resembling the one he knew.

Chinese medicine, observed another Jesuit, also used the blood of wild boar, musk, deer, and gazelles. A stag's blood, drunk warm in autumn, revived a debilitated temperament, cured inveterate kidney illness, stopped pneumonia-induced spitting of blood, restored impoverished blood, and reinvigorated the overworked official or the woman weakened by blood loss following delivery. The *Bencao gangmu* recommended it to promote smallpox eruptions, but the formula was so complicated, and presupposed such knowledge of Chinese pharmacy, that the priest dared not attempt translation (Anonymous 1782). In the United States one found references to the medicinal use, not of the blood of deer and elk, but of their hooves. Stearns (1801) recommended roasted deer's foot oil for asthma.

Lambert (1750, vol. 11) wondered whether *tchucha* was the cinnabar described by Dioscorides as full of mercury. Powdered and used in cordial, it reestablished vigor, and it was admirable against convulsions and malignant illnesses in children. Jesuit Fr. Cibot compared cinnabar and quicksilver, or *ling-cha*. Chinese medicine from the third century BCE, he wrote, considered cinnabar dangerous, to be used internally only in extraordinary circumstances. The dictionary of drugs *Pin-ouei-tsin-yao* described it as "a little cold by nature; its *qi* is weak, it is the *yang* of a joint *yin*. Its principal virtue is to protect the heart and calm one's spirits" (Cibot 1786, 309). Cibot, too, hesitated to provide formulas, given that few Europeans knew Chinese pharmaceutical measures and procedures. He did say that cinnabar pills were recommended in times of plague. Moreover, if one evaluated the Chinese ability to sublimate the mercury in cinnabar by what had been imported from Canton, one would be misled, as that was the type used in red paint.

European chemists had mocked missionary reports of mercury extracted from plants. Chinese texts, however, all agreed on this point. "We have preferred to trust their evidence in a matter of fact," Cibot (1786) wrote, "than the infallibility of a science which, after all, could still be behind in many articles on the natural history and arts of East Asia" (313). Learned Chinese administered quicksilver in conserves, in fruit pulp, or in decoctions. Cibot detailed one restorative, involving six-month-old hens fattened for a month with grain and mustard seed. "Then after having made them fast for two days to void them, one feeds them a paste in which one has crushed mercury that has been well purified; then one carefully collects the excrement, which one dries, and which one then gives in an appropriate manner according to the illness" (314).

The *Mémoires* included an article on *lin-tchi,* a mushroom referred to in France as *agaric,* administered as a cordial and stomachic. The Chinese used its ashes to staunch bleeding. Those who performed "amputations on men trying to enter the inner palace"—eunuchs—coated the "singular wound" with it (Anonymous 1779e, 502).

Mugwort was used medicinally in both Europe and China. The revised Culpeper (1792) identified it with Venus and, hence, women's disorders. He recommended an ointment of mugwort and hog's grease to reduce growths on a patient's neck. Either fresh or as a juice, it offset overindulgence in opium. Three drams of powdered leaves in wine helped sciatica; a decoction with chamomile and agrimony, used topically, treated sinew pain and cramps. Brookes recommended it for women's disorders, suppressing menses, and difficult labor. Stearns prescribed it to prevent hysteric spasms, and for sciatic complaints.

Regarding Chinese uses, a single Jesuit wrote, "They only use the leaves and seeds of mugwort here; they attribute to the former the same virtues as we do for the illnesses of the sex and of women in labor, but we have not seen that we might make use of its juice while it is still green, as they do here, for sudden spitting of blood" (Anonymous 1780a, 516). He emphasized Chinese attention to locating where the most efficacious mugwort grew. "It is surprising," he wrote, "that with all our knowledge about botany, we have yet to know where in France the best plants grow that are used in our medicine. If they have more strength and virtue in one place than another or, even more, if they do not have force and vigor except in certain places where the sun and the climate are more favorable to them, as they have always claimed here [in China], would that not merit our paying attention to it?" (515). Moreover, might the Chinese assign greater virtue to an herb than did Europeans, due to where it grew (516)?

Then there were plants without known European equivalents, like *Chirma,* which Lambert described as blooming in spring and growing three or four feet tall. Its roots were sudorific, countering poisons, miasmas, and heat-related problems. *Ko-ken* treated fevers, migraines, colds, and children's illnesses from overheated blood. *Choyo,* peony root, addressed blood impurities, illnesses due to humidity, cankers, dysentery, and discomfort before and after labor. One found *Kin in hoa* everywhere, with its golden or silvery flowers. It treated abscesses, cankers, ulcers, and poisons. *Tchi tiao teou,* a kind of pea, relieved dropsy. *Santsi* grew in the mountains of Yunnan, Guizhou, and Sichuan. The stems and leaves, gathered in midsummer and ground with lime, were dried and used for sores. The juice, mixed with wine, cured the spitting up of blood, but only in summer (Lambert 1750, vol. 10).

Tam-coué (danggui), an oily aromatic root, nourished blood and circulation. It did not rot during shipment, if one avoided smaller merchants: "They cut the root . . . into very small pieces, which they sell at retail. It is why, if European merchants wished to buy Chinese drugs in Canton, they should only get them at the large stores, and not in the stalls, where the roots are sold only in little sections" (Lambert 1750, 11:11–12). Lambert criticized Chinese physicians for not developing salts, acids, or alkalis to assay drugs' active ingredients. Those who prescribed *Tam-coué* did not know its full potential, because they could not analyze it. "The most singular plant growing in China," he added, "is the *Hia-tsaa-tomchom,* which means that during the summer it is an herb, but when the winter comes, it becomes a worm" (11:1–2). One stuffed five drams into a duck's belly, cooking it over low fire, then removed the drug, whose virtues had entered the meat, to be eaten twice daily for ten days.

Grosier cataloged elephant flesh, gall, skin, bones, and ivory, along with sea horses and crabs. Lambert discussed elephant gall, citing a case involving the Kangxi emperor's grandmother, whose eye disease court physicians had failed to cure. Finally, one feigned recalling that elephant's gall might serve. The emperor immediately had an elephant killed, but after cutting up the liver and parts surrounding it, the doctors found nothing. The emperor, informed of the failure, charged the doctors with laxity (and stupidity), and summoned the imperial scholars. They, too, found nothing. Finally, one scholar appeared, saying they had sought the gall in the wrong place, "in the liver, where it was not—that the liver of this animal moved throughout the body, according to the different seasons; that in that case, it must be in such and such a leg." The gall was found, and the scholar immediately promoted to the rank of imperial scholar (Lambert 1750, 10:121–126). Sue (1796–1797a) repeated the story, commenting that it said little for Chinese anatomical knowledge because elephants had no gallbladder. He included another ophthalmic cure, from d'Entrecolles: One wrapped a sheep's liver in a water lily leaf, sprinkled with saltpeter. The bundle was steeped slowly and stirred often. One held one's head over the pot, covered by a cloth, keeping one's eyes open so the fumes would dispel morbid humors.

Lambert (1750) reported a deep natural well near Canton, with unusually clear water. One soaked the skin of a black ass in well water for five days, then scraped the skin, cut it into small pieces, returned it to the water, and simmered it. The residue was strained, dried, and molded into a gum, called *Ngo-kiao* (vol. 11). Imitations were made from the hides of mules, camels, horses and, sometimes, old boots, "and because one finds almost as many simpletons and dupes who buy it as there are rogues and knaves to sell it, there is much demand for it." The authentic product was, however, easily recognized: it neither smelled nor tasted bad, but was crisp and friable, and only came in black or reddish-black. Decocted with other herbs, it dissolved phlegm, restored blood, maintained the bowels, strengthened an infant in the womb, dissipated winds and heat, stopped bloody flux, and provoked urine (11:14–16).

The *Mémoires* published a natural history article on plants and trees of China (Anonymous 1778), the anonymous author adding cursory medicinal applications. *Mou-li-hoa,* for example, was a jasmine whose berries treated burning in the chest, constipation, and urine retention. Ashes from the flowers stopped nosebleeds; infusions treated stomachache and colic. *Yu-lan* was a tall, beautiful tree with medicinal fruit pulp. After being softened in warm water, the pulp was dried in the shade, powdered, and taken instead of tobacco, soothing migraines and clearing the nasal passages. Infusions relieved chest congestion.

According to Jesuit Fr. Térence's Chinese herbalist, the fruit of Chinese water lilies, *Lien-pong*, treated colic caused by an abundance or thickening of blood. Cooked in wine, it eased the aftermath of labor; in water, it countered poisonous mushrooms. The seeds strengthened the chest, soothed hunger, fortified the elderly, and were a remedy against dysentery, kidney problems, and women's illnesses caused by thickened blood. The root promoted blood circulation, fattened those who used it regularly, sweetened bile, and facilitated digestion. When pounded and applied as a poultice, it was good for all wounds (Anonymous 1778).

Unlike these Jesuits, the Macartney party showed little interest in Chinese *materia medica*. Gillan (1962) expressed passing awareness of an herbal text but thought it related more to "agricultural and culinary purposes than to medicine" (279). In addition to ginseng, rhubarb, and China root, Barrow (1804) listed animal and mineral ingredients—"snakes, beetles, centipedes, and the aureliae of the silk worm and other insects . . . saltpetre, sulpher, native cinnabar, and a few other articles" (230). Yet apart from some members' general interest in botanical specimens, and despite the fact that Staunton, Gillan, and one other were physicians, the party exhibited no interest.

Foreign Mud

Two drugs, opium and ginseng, represented large shares of the China trade. Looking to recover silver spent on tea, British East India merchants began shipping opium, obtained through India, to pay for tea, silk, porcelain, and other goods. The Chinese government prohibited the trade in 1729, calling opium "foreign mud" and "vile dirt." However, European and, eventually, American drug runners—financed by trade companies and abetted by corrupt Chinese officials—flouted regulations. Complicating matters, opium also entered China for medical use, making it harder for honest officials to differentiate between legitimate and illegitimate shipments.

Opium had earlier been mostly *madac*—crude opium dissolved in water, boiled, strained, reduced, and mixed with tobacco leaves. Eventually, smoked in its pure form, its use became widespread (Spence 1975). Barrow (1804) described the governor of Canton's rhetoric, "that foreigners, by the means of a vile excrementitious substance, derive from this empire the most solid profits and advantages," only made worse by his countrymen's pursuit of "this destructive and en-snaring vice, even till death." And yet, alleged Barrow, the same gover-nor "very composedly takes his daily dose of opium" (102–103).

The European analogue was alcohol. In England, the poor con-sumed staggering quantities of gin. The rich drank brandy and port. Samuel Johnson, Oliver Goldsmith, and William Pitt, for example, were regularly drunk. (Johnson on one occasion was alleged to have consumed thirty-six glasses of port, without getting up.) In 1789 one rural French parish with four hundred residents had eight taverns, as well as smaller cabarets (Weber 1971).

Panax Ginseng, Panax Quinquefolium

In 1739 surgeon John Kearsley wrote from Philadelphia to antiquarian Peter Collinson about ginseng, which he had expected "to find in this Latitude, as it is parallel to that part of Tartary where this Plant is found" (Appleby 1983, 132). He had provided a picture to Quaker naturalist John Bartram (1699–1777), who located it in multiple sites. Indeed, on July 27, 1738, Benjamin Franklin's *Pennsylvania Gazette* had announced, "We have the pleasure of acquainting the world, that the famous Chinese or Tartarian Plant, called Gin seng, is now discovered in this Province near Susquehannah" (Berkeley 1995, 401–402). Bartram shipped ginseng specimens to Collinson, who sent a parcel with a friend to China, "to see how they approve of it, and to find what price it bears; but my friend is under promise not to discover that it is *Ameri-can*, for if they know that, they are so fanciful, it may not be so good as their own" (Appleby 1983, 134). London's Royal Society members also sought samples. By midcentury, a ginseng trade had emerged be-tween Philadelphia and England, with merchant James Pemberton commenting that "small parcels" of the root were commanding "a very advantageous price in London" (Goldstein 1978, 22).

Following Fr. Lafitau's earlier discovery of Canadian ginseng, the French began exporting it to China and Europe. Fetching two francs in Quebec, it resold for twenty-five in Canton. In 1752 the export's rep-utation was damaged by a French shipment that had been gathered out of season and badly dried. Excessive collecting threatened to de-stroy the stock. Traveler Peter Kalm observed, "at present there is not a single plant of it to be found [around Montreal], so effectually have they been rooted out" ([1770]1964, 435–436). In 1764, Collinson deplored the ransacking, saying that "the market in China [had been] glutted with this root, which had been artfully concealed and prepared by the Chinese, and sold under secrecy to the great people for true Chinese Ginseng, but its great plenty soon discovered the cheat, and then it sank to nothing" (Appleby 1983, 134). Ginseng periodically disappeared from export lists to England, as in 1772, but it reappeared in 1783. In December of that year, the Boston ship *Harriet* carried a load of ginseng to the Cape of Good Hope, trading it for tea from the captain of a British East India Company ship, and returning to Boston early in 1784 with reports of a significant profit. The news laid the groundwork for the subsequent voyage of the *Empress of China* (Goldstein 1978).

French *materia medica* books included discussions. M. Dienert (1765) listed ginseng under cordials. M. Liutaud (1768) characterized it as famous among the Chinese but noted, "As we have this medicine only in small quantities: and [because] it is at an excessive price, there are few occasions in which one can prescribe it; which makes it useless to examine whether, among the number of species of medicine of the same genre, which are well known and more common, as many virtues are to be found as in ginseng. One prescribes from two scruples up to a gross and a half, to make an infusion: it is prescribed in substance, from fifteen grains up to a half-gross" (230).[18] Still, he added, it grew naturally in the part of America called "Canada."

In England, the *Gentleman's Magazine* recommended digging up and curing ginseng "in the Chinese manner" (Anonymous 1753, 209). In 1769 British doctor William Heberden described that method, informed by a John Burrow Esq., who got it from a "Mandarin [from] that part of Tartary where the Ginseng is gathered and cured." One collected roots when the plant was not in flower, washed them carefully, and boiled water in an "iron torch" (a "flat stewpan"—possibly a wok), adding the root for three or four minutes. It was wiped clean, placed in a clean "torch" over low fire, and turned occasionally, eventually yielding pieces "dry enough to sound like a piece of wood when dropped upon a table" (Heberden 1785, 35–36).

By midcentury, ginseng had been found in Massachusetts and New York; later it was found in Vermont. American traders shipped it to London brokers. "Sang diggers" traded roots for rum, tea, and porcelain. Robert Johnston—surgeon on the *Empress of China*—provided over thirty tons from Pennsylvania for the ship's cargo. The success of the *Empress*'s voyage generated widespread enthusiasm toward the Chinese and toward the prospect of strengthening Sino-American trade partnerships. Chinese merchants were warmly described as "respectable men, exact accountants, punctual to their engagements, [who] value themselves much upon maintaining a fair character" (in Goldstein 1978, 69). In 1785 Thomas Jefferson wrote to John Adams that he foresaw supplying Portugal, to meet demand in the East Indies (Jefferson [1785]1971). Sir Joseph Banks wrote in 1786 to Bartram's cousin Humphry Marshall with instructions regarding collection and preparation. Marshall dispatched his physician nephew Moses, who traveled into the mountains, more accessible supplies being exhausted. Daniel Boone in 1788 dug "sang" in the Allegheny Mountains of Kentucky and West Virginia. His plan to transport twelve tons by water to Pittsburgh and then by wagon to Philadelphia, ran aground with his barges on Ohio River sandbars, waterlogging and ruining his stock. Nevertheless, he stayed in the trade, crediting it for part of his fortune. John Meares hoped to acquire ginseng in the Northwest, thinking the quality there closer to the "Tartarian," one picul (133.33 pounds) of which sold for $3,000, in comparison with the *Empress*'s cargo, which sold at $150–$350 per picul. With the glut, prices fell from $190–$400 for 800 piculs in 1799–1800, to $120–$200 for 1,600 piculs in 1800–1801, and to $50–$80 for 1,700 piculs in 1801–1802 (Gibson 1992; Nash 1898; Appleby 1993).

Collinson thought American and Chinese ginseng might be identical. Linnaeus bestowed the name *Panax* (panacea) on the Chinese variety in 1753, but not until 1842 would botanist C. A. Meyer identify five distinct species. Chinese ginseng would remain *panax ginseng;* the North American variety was designated *panax quinquefolium.* M. Valmont de Bomare's *Dictionnaire raisonné universel d'histoire naturelle* (Universal Reasoned Dictionary of Natural History, 1775) provided detailed comparisons of "gens-eng" and "ninzin." Chinese physicians, he commented, "have written entire volumes about this specific, which they decorate with the titles *Spiritous Simple, of the Pure Spirit of the Earth* and *Recipe of Immortality*" (Valmont de Bomare 1775, 4:64). Because Chinese ginseng retailed through customhouses controlled by the emperor, Europeans could purchase it only through these channels at higher prices, "and in particular [from] the Dutch East India Company, which sells almost all the ginseng consumed in Europe" (4:68).

Some wondered whether ginseng was the European mandrake, or "mandragora," described by Greek writers. The former—"narcotic, cooling and stupefying"—was ruled out. However, Lafitau had thought that the mandragora discussed by Theophrastus might have been a species now lost, whose effects resembled those of ginseng, reinserting the latter into European medical history. Grosier (1788) devoted roughly half a chapter to ginseng's appearance, cultivation, collection, and price. He reprinted Lafitau's letter, awarding the honor for most accurate description to Jartoux (1:534).[19]

Sloane experimented with prescriptions in Du Halde—one of the few explicit adoptions of Chinese herbal formulas. The *Compleat English Dispensatory* classified ginseng as one of the "Nervous Simples," which affected the nerves, and produced an "immediate effect on the spirits . . . so that the sensations at the head, stomach, or heart, become forthwith much more lightsome and agreeable than before," although few physicians were said to employ it (Quincy 1749, 54, 67–68). In 1750 Fothergill suggested that ginseng was not frequently used in England, although he recommended it for impotence, chronic colds, and illnesses among the elderly (Appleby 1983). John Bell reported having "heard many stories of strange cures performed by it; that persons, seemingly dead, have, by its means, been restored to health." He subscribed to the root's powers, although unable to replicate them. "If it really has any extraordinary virtues," he reported, "I could never discover them, though I have made many experiments on it, at different times" (Bell 1965, 186).

William Cullen (1710–1790)—an Edinburgh-based teacher of many American doctors, including Benjamin Rush—wrote, "The weakness of its sensible qualities gives it no foundation for a place in medicine," conceding only that it made "a safe masticatory" (Cullen 1773, 276). He later expanded his remarks:

[Ginseng] has now for many years been well known in our shops. It is a very mild aromatic, with some sweetness; but these qualities are so weak, that nothing but a popular notion among the Chinese, and the great price put upon it by them, would ever have engaged our attention to it as a medicine. We are told that the Chinese consider it as a

powerful aphrodisiac; but I have long neglected the authority of popular opinions . . . I have known a gentleman a little advanced in life, who
chewed a quantity of this root every day for several years, but who acknowledged that he never found his venereal faculties in the least improved by it. (Cullen 1789, 2:161)

Its being "well known in our shops" may have referred to popular use
rather than physician prescription. Indeed, M. Desbois de Rochefort,
in his *Cours élémentaire de matière médicale* (Elementary Course of *Materia
Medica*, 1793), classified ginseng among nourishing tonics but argued
there were others that were as good or better, writing, "We also have indigenous tonic roots" (2:25).

Americans regularly identified ginseng with different Native American tribes. Bartram (1957, 364), for example, reported: "The Lower
Creeks, in whose country it does not grow, will gladly give two or three
buckskins for a single root of it," using it for stomach disorders, "a dry
bellyache, and disorders of the intestine, colic, hysterics, etc." European immigrants and enslaved Africans adopted it accordingly, later
slave narratives describing ginseng leaves used as herbal wrappings
(Wood 1978). Kalm (1964, 435–436) observed ginseng planted in Canadian kitchen gardens "for curing asthma, as a stomachic, and promoting fertility in women."

Stearns's *American Herbal* placed ginseng in Canada, Vermont, and
Virginia. Stearns reviewed other authors: Dr. Wallis classified it as a
stimulant, and Dr. Healde, as an antispasmodic. Healde added that the
Chinese esteemed it as a restorative, sometimes using it for convulsions, while Dr. James said they decocted it for consumptive cases and
other debilities. Stearns used it for "coughs, consumptions, and spasmodic disorders." Decoction, he added, entailed "boiling two drachms
of the sliced root, in a quart of water, till but eight ounces are left. The
liquor is then to be sweetened and drank. When the decoction is gone,
boil the roots a second time in a quart of water, for they will always
bear two boilings." One drank two ounces a day, morning and evening;
if eating the root itself, one took "a scruple, twice a day" (Stearns 1801,
157–158). Stearns indicated no awareness that the Chinese often
boiled herbs twice, for two doses. Encounters with Native American
uses of ginseng surely contributed to its introduction into Western
materia medica. Still, ginseng's reputation in China, coupled with com-

mercial prospects, accelerated its export and introduction into Western practice, to the point where it became "well known."

Medical Exchanges

Just as efforts were made to collect Chinese medical texts and herbals, so books on Western medicine reached China through French and Portuguese Jesuits in Beijing and Macao. They included Robert Smith's *Complete System of Opticks* (1738), along with the works of William Harvey, Herman Boerhaave, Lorenz Heister, and various Portuguese authors. A Chinese official visiting the French Jesuit library in the early 1750s was struck by the extent of the collection. Following the expulsion of the Jesuits from Macao and the seizure of their possessions in 1762, the 4,200 sources in the library were dispersed, and pharmacy contents were sold off for a pittance (Boxer 1974).

Small numbers of Jesuits served as physicians and surgeons at court, although they left few records. Among them were Frs. Rousset and Giovanni-Giuseppe da Costa (1679–1747). A Dutch physician was mentioned in 1635. Surgeon Emmanuel de Mattos (1725–1764), arriving in Beijing in 1751, also provided medical care (Standaert 2001), remaining a lay brother to be more available to patients. In contrast, British surgeon Abraham Leslie alienated both the Chinese and his own colleagues by lending money at high interest to Chinese merchants and seizing property when one of his debtors went bankrupt. He was arrested in 1781, resurfacing in India in 1783 (Wu 1931). Brother Louis Bazin (1712–1774) spent the last six years of his life in Beijing. Engaged in providing care, these physicians neither translated texts nor studied Chinese practices in any publicized ways.

Amiot (1791b) praised his own Chinese doctor. "As it is to him that I owe the health I enjoy today," he wrote to a European physician who had sent questions. "I do not need to tell you . . . how he has conducted himself on my behalf, to give you an idea of what he knows how to do" (vi). In relaying responses to questions sent from Europe, Amiot asked for clarification when he didn't understand the explanations, admitting that some points might still have escaped him. His doctor, in turn, was gratified by the European physician's interest. "He must be very able," Amiot quoted him as saying: "as he is not presumptuous, and thinks that one can find lights among foreign people with which to illuminate his own art. I wish with all my heart that our occupations, his and mine, permitted us an ongoing correspondence. I would devote myself to it with the greatest pleasure, persuaded that it would turn to the advantage of the art, and that it would contribute to the easing of human suffering, in the regular exercise of our profession" (xi). Through Amiot, the Chinese physician sent a compounded powder for migraines, which one took like snuff. Amiot hastened to add, "I am the living proof that my doctor is hardly a charlatan, as without his aid, I should have been dead long ago" (xi).

Members of the Macartney party sought help from a Chinese doctor. Staunton described care provided for a servant afflicted with dysentery, who "was induced to consult a physician of the place, who, to the doctrine of the pulse, added a discourse upon the different temperaments of the human frame, and unluckily attributing his patient's suffering to the predominance of cold humours, prescribed for him strong doses of pepper, cardamoms, and ginger, taken in hot show-choo or distilled spirit; a medicine which so exasperated all the symptoms of his disorder, that he had much difficulty to escape alive to Pekin" (Staunton 1797, 2:101). Macartney's valet Anderson, however, reported the incident differently:

> I was witness, in one instance, to a skillful application of it, in the case of John Stewart, a servant of Capt. Macintosh, who, on our return from Jehol, had been seized with the dysentery, which increased so much on the road, that at Waunchoyeng, there were not hopes entertained of his being able to leave that place . . . [A] Chinese physician was called to his assistance; when the man's case was explained to him by Mr. Plumb, in the presence of Sir George Staunton. The physician remained a considerable time with his patient, and sent him a medicine, which removed the complaint, and restored him to health. (Anderson 1795, 194)

The accounts prove irreconcilable. We do not know what role social location played in the assessment. Was the valet more inclined to be credulous, or was he a more faithful witness to the experience of a peer? Staunton, himself a physician, may have judged his Chinese counterpart more stringently. Perhaps it was pique at not having produced a cure himself. Stewart provided no account, but the presence of these two illustrates the disparate reports entering the West, sometimes regarding the same subject.

Burning with Moxa

European physicians continued to classify Chinese moxibustion as cautery. Leading promoters of the day included French surgeons Claude Pouteau (1724?–1775), Baron Pierre-François Percy (1754–1825), and Jean-Baptiste Blanc. Occasional dissertations appeared, like that of Jean Gieulés. A surgery text by Lorenz Heister (1638–1758) remained in print, and surgeons François Dujardin and Gerard van Swieten (1700–1772) folded discussions of moxibustion into their own widely read works.

Genre conventions structured the discussions. Medical writing legitimized innovation by detailing a practice's lineage, supported by new case experience. In relation to moxa, Pouteau (1783) cited Hippocrates, while Blanc (1799–1800) added Galen. Celsus, too, had recommended therapeutic fire. Through Hippocrates, it traced to the Scythians. Prosper Alpini's *De medicinae aegyptorum* (1591) documented Egyptian use, while Pouteau (1783) hypothesized that the Egyptians got it from the Arabs. Linnaeus added Laplanders. Fabricius of Aquapendente had employed moxa, as had Marcus Aurelius Severinus, a celebrated surgeon of Naples. Pouteau also cited Albucasis, "our celebrated Paré," and Matthias Glandorp. Blanc added Lancisi of Rome and Vallesius, both of whom used it during epidemics. Quoting ten Rhijne and Kaempfer, Percy (1792) wrote: "This operation . . . is even more delicate than one might commonly think, which is why some peoples, such as the Chinese, attach such importance to it, trusting its execution only to a certain order of physicians . . . others have mixed religious principles into it, and have charged this part of the healing art only to priests who perpetuate among themselves the custom and right to practice it" (69–70).

The chapter on moxa in Johann Pechlin's *Observationum physico-medicarum* (1691) and Matthew Purmann's *Chirurgia curiosa* (1706) expanded the available Western literature. Few foreign observers provided more current details, although Barrow (1804) exhibited general familiarity: "Sometimes, after puncturing the part with silver needles, they set fire to the leaves of a species of Artemesia upon it, in the same manner as the Moxa in Japan is made use of to cure and even prevent a number of diseases, but especially the gout and rheumatism, the former of which is said to be unknown in China" (354). He had not, however, observed it. Diplomat Carl Peter Thunberg (1795) commented on moxa's preventative uses: "Every one makes use of it, old and young, children, rich and poor, and even the prisoners themselves" (4:74). Gieulés (1803) cited ten Rhijne and Kaempfer, too, reporting that "one only saw men covered with pock-marks and scars which the impression of this caustic leaves" (6–7).

Pouteau was regularly credited with rescuing moxa from near oblivion. He suggested that, with the discovery of the circulatory system, ancient practices had been rejected "and the application of fire was relegated to the people who remained in deep ignorance about new discoveries in medicine" (Pouteau 1783, 215). But, he concluded, history furnished a thousand proofs of its value. Blanc suggested that resistance occurred because, as his teacher said, "remedies—like boots— often go out of fashion" (Blanc 1799–1800, 9–10). There was also patients' fear, although Pouteau (1783, 217) recommended ignoring it: "Their pains are so cruel, that the most active burning will be weak in comparison." Still, Dujardin felt compelled to assert that moxa was not as painful as one might think—even children tolerated it.

The ancients had used boiling water, hot oil, or heated metals. Percy knew the Chinese used artemesia, while Dujardin paraphrased ten Rhijne and Kaempfer on how to use it:

> [One forms it into] small masses in a pyramid shape, slightly larger than a pea; sometimes one wraps this vegetal fleece in a paper, and compresses it in one's hand, so as to make it more uniformly crushed; one then cuts it into large capsules about as big around as two writing quills, which one applies with the ends of one's fingers to the sick or painful spot, which is to be burned; the top of this tow is lit with a match or some flammable matter. In China, the rich carry luxury even into their remedies; they use a lit stick . . . made of musk, powdered aloe, and other aromatics proper to delight the sense of smell. The fire, which burns through the tow fairly slowly, does not immediately reduce it to ashes; there remains at the base a small segment in such a way that the skin is drawn without violence, and from it there is raised a small blister or pustule: most often, the remains of the fire are no more than an ashy spot. (Dujardin 1774, 89)

Nicolas Culpeper's updated *materia medica* reported, "The moxa, so famous in the eastern countries for curing the gout by burning the part affected is the down which grows upon the underside of this herb" (Culpepper 1792, 1:437). Pouteau (1783) suggested using "the cotton of the Arabs and the Egyptians, the moxa of the Japanese, or the raw linen of Hippocrates" (1:280). Percy (1792, 76–77) fabricated small cardboard cylinders, substituting cannon-wick for cotton—an idea borrowed from Fabricius; saturated with saltpeter, the wick burned better.

Physicians concurred that one should avoid burning moxas on delicate skin, cartilage, tendon, or bone. Sites like the testicles, Pouteau (1783) explained, required placement "in the closest area, considering the direction of the nerves" (1:281)—suggesting that nerves conducted the heat. Point location was left to experiment and experience, although pain-point application prevailed. Dujardin (1774) printed ten Rhijne's four plates. Readers could observe points lying along channels connected to other parts of the body. In theory they could experiment, testing points to learn their effects.

The anonymous English author of a 1775 article on Chinese "cautery" cited merchant-visitor Hwang-a-tung:

> [He,] at present in London, happening to be at the house of a gentleman there, who, among other Chinese articles, had in his possession a drawing representing a naked man, with straight lines in different parts of the figure, was asked what these meant? He replied, that such figures were intended for the younger practitioners in physic, to teach them to what parts of the body the cauterizing pin should be applied, in order to remove a disorder in other corresponding parts. The Chinese practitioners attribute very great powers to the actual cautery, and have frequent recourse to it. He, at the same time, shewed a scar near the first joint of his thumb, where he had been cauterized for a pain in his head. (Editor 1775a, 216–217)[20]

The logic behind applying moxa at one point, to remove a disorder at another, still remains largely unexplored.

The availability of this knowledge resurfaced in Sue's treatise on the state of surgery in China. "The doctors of China and Japan," he wrote, quoting Dujardin, "distinguish according to queer figures, which are part of their art, the places where one should apply moxa, and it is above all in this that their science and their ability consist." He added that without the plates in Dujardin such details could not be well understood (Sue 1796–1797a, 41). Yet neither Sue nor the other surgeons who discussed moxa documented experiments involving the points marked on the diagrams. Little consensus obtained regarding the number of moxas to apply, whether to burn several at the same point, or whether a superficial burn sufficed.

Broadly speaking, moxa was used to treat pain, including gout. According to the ancients, wrote Pouteau, *"ignis firmat partes"*—fire strengthens the parts. However, if one applied moxa to gout at its most common point (the feet), pain often relocated to the knees, abdomen, or other locations. If it seemed stationary, fire remained the most active agent (Pouteau 1783, 1:264–265). Both Pouteau and Blanc recommended moxa for sciatica, Pouteau providing cases. Twenty-two-year-old waiter Perruquier had tried other treatments unsuccessfully (Pouteau 1783, 1:206). Sister Françoise Gervais, at thirty-six, suffered from sciatica. Blistering agents, warm mineral baths, and even opium had failed. Moxa worked, to varying degrees. "Rheumatism"—a broad heading applied to different kinds of pain—responded to moxa in five cases cited by Pouteau, one involving himself as a patient. He added the cases of a coachman's aching thigh, a washerwoman's painful foot, and others, like Mme Dumas's weakness, to which he applied "the arabic burn." Blanc reported treating paralysis and vertebral pain, and restoring tone to the lungs. Both doctors acknowledged that moxa was often a remedy of last resort. M. Dubois (1803) used it to treat a loss of speech resulting from fever.

Some physicians pondered how moxa worked. Van Swieten—who had reorganized the University of Vienna's medical faculty, carrying on the work of his teacher Boerhaave—assumed that moxa's "action" lay in its effect on the nervous system. Unlike many other writers, he recognized that points of application could differ from the site of the pain, but concluded that this meant the nervous system required further mapping. He also acknowledged the experiential basis of Chinese and Japanese physicians' expertise. Pouteau (1783) wrote that he had not bothered much with theory. Was outcome not the issue? One used quinine for fevers, mercury for venereal diseases, and opium for pain, without knowing why they worked. With rheumatism, however, he posited that fire vitalized the vessels capable of breaking down the corrupt humor, mixing it with fatty juices and facilitating its elimination

(1:280). He also speculated that fire functioned as a counter-irritant. Fire's action upon the nerves was that of "an agent which is the soul of all nature" (1:277). Moxa was also classified with blistering agents because one frequently promoted infection in the resulting burn, as with other cauterizations.

Percy (1792) described fire as a fluid, having a single nature. It penetrated the body, distributing itself evenly, although "some arrive at this equilibrium sooner and others later, as the thermometric experiments of Dr. Franklin have demonstrated" (26). Blanc added that since the ancients it had been known that the primitive effect of fire fortified solids, and resolved, divided, and alleviated thickened fluids. (An expanding medical language of fluids was gaining prominence.) Moxas summoned the corrupted humors with which underlying parts were impregnated, to the part subject to fire's action.

Infrequent correspondences aside, relatively little new information appeared during this period about moxa as used in China. Moreover, cautery was already so identified with European practice that doctors promoting it often cited the Chinese only as evidence that China, like other ancient systems, employed therapeutic heat. The function of this authority was to buttress a practice they traced to the early days of European medicine. The adoption of a name identified with Chinese practice therefore does not mean that these surgeons thought of themselves as adopting a Chinese practice, even as they listed the Chinese among the originators.

Acupuncture

Western surgeons, often identified with minor surgery, sought to elevate their status. In 1745 the London Company of Surgeons, formerly affiliated with barbers, formed an independent organization. The growing number of hospitals contributed to developments in surgical techniques. By 1794 many medical schools also taught surgery. By 1800 surgery had its own journals, in England its own college, and in general a rising social standing. Because acupuncture involved puncturing the skin, it continued to be classified as surgery. Surgeons' own relatively recent elevation in the field of Western medicine may have informed more critical responses toward what looked like counterparts of the lesser forms of their art among the Chinese.

Without Recourse to Bleeding

Thunberg observed that some Chinese physicians practiced surgery and "frictions" (massage), which Sue suggested attempting in Europe, to improve humoral circulation. Sue also cited a Chinese work on treating wounds, which was translated into Latin and housed in the French national library.[21] Most European authors, however, focused on what they perceived as deficiencies in Chinese practice. Although acknowledging Chinese practitioners' skills in cutting corns and nails, cleaning ears, applying plasters to sores, and performing castrations— the type of task identified with Western barber-surgeons—Gillan (1962) wrote, "I never heard of blisters, cupping or scarifying. Amputation they never perform" (283–284).

Resistance to bloodletting drew exaggerated attention. Only Bell (1965) provided a sympathetic explanation: "They compare a fever to a boiling pot, and chuse rather to take the fire from it than diminish the quality of liquor it contains, which would only make it boil the faster" (185). Dujardin contemptuously cited a "Monsieur de Malon," who castigated bloodletting, using the Chinese as counterexamples. De Malon (1766) wrote, "One heals [in China] perfectly well without recourse to bleeding. One scarcely sees paralytics there, asthma is even rarer, and the elderly of one hundred and more are quite common" (140). But as bloodletting would not be strongly challenged in the West for some time, Chinese attitudes continued to fuel a growing bias that intersected with the racializing of the Chinese. Barrow (1804), for example, claimed that the Chinese feared sharp instruments, even as he acknowledged that "they are in the practice of drawing blood by scarifying the skin, and applying cupping vessels" (237). He failed to acknowledge his own contradictions.

In 1786 Sue sent nine multiple-part questions to Beijing. Fr. Raux returned the replies of a Chinese physician, which reached Sue in 1790. "One will see," Sue commented, "that the Chinese have made great progress in an art that is as useful and even as necessary as surgery" (Sue 1796–1797a, 123–124). Sue had asked the following sorts of questions:

How did the Chinese set fractures and dislocations? How long did they keep them bound? What medications did they use?

Did they practice trepanning for head wounds? With what instruments?

Were they subject to hernias or prolapsed organs? Did they bandage them, or operate?

Did they have remedies for gangrene? Did they amputate?

Did they have cataracts and other eye maladies? Were there operations for such cases?

Were they familiar with aneurisms or arterial tumors? Did they tie hemorrhaging arteries or cauterize them?

Did they sew wounds, or only bind them?

Did they open the bladder to extract stones? If not, how did they remove or destroy them?

In deliveries, did they ever use hooks or other instruments?

Raux replied that fractures and dislocations were almost the only surgery in which the Chinese were experienced. His physician consultant had written four copybooks on the subject, with figures illustrating procedures and instruments. "My affairs have not permitted me to put his work in a state such that it can be sent by ship this year; I propose to send it next year" (125). To Sue's regret, he never did.

Trepanning had not been used since Han doctor Huatuo, whose secrets died with him. A Jesuit father, however, performed it on a sheep, exciting the Kangxi emperor's admiration. The event was recorded in the *Lettres curieuses* (Sue could not find it).

The Chinese experienced hernias, but doctors used neither bandages nor other external remedies. They recognized seven types, treating each primarily for pain.

Amputation for gangrene was unknown—the Chinese doctor was surprised to hear of it. If gangrene first appeared as a tumor, they pierced it with a needle to expel the blood or pus, and then applied a piece of beef.

Although not familiar with "true cataracts," they knew many eye diseases. After determining the source of the problem, they used remedies to strengthen the related "intestine" [*zangfu*] to remove the inflammation. Water flowing from a crag in Tartary was said to be a sovereign remedy.

They knew about arterial tumors, differentiating between various kinds. Physicians neither tied them off in cases of hemorrhage nor cauterized them. Instead, if related to fractures or bruises, a remedy of incense and melted alum was applied. Internal remedies included juice pressed from ginger, or sesame oil.

When treating a wound, they rarely sewed it, but bound it with bandages, having the patient lie on it to expedite its closing.

Problems with "the stone" were practically unknown, which they ascribed to tea drinking. Nevertheless, medical books did contain a remedy consisting of an ounce of *han tsao* (licorice), a tenth of an ounce of *tschou-cha* (cinnabar), and six ounces of *joa-chi*. One ground everything to a powder, added a little *houpa,* and put three-tenths of an ounce in water from cooking rice. Raux sent samples. "I do not know what became of these drugs," Sue grumbled in parentheses (130–131).

Delivery rarely led to accidents, and involved midwives, who used their hands. If the mother's tongue looked black or violet, they could tell the child had died and gave remedies to expel it.

Sue concluded that because many of these responses were so concise, he still could not fully evaluate Chinese surgical knowledge. He sent European works related to the topics he had raised, posed additional questions, and requested the copybooks on surgery. "I have still not received a response," he wrote, "and it is more than likely that I will not receive one until after the peace, which will allow for the reestablishment of a correspondence that the events of the revolution have interrupted" (132–133). No further correspondence appeared.

Acupuncture, or Acupuncturation

In 1757 physician Xu Daqun described acupuncture as a lost art, "for there were then left very few experts in it, and young physicians were at a loss to find teachers to instruct them in it." He suggested ten reasons for the decline—among them, that doctors and patients now preferred prescriptions and medicines (Unschuld 1990, 31). Acupuncture's continued diminished status was another. Nevertheless, the practice continued to draw some attention in Europe. Heister ([1743]1759), for example, wrote: "Somewhat a-kin to Scarification is the famous Operation of the *Chinese* and *Japonese,* termed Acupuncturation. Those Nations rejecting Scarification and Phlebotomy as pernicious, have Recourse to their Acupuncturation and Cauterization . . .

The first of these Operations they perform with a large Gold or Silver Needle . . . which they strike into the Flesh, either with their Hand or the little Hammer" (1:334). A "scarifactor" or scarificator, was an instrument with multiple small blades that were tapped into the skin to produce bleeding. A glass cup was sometimes heated from within to create a vacuum and placed over the incisions to accelerate bleeding. One of Heister's plates depicted not only a scarificator but also other methods for piercing skin, drawing blood, amputating appendages, and cauterizing—among them, an acupuncture needle and case, and a burning moxa cone (see Figure 17). The very grouping illustrated how he conceptualized both modalities. Heister wrote, "I do not know that the Practice [acupuncture] has been received by any of our *European* Nations: And therefore, as the Process is so much abhorred, we shall not here give a prolix Account thereof." Nevertheless, he characterized the Chinese as "judicious," and referred his readers to ten Rhijne and Kaempfer, "Spectators of the Operation" (334).

Heister's *Chirurgie* introduced generations of surgeons to acupuncture, establishing ten Rhijne and Kaempfer as authorities while positioning acupuncture within Western surgical frames of reference. Sim-

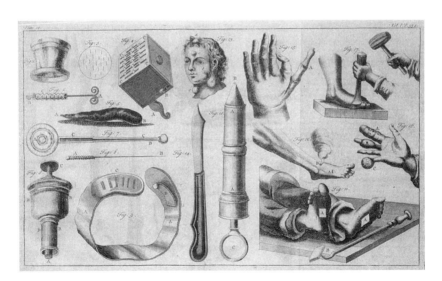

Figure 17. Surgical methods. Lorenz Heister, *Institutiones chirurgicae*, 1739. Courtesy of the Boston Medical Library in the Francis A. Countway Library of Medicine.

ilarly, Dujardin's (1774) chapter on Chinese and Japanese surgery relied on ten Rhijne. William Black's history of surgery praised ten Rhijne and Cleyer for "explaining the medical practices of various remote Nations," and cited Heister (Black 1782, 239). Vicq-d'Azyr wrote a treatise (1805) based on ten Rhijne and Kaempfer. Most European writers relied almost exclusively on these three sources, citing, quoting, and cribbing from them into the nineteenth century. Sue was one the few surgeon-authors who proved familiar with medical discussions in Martini, Kircher, the *Mémoires,* Du Halde, and Grosier, or who exhibited awareness of the Chinese medical texts in Paris's national library. Jesuit publications, he concluded, suggested that China provided few resources for surgical illnesses or related operations. "Everything is reduced to several topics," he complained, "pricking with needles, the application of moxa" (Sue 1796–1797a, 43).

Dujardin lifted directly from ten Rhijne and Kaempfer on acupuncture implements:

> To practice the puncturing, they desire that the needle be long, well sharpened and round; the handle should be turned in a spiral; the material is almost always gold, rarely silver, and never another metal.
>
> The mallet must be of ivory, ebony, or some other very hard wood; it is polished on the two sides, but pierced with shallow little holes, like a thimble, to receive the head of the needle; the handle is grooved along its length to serve as a holder, and it is secured by a silk ribbon, fastened to the end of the handle. (Dujardin 1774, 95)

Thunberg (1795) reported that needles had to be nearly as fine as a hair, and were made of gold or silver by artisans trained "to give them the temper, pliability, and fineness, which it is requisite for them to have" (4:75). Sue quoted Jesuit Fr. Poirot: According to people in Beijing, some practitioners introduced needles as long as half a foot without pain or danger. "But I have not seen it with my own eyes," noted Poirot, "and I don't have faith in the eyes of the Chinese" (Sue 1796–1797a, 50).

In 1802 Mr. W. Coley—"a surgeon from Bridgenorth"—published an article on "acupuncturation" in the *Medical and Physical Journal.* He had read Kaempfer, reprinted in *The Modern Part of an Universal History from the Earliest Account of Time* (Authors of the Ancient Part 1759)— "the best account I have seen of the acupuncture" (Coley 1802, 236–

237). He included Kaempfer's description of the "copper tube, of the bigness of a goose-quill," the gauge used to control the depth of insertion (238).

Point location presented a challenge. Dujardin (1774) described training mannequins: "The places that must be pricked are designated by green points, and those that must be burned, by red points" (91). Vicq-d'Azyr (1805) referred "those who desire a detailed knowledge of the parts of the body upon which the Orientals practice acupuncture" to meridian diagrams (137). Neither he nor Dujardin understood the connections between specific needling formulas and particular illnesses. Cibot (1782) explained only that acupuncture's "great secret is to know where one must stick the needles, in how many places, and the manner of inserting and withdrawing them" (262). Thunberg (1795), paraphrasing Kaempfer, designated the stomach as the site where "several small holes, often to the number of nine are made . . . but other fleshy parts of the body likewise may be selected for this operation." He added, "The bony parts are carefully avoided" (4:76).

Sue recommended two Chinese books in the French national library. *"Tum-Gin"* contained figures illustrating treatment points for men's and women's bodies. The other was in manuscript form. Sue quoted a M. Fourmont, who was sure that some Europeans practicing surgery in China also used acupuncture.[22] Through Dujardin, Sue knew ten Rhijne's diagrams, noting that Dujardin had also described where and how to place needles, as well as the type to use. Like many medical authors, Coley "transcribed" texts he found instructive, including Kaempfer on abdominal points for "senki," a form of colic described by both ten Rhijne and Kaempfer as common in Japan (Carrubba and Bowers 1974, 397). Coley added that benefits accruing from acupuncture in relation to "distemper" had led others to apply it indiscriminately to points where moxa was ordinarily used. By avoiding nerves, tendons, or blood vessels, "others have cured their patients by it, without putting them to the excruciating torture which attends that of *Moxa*" (Coley 1802, 237–238). It is not clear who these "others" were, but the remark suggests prior, unrecorded experimentation with acupuncture. As for technique, Dujardin (1774, 95) quoted ten Rhijne's explanation that the needle should be inserted "by turning it with the thumb and index finger, or driving it in lightly with the mallet, according to the nature of the illness and the structure of the part upon which one is operating." Thunberg (1795, 4:75–76) knew that one "twirled [it] round between the fingers."

Vicq-d'Azyr reviewed ten Rhijne's list of applications for stomach disorders; hysterical or hypochondriacal attacks; lippitude, early cataracts, fevers, illnesses caused by worms, tetanus, convulsions, tumefaction of the testicles, gonorrhea, and rheumatism, and repeated the saw about needles inserted into the abdomens of pregnant women. Thunberg related acupuncture to expelling wind. In Gillan's description of Heshen's case, the Chinese doctors attributed the problem "to a malignant vapour or spirit which had infused itself into, or was generated in, his flesh, which shifted itself from place to place, and always excited pain, inflammation, and swelling in the part where it fixed itself . . . the method of cure was to expel the vapour or spirit immediately: and this was to be effected by opening passages for its escape directly through the part affected" (Gillan 1962, 85). Coley, too, explained that acupuncture released "morbific matter, giving it a proper vent" (Coley 1802, 236–237).

Using needles to expel a vapor or wind was usually identified in Europe with eliminating excessive fluids or "winds," as in gas. Surgeon Samuel Sharp, for example, commented: "The method of pricking the Intestines with a Glover's large Needle in order to restore them, by discharging the Wind, and diminishing their Bulk, is condemned by all the Moderns, tho' not upon unexceptionable Grounds; for I think it is not true, that a Number of Punctures, sufficient to evacuate a Quantity of Air, will be pernicious to the Intestines" (Sharp 1761, 24). Coley pointed to tympanites—abdominal swelling due to gas, relying on Benjamin Bell, who recommended perforating the abdomen to discharge air when all else failed, and Dr. Darwin, who suggested a "glyster-pipe" to open the sphincter. The use of acupuncture for *senki* seemed, to Coley, potentially simpler, and he encouraged English surgeons to consider it.

Fothergill (1772) also employed a scarificator to treat dropsy (edema), to drain "a large quantity of water . . . without risk of inflammation, or deterring the patient from a repetition if necessary" (121). The related practice of "tapping" involved inserting a needle to release lymphatic fluid. Physician Richard Wilkes recalled Sydenham's aversion to such applications. Wilkes himself advocated pricking affected parts several times a day "till all the water is discharged" (Wilkes 1775, 282). Such practices were sometimes called "acupuncture."

Regarding how acupuncture worked, van Swieten hypothesized: "[It seems] to stimulate the nerves and thereby to alleviate pains and cramps in quite different parts of the body in a most wonderful way. It would be an extraordinarily useful enterprise if someone would take the trouble to note and investigate the marvelous communion which the nerves have with one another, and at what points certain nerves lie which when stimulated can calm the pain at distant sites. The physicians of Asia, who knew no anatomy, have by long practical experience identified such points" (in Lu and Needham 1980, 293). His speculations took seriously the practice of treating points at a distance from the afflicted site, and attempted to establish links with anatomical knowledge. The nervous system allowed him to do so, bypassing the meridians.

Dujardin (1774) assumed that the principles underlying acupuncture "could only be the result of an infinite number of experiences endlessly multiplied" (92). He suggested that needles—rather than expelling harmful influences—brought "a greater influx of humors into the irritated part." The other active factor, he thought, might be "the imagination, dispenser of as many blessings as of physical illness" (47). Classifying acupuncture with irritants and stimulants, Vicq-d'Azyr (1805) refused to credit that one would pierce a pregnant woman's womb. "It is easy to judge by this account," he wrote, "that the system of good standing among the peoples of China and Japan, concerning these alleged harmful humors which they think to release through *acupuncture,* without being more ridiculous than as many other systems, has no basis" (139). That is, he assumed that the modality's virtues must be exaggerated.

Dujardin (1774) remained ambivalent. "What they say of anatomy is most often the work of the imagination; thus, all knowledge which they deduce from it could not be very solid" (7). He resorted to the metaphor of "a harmonic machine, like a type of lute" (83), whose parts rendered different sounds through the nerves, veins, and arteries. According to ten Rhijne, the deeper "sympathy" between these parts was unknown to European doctors. Dujardin concurred: "Among us, the study of the parts has made [us] neglect the practical science of the whole, or this agreement of the parts among themselves, so well observed by Hippocrates and by all the true physicians: in this alone, the medicine of the Chinese, as empirical and imperfect as it is, even in this respect is worthy of some attention" (94). While questioning Chinese theory, Dujardin nevertheless used its example to critique a European lack of holism, in which the body should be conceptualized as a machine, understood as a whole, with interconnected parts.

Grosier (1788) was unabashedly impressed by "one of the most extraordinary operations which can be employed in the healing art." It was the reported efficacy that captured his attention, its "numberless cures" appearing "almost supernatural" (2:488). Still, according to Vicq-d'Azyr (1805), acupuncture had not entered European practice. "It is up to those who know the animal economy well, and who have meditated profoundly on the nature of illnesses," he editorialized, "to decide whether we should regret that this intervention is never used by us" (139).

In reviewing resources to which Western physicians of this period had access, we find treatises on pulse reading, explanations of *qi*, diagrams and figures of moxibustion and acupuncture points, lists of treatable conditions, discussions of technique, and even preliminary analogies to help bridge cultural divides. Some authors had access to many, if not most, of these sources. The one missing piece, by which they might have actually tested the *qi* paradigm and meridian system, was the link between diagnoses comprehensible to them and specific needling formulas. Throughout the eighteenth century, this knowledge gap functioned as an apparently unbridgeable chasm.[23]

Vital Principles and Imponderable Fluids

Despite the fact that medical authors attempted to explain acupuncture's "action," most Western scholars—whether because they were immersed in their own theories or because they did not include China-related sources in their research—did not make the connection with current thinking about vitalism. Not until the early nineteenth century would acupuncture be linked to these ideas, the most important being theories of subtle fluids, especially electricity and magnetism. Yet developments during this period would later influence discussions of acupuncture. Conceptual parallels between meridians and *qi*, on the one hand, and emerging ideas about electric, magnetic, and nervous fluids, on the other, are striking, although they generally went unnoticed at this time.

The term *fluids* had long been used in relation to humors and expanded to encompass other intangible but dynamic phenomena. Boerhaave, for example, had emphasized the need to understand the properties of fluids. As noted earlier, Newton hypothesized an aetheric medium permeating and surrounding matter, underlying all vital forces. Others translated this single fluid into separate ones corresponding to light, heat, gravity, electricity, and magnetism. Benjamin Franklin assumed that an electrical fluid pervaded both earth and atmosphere. As a fluid, it was "elastic," meaning it could expand and spread. It was also "subtle," able to penetrate openings between particles of matter. Eventually, electricity was recognized as an "imponderable" fluid: it could be neither weighed nor measured with precision. The amounts contained by separate bodies changed ceaselessly—as when Luigi Galvani (1737–1798) of Bologna observed that, if a connection is established between an "electric machine" and a frog's legs, convulsions result from the transfer of fluid he called Galvanism, or Animal Electricity. Galenism had endowed European medicine with the idea that the brain produces "animal spirits," which flow through the nerves to animate the muscles. Accordingly, nerves were assumed to be hollow, some anatomists conceptualizing the body as a system of tubes and fluids. With the second English edition of Newton's *Opticks* (1718), animal spirits were increasingly discussed as "nervous fluid," linked conceptually with electrical fluid.

Such discussions prompted theorizing about medical applications. Disease was conceptualized as a result of disruptions in electrical fluids; the removal of such obstacles would restore health. Electricity was applied to problems associated with obstructions in the nerves— "palsies, gutta serena, epilepsies, and the like" (Elliot 1786, 212). The largest category encompassed varieties of pain—aching heads, teeth, stomachs, toes, and lower back, sore throats, rheumatism, gout, lumbago, and sciatica. Eye inflammations, cataracts, *fistula lachrymalis,* and even blindness were pronounced potentially curable, as was deafness.[24] Lameness and paralysis, including tetanus, palsy, wasted muscles, and loss of movement, along with weakness and vertigo were included. (Benjamin Franklin [1758] treated paralysis and palsy with electricity, but observed few lasting effects.) So were convulsions, contractions, and epilepsy; fevers—ague, peripneumony, pleurisy, and intermittents; obstructed fluids—dropsy, blocked menses, and suppressed urine; hemorrhoids, other inflammations, and felons. There followed catalogs of catastrophes: burns, scalds, chilblains, hemorrhage, bronchocele, chlorosis, cramping, ganglions, gravel, hysterics, leprosy, madness, quinsy (inflammation of the throat), rickets, ringworm, scrofula, shingles, smallpox, spasms, heart palpitations, measles, Saint Anthony's Fire, Saint Vitus's dance, diseased testicles, cancers and tumors, ulcers and abscesses, and wounds that wouldn't heal, wens, and even cases of "suspended animation" from drowning or hanging.[25] Long-standing conditions responded less well, although there were exceptions. This compendium of conditions thought responsive to medical electricity very likely laid a foundation for how later generations of surgeons would conceptualize and test acupuncture.

Hypothesizing about medical electricity's "action," John Becket (1773) thought it produced a vibratory motion throughout solids and fluids, accelerating the latter's circulation. Tiberius Cavallo (1781) described it as a mechanical stimulus. Jean-Paul Marat (1784) conceded that it produced a small acceleration in the pulse and an equally faint increase in one's temperature. T. Gale (1802) inserted cosmic dimensions: "I believe the Millennium as at the door," he wrote, "and that this ethereal fire will be as conspicuous a mean of purifying the body from disease on that day, as the fire of the spiritual kingdom will be, in purifying the souls of men" (68–69).

Properties ascribed to electricity were likewise assigned to "magnetic fluid." Franz Anton Mesmer (1734–1815) conceptualized what he called "animal magnetism," which, when imbalanced, generated illness. One restored balance by transmitting magnetic fluid from practitioner to patient, a process usually involving the practitioner's passing his hands over the afflicted area. The French Academy of Sciences established a commission, which included Vicq-d'Azyr and Franklin, to investigate. In 1784 the commission failed to find that Mesmerism yielded consistent outcomes, ascribing them, instead, to the power of the imagination. Nevertheless, Mesmeric practice persisted both in Europe and, eventually, in the United States.

In 1798 Elisha Perkins, a Connecticut surgeon, patented a device he called "tractors"—two pointed metal prongs that one infused with electrical fluid by stroking them. Perkins claimed success in treating a large subset of the problems for which medical electricity had been judged effective. Charles Langworthy (1798), a supporter, noted that not only had Perkins demonstrated the tractors to Congress; even George Washington had bought a set. Critics dismissed the effects as also deriving from the imagination (Haygarth 1800), comparing tractors with Mesmerism (Editor 1802).

Generally the Chinese were viewed as having no theories of electricity or magnetism. (For this reason, Bertin arranged for his Chinese protégés to learn about the former.) According to Fr. Lambert, Chinese doctors treated tumors with lodestones, putting iron filings in strong vinegar and boiling the mix several times. One then removed the filings and passed a large magnet over them, attracting them to its surface. Both magnet and filings were said to be the effective element against inner poisons causing the tumor. Some years later Barrow (1804) pronounced, "Of pneumatics, hydrostatics, electricity, and magnetism, they may be said to have little or no knowledge" (238). A Doctor Dinwiddie delivered lectures on electricity to European residents in Canton, which the Macartney party attended, as did some local Chinese who spoke English. They were impressed, Staunton (1797, 2:227) suggested, although they did not always understand the lecturer's explanations.

Religious Healing

In writing about Chinese religious specialists, Jesuit observers struggled to sift out what they viewed as potentially useful medical information from what they could only condemn as superstition or idolatry. Practices involving divination particularly troubled them.

Calculations of Destiny

Grosier detailed geomantic practice *(fengshui)* and tensions resulting when neighbors positioned houses at unfortunate angles relative to others' dwellings. If legal proceedings failed, the plaintiff might mount a clay dragon on his roof to deflect harmful influences. Even the Jesuits found themselves implicated, after building a church overlooking a local governor's palace. The governor placed a dragon on his roof and erected a three-story protective façade. One suspects

Grosier of unholy amusement in narrating subsequent events. The governor's successor developed a chest disorder, yielding a thick, whitish phlegm that was blamed on the whiteness of the façade. Retainers covered the wall with black paint, "in hopes that they would then produce a quite different effect: the mandarin, however, died; and it was concluded, that the useful precaution had been taken too late" (Grosier 1788, 2:257). The story reiterated long-standing associations between *fengshui* and illness.

Grosier also described itinerant practitioners of *suan ming* (*xuanming,* to calculate fate). Many of these practitioners were blind. Their diagnoses generally identified an offended god. "The remedies they prescribe, the speedy efficacy of which they always warrant, consist in appeasing certain evil genii, by sacrifices, and by the prayers of some bonze" (2:253). Barrow (1804) described them as "known by a wretched squalling flute, on which they play . . . By being made acquainted with the day and hour of a person's birth, they pretend to cast his nativity, which is called swan-ming, or the art of discovering events by means of numbers" (325). To Barrow's amazement, his ignorance of the practice made it difficult to persuade court officials he knew anything about the astronomical instruments among the embassy party's gifts for the emperor.

Grosier (1788) described temple divination:

> Upon the altar which supports [the] idol, there is always a kind of horn, filled with small flat sticks, about half a foot in length, upon which are traced a variety of unintelligible characters. Each of these small sticks conceals an answer. After a great many prostrations, and other preliminary ceremonies, the person who consults, lets fall, at random, one of these small sticks, the inscription of which is explained by the bonze who accompanies him. When no bonze is present, they have recourse to a paper fixed up to the wall of the pagoda, to discover the enigmatical meaning of the word. (2:254–255)

Pilgrims consulted about health, journeys, and other life events. Barren women rubbed "the bellies of certain little copper gods," hoping for conception and children (Barrow 1804, 324). Other divination practices included physiognomy, palmistry, dream interpretation, spirit writing, an analysis using the written characters of a person's name, and, of course, the Classic of Change *(Yijing)*. Indeed, Barrow added, "The practical part of Chinese religion may, in fact, be said to consist in predestination" (325), all of which could be turned to inquiry about illness and health. Like earlier observers, he failed to understand the premise of a cosmological network of interconnected phenomena, knowable through readings of its different parts.

Humans Immortalized

The missionaries tried to differentiate for their readers between Chinese longevity and immortality practices. Cibot (1788) railed, "The ridiculous efforts of the superb *Tsing-chi-hoang* [the emperor Qin Shihuang] to find the drink of immortality, caused the true knowledge of the first ages about drugs and their nature, about remedies and their uses, to be neglected" (364). The Chinese did not fully feel their loss, he continued, until civil wars left the country "covered by the shadows of magic, superstition, prejudice, the most lamentable ignorance, and finally, idolatry, perennial source of all sorts of evils" (364). Nevertheless, books like the *Liji* (Book of Rites) and the *Zhouli* (Book of Zhou) provided details regarding how to care for one's aging parents. "The article on nourishment is singularly remarkable, in that it indicates not only the correct season during which to eat each food, but also the seasoning, the cooking that suited them; what is very worthy of remarking, what the other things are with which one can or cannot eat them" (368). Such practices contributed to long life in natural ways. From earliest times, added Amiot, the Chinese had men devoted to curing illnesses, the most ancient being Shennong, the Divine Husbandman. He was not, however, a god. Men like him, "immortalized for their wisdom and their virtues," were honored with secondary cults (Amiot 1791b, 13). Sue (1796–1797a) pointed to mythic rulers like Yu and the Yellow Emperor, quoting from physician M. Clerc's *Yu the Great and Confucius* and praising Yu's medical knowledge and attention to public health.

In contrast, some impeccably moral individuals were believed to become *xian,* or immortals. Persons guilty of slight defaults turned into *shen,* or spirits, with "superior and subaltern" degrees, the first governing the second. Subalterns who failed to fulfill petitions were demoted, with no recourse for improving their lot aside from reincarnation (Amiot 1791a). "One reproaches their little talent, their

inattention or their idleness; one injures them, one brings oneself
sometimes even to strike and smash the statues that one had assigned them as a dwelling" (218). Criminals, or those who had been
unjust or vicious, became ghosts, condemned to frequenting tombs,
mines, the surface of marshes, and infected places. The exhalations
of rotting cadavers served as their food. It was they who made people sick.

Chinese immortality practices continued to draw censure. "The majesty of the throne has not saved several emperors from the stupidity of
believing in it," jibed one Jesuit (Anonymous 1779a, 441). Voltaire
commented on "charlatans who resemble our alchemists," for whose
elixirs various emperors had paid great sums. "It is as if the Asians believed that our kings of Europe have seriously sought the *fountain of
youth,* as known in our ancient Gallic novels" (Voltaire 1878, 2:432).
Cornelius de Pauw (1795), private reader to King Frederic II of Prussia, wrote that the Chinese had inherited the "superstitious folly" of researching a "drink of immortality" from the "Tartars" (1:321), whom
he appears to have identified with both Mongols and Tibetans. The
idea of rebirth, he speculated, must have given rise to the idea of possible immortality. He concluded that "China possesses no chymists; and
nothing more is found in the pharmacies of that country, than herbs,
grains, and roots" (1:328).

Barrow (1804) speculated that such elixirs contained opium and
other drugs, providing a temporary stimulus, "and the succeeding lan-
guor requiring another and another draught, till, at length, the excit-
ability being entirely exhausted, the patient 'puts on immortality'"
(313–314). He quickly added, however, that it was no more ridiculous
than "the Perkinses . . . with an innumerable host of quacks, whose in-
decent advertisements disgrace our daily prints" (314). Why mock the
Daoists, when one could point to greater follies at home, like Perkins's
tractors?

Amiot (1791a) translated *dao* as "virtue, science, reason, doctrine,
perfection, path, way," and *daoshi* (master of the Way) as "master in the
science of sciences" (209), adding that the Chinese had always pursued occult sciences. Grosier (1788), who classified such practices and
practitioners among "other Chinese superstitions," added women and
the lower classes—believers in fox, cat, ape, tortoise, and frog spirits.
"For this reason, when they fall sick, they consult no other physicians

but the *Tao-ssé*," who made a "frightful din and noise" to banish the spirit afflicting their patient (252–253). W. Winterbotham, a member of the Macartney party, described how *daoshi* ritually distributed small pieces of paper with "magical characters," for talismanic and therapeutic uses (Winterbotham 1796). Barrow (1804) knew that they functioned as "a kind of doctors, and make plaisters for a variety of purposes, some to draw out the disease to the part applied, some as charms against the evil spirit, and others which they pretend to be aphrodisiac" (232).

Criticisms of *daoshi* paled in comparison with aspersions cast on Buddhist monks. Winterbotham (1796) vilified them as widely despised, "men without character, brought up from their infancy in effeminacy, luxury, and idleness." He claimed they purchased children to swell their ranks and feigned humility (2:98–99), and retold an anecdote from a Jesuit letter: A Chinese physician's daughter entered a Buddhist temple with two companions. Smitten, the abbot ordered her abduction. Her father appealed to the local "Tartar general," who was told that "the god Fo," enamored of the young woman, had spirited her off. Unconvinced, the general searched the temple, finding the maiden among other kidnapped women. He rescued them all and burned the temple (2:103–104). The story circulated internationally, later resurfacing in *Boston Weekly Magazine* (Anonymous 1804). It was not an event from history, but instead a trope from Chinese fiction, reflecting popular suspicion of Buddhist celibacy.

Such condemnations had parallels among the Chinese. In 1768 panic erupted throughout the lower Yangzi provinces, related to fears of sorcery. Queues (braids) were reported mysteriously clipped, and souls stolen—a loss that could cause disease, especially among children. Wandering Daoist priests and Buddhist monks were blamed, their outsider status making them the living equivalents of dangerous forces like ghosts. Mobs sometimes beat suspects to death and burned their bodies (Kuhn 1990). At the same time, the Buddhist White Lotus sect drew followers, in part because some of its leaders were healers. Their abilities were construed as evidence of spiritual authority, as were the protective and therapeutic amulets, charms, medicines, sutra recitations, herbs, and acupuncture they offered (Naquin 1985). In the popular Chinese imagination, Buddhist monastic identity thus fluctuated between the vilified and the protective.

Postures Called *Gongfu*

Among practices touted for extending one's life was *gongfu*. Amiot complained that the Chinese had long been deceived into thinking that these "singular postures" constituted a religious exercise that cured infirmities, released the soul from the power of the senses, prepared one to interact with spirits, and opened the doors to immortality. Attempting to uncouple the physical movements from their religious objectives, he relocated *gongfu* in ancient medical theory and practice, independent of the *daoshi*.

He had more difficulty explaining the breathing exercises. For that, one had to observe someone schooled in the practice. What little he could describe, he owed to a Christian convert who had done *gongfu* while "still an idolater" (Amiot 1779, 445). Focusing on the "physical and medicinal part" (444), he described postures to be done in relation to particular maladies. "The morning is the true time for *gongfu*," he wrote. "After a night's sleep, the blood is more reposed, the humors more tranquil, and the organs more supple" (445). Herbal teas enhanced the effects. Following one posture, for example, one imbibed an infusion of cinnabar and alum in cold water. He included illustrations (see Figure 18).

According to the Chinese, Amiot added, the body's mechanism was hydraulic (he drew no connection with parallel assertions from European physicians). Health resided in a dynamic equilibrium that modified the movement and reciprocal action of blood, humors, and spirits—claims that, on their own, European doctors would have accepted. *Gongfu* practitioners attended to sympathetic correspondences between different parts of the body, and to the actions and reactions of the organs of circulation, the secretion of humors, and the digestion of food. Amiot decided not to dwell on these aspects because, short of knowing Chinese medicine in depth, "one would clearly run the double risk of distorting an estimable system, and of not being understood" (449). If *gongfu* had medical value, he concluded, European doctors did not need Chinese physicians to deduce or perfect it. Rather, he proposed "that they examine whether the medical part of the *daoshi's gongfu* is really a practice of medicine of which one might make use, for the relief and cure of some illnesses." If so, he would feel compensated for the trouble he had taken with a subject "so tiresome for a person of my state, and so foreign to my studies and occupations" (442).

Over time, his views changed. In a 1783 letter to "Mr. Desvoyes," Amiot admitted to having viewed *gongfu* as "remedies only for those who were [already] well; but who, overworked and believing themselves ill, thereby cured themselves at little cost, by simply entertaining their idleness" (Huard 1978, 62).[26] Having discovered Mesmer's theory of animal magnetism, however, his opinion had undergone a revo-

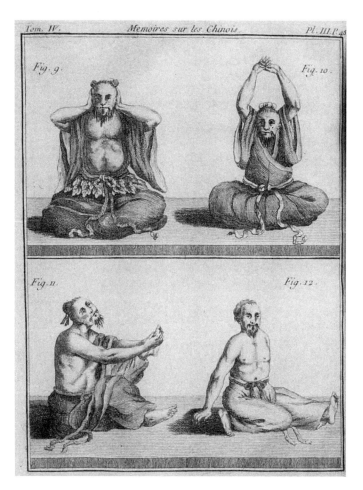

Figure 18. Gongfu of the Daoist monks. Amiot, *Mémoires concernant l'histoire, les sciences, les arts, les moeurs, les usages, &c. des Chinois,* vol. 4, 1779. Widener Library of the Harvard College Library.

lution. "What you tell me of the wonders worked at your Mesmer's place opens my eyes," he enthused, "and I already glimpse, as though through a cloud, that it could as well be of Chinese *gongfu,* as of Mesmeric medicine" (62–63). If anything, he thought, the Chinese principles more accessible than Mesmer's.[27]

Instead of equating *yin* and *yang* with humoral theory, as had so many European observers before him, Amiot was perhaps the first to propose magnetic theory: "For animal Magnetism and its two Poles, I substitute very simply *Tai-Ki* [*Taiji*], *yin,* and *yang* . . . The order that reigns in nature, its power—of which our weak constitution does not know the limits—its marvelous fecundity, the astonishing variety of its productions . . . is only the effect of the conjunction of *yin* and *yang* combining with each other, following the rules of harmony" (Huard 1978, 64–65). Excess or deficiency in either *yin* or *yang* led to false harmonies and disorder, from which was born illness. To restore harmony and health, one discerned which was the case and rectified the surplus or lack. Mesmer's practice, Amiot suggested, amounted to knowing the state of *yin* and *yang*—a paradigm that Amiot appeared to embrace: "What perhaps seems to you an unintelligible jargon, is for me a language as luminous as that of your Newtonian and other philosophers when they speak of principles of attraction, of Electricity, of the movement of Magnetism, of the turning of planets etc. . . . For thirty years, I have only heard *qi, yin,* and *yang* spoken about; I should be familiar with these terms which are the key to all the sciences here. There is nothing that one can explain except by using them opportunely, and provided that one forms an accurate idea about them, one is not at a loss for anything" (67–68).

Amiot's long experience in China led him to insist on the reality not only of *yin* and *yang,* but also of *li,* the "unknown principle" of the various gravitational theories (69). *Li* could well function as the foundation upon which rested all other truths related to the physical order. As the ordering principle of the *Taiji, li* was the "universal agent," simultaneously corporeal and invisible, "which influences everything, to which everything is obedient and which, since the first moment of its existence until the one when it must cease to be, acts constantly according to the simplest possible laws, has produced and will produce without stopping, all the secondary causes that constitute the vast universe, like the physical Agents that are necessary to conserve and maintain it in order" (74). Admitting that Bertin might not understand, Amiot insisted that he was communicating as clearly as possible.

Amiot speculated that *gongfu* dated back to Shun, Huangdi, and Shennong, and that some doctors must still practice it. "If there were only two or three in the vast precinct of Beijing," he added, "I would unearth them, and I would render you an account of their operations, of their manner of operating and the principles upon which they are based" (63). In another letter, written in 1784, he suggested that what Mesmer had said about animal magnetism had been said four thousand years earlier about *yin-yang.* "This fluid which is universally spread out and contained in a way so as not to suffer any vacuum, whose subtlety does not permit any comparison, and by its nature is susceptible of receiving, propagating, communicating all the impressions of the moment, is none other than the yin-yang of the Chinese" (Huard 1978, 81–82). It was this reality, he thought, that Shennong had recorded in the hexagrams appearing in the *Yijing,*[28] and that the *daoshi* transmitted to their initiates. Those who learned to attune themselves to the *yin* and *yang* within themselves could direct both through "the fluid of the same nature that fills space," extending out to distant phenomena and returning to transmit an awareness of what they had touched upon at a distance. Such men seemed able to know what occurred far away, "as though it were happening before their eyes" (83). Nor did Amiot dismiss the possibility.

In 1790, again writing to "Desvoyes," Amiot began by asserting his confidence that his benefactor's good wishes were largely responsible for his own vigor, freedom from pain, and general rejuvenation. Describing himself as looking more like a man of forty or fifty than of seventy-three, Amiot insisted that if Desvoyes were to extend this same "strong volition" even once a year, he might anticipate becoming "completely young before having reached the age of eighty years" (Huard 1978, 84). It was an expression of what we now might call "distance healing."

The letter also detailed Amiot's experience with "magnetizers"—not individuals with special salons, as in Europe, but street barbers available to any laborer able to pay thirty cash for an hour's treatment. Initially, Amiot had observed such practitioners while walking near a Jesuit country retreat house. "Whoever might have told me then that a similar spectacle would one day be the subject of my most profound meditations and would lead me by degrees to the true principle of the true Physics" would have seemed a visionary to him, he admitted. Only after having been "initiated into the science of Magnetism" did he discern core analogies (88).

The subject sat on a low bench. The barber washed and rubbed his head, to soften the hair and shave him. Such preliminaries served additional purposes: "All the nerves of the human body, they say, end in the head, or to put it more correctly, have their root in the head; the *qi,* or the agent, before circulating in the nerves and penetrating them, must above all, be concentrated in the head to be able from there to spread into the other parts of the body, following the direction that one indicates for it" (88–89). By shaving the head, one concentrated the *qi,* before directing it in ways that would effect a cure. The barber then stood before his client, meeting his eyes to establish a harmony. Placing his hands upon the newly shaved head, he palpated, tapped, and struck it lightly; pressed the nerves around the temples; lightly massaged the eyelids; and worked the muscles of the neck. He then pinched, rubbed, shook, and pressed the muscles of the shoulders, arms, hands, and thighs. To the observer, noted Amiot, it might seem that the magnetizer was diverting "the spirits and humors from their ordinary path" rather than harmonizing them. It was during the last part of the treatment, however, that the "beneficial *qi*" restored equilibrium.

The barber again stood before his client, fixing his gaze. He then passed his hands several times before the client's face, "in the way he would do if he wished to chase Flies and finishes by pinching him at the root of his Nose, precisely between his two eyes, then standing all of a sudden behind him, he proceeds to *tapping* [*tapotement*], forgive me this term, it expresses the thing better than *percussion* or everything else I could substitute for it." The tapping—mixed with open- and closed-handed percussive movements—moved from the head to the shoulders, arms, and legs, much as one might perform a piece of music. "One would think one is hearing a concert," wrote Amiot, "for which there are no instruments except the two hands of the magnetizer and the body of the magnetized" (90). Clients left filled with "such a state of well being that they scarcely recognize themselves" (91). The single risk lay in the state's lasting for only hours. When pain from sciatica or gout returned, one could return, but one could also become overly accustomed to the post-treatment state and unable to do without it.

As noted earlier, *qi, yin,* and *yang* did not generally enter European discussions of vitalism. Only Amiot connected them with Mesmerism. In a letter published in 1791 he continued to speculate that animal magnetism was simply the corollary of healing practices rooted in *yin-yang* theory (Amiot 1791b). Yet the setbacks that had undermined Mesmer's credibility in much of Europe appear to have created little incentive to pursue the tantalizing connection hypothesized by the Jesuit. The longer letters to Bertin remained unpublished, the potential connection unexplored.

China continued to function for many as a standard of inspiration politically, philosophically, artistically, and, for a few, medically. At the same time, shifts in the balance of power—the disenfranchising of the Jesuits, conflicts between the French and the British, the effects of British imperial expansion coupled with American independence, the French Revolution, and destabilizing rebellions in China—contributed to a gradual sea change in perceptions of, and reports about, the Chinese and their practices. So did a growing emphasis on constructs of rationality, invention, and progress, as these informed understandings of science and social order.

Racialized typologies, while still including nuanced subdivisions, increasingly reified first four and then five color-based categories that took "yellowness" for granted, and positioned all colors relative to the constructed superiority of Caucasian whiteness and beauty. Long-standing tropes representing the Chinese as suspect, cruel, and untrustworthy gained momentum in popular imagination, challenging concurrent representations of friendship, collegiality, and mutual respect.

The spirit of chinoiserie did not die. Some authors who produced the most censorious comments had themselves been inspired by that very spirit, as was Lord Macartney. Years later, John Barrow differentiated between "the lowest class who mingle with foreigners" and "the respectable class of society." Of the latter, he wrote, "With regard to these and the upper ranks, I must say that the impression left on my mind, and mostly on the minds of my companions, was—that in our estimation of the character of the Chinese, on leaving England, we were far from doing them that justice which, on a closer acquaintance we found them to deserve" (Barrow 1847, 133). And yet, with the waning of long-term Catholic missions in Beijing, Western encounters with the Chinese were increasingly restricted to the southern seacoast, mercantile groups, and the poor. Where Catholic missionizing had, to varying degrees, found ways to accommodate to Chinese religious practices, Protestant versions would prove less able to do so, intensifying the foundations for censure.

Nevertheless, a considerable amount of fairly accurate evidence about Chinese healing systems reached European audiences. Sue's summary of Chinese surgery, with its comprehensive allusions not only to medical literature but also to a wide range of missionary narratives, demonstrates that such knowledge was, at least in limited circles, comprehensively available by the time the *ancien régime* was coming to an end in France. An even more encompassing summary appeared in Louis-François Delatour's *Essais sur l'architecture des Chinois, sur leurs jardins, leurs principes de médecine et leurs moeurs et usages* (Essays on the Architecture of the Chinese, Their Gardens, Their Manners, Their Principles of Medicine, and Their Customs), published in 1803.

Delatour (1803), largely dependent on Jesuit accounts, summarized the state of Western knowledge regarding "Chinese medicine." His review included discussions of vital heat and radical moisture, Chinese pulse taking, the rejection of bloodletting "which they call the remedy of the barbarians" (255), medicine consisting mostly of decoctions of simples, the avoidance of violent remedies, theories of circulation, smallpox, eye diseases, forensics (the *Si-yuen*), *gongfu,* and detailed reviews of herbs.[29] He excerpted and summarized from William Temple; Du Halde, Le Comte, Cibot, Amiot, d'Entrecolles; Cleyer, Boym, Solano, Nihell, and Bordeu on pulse; de Pauw; and Sue on surgery. He cited Gillan from the Macartney embassy, and included a detailed alphabetized and annotated list of Chinese *materia medica,* drawing on Du Halde, the *Mémoires,* and Buc'hoz. Unlike Sue, Delatour devoted little attention to acupuncture, commenting only that "the puncture of a needle, consists of pricking the small branches of the arteries with prepared needles. Blood should not come out of these pricks; one cauterizes them with small balls of mugwort, which one burns upon them. They number incredible cures effected by this singular medicine, but its great secret was to know where one had to stick the needles, in how many places, and the manner to insert and withdraw them" (262). He quoted from a 1786 letter of Amiot, in which the priest described needles as used to cure pain caused by blocked sweat, drafts, or winds, or by the lack of the circulation of the spirits [*yin* and *yang*] (363). Like Amiot, Delatour discerned potential connections between *gongfu* and Mesmerism. Unlike Amiot, he thought both absurd. "If these ridiculous and extravagant attitudes," he wrote, "were to come to the knowledge of the Mesmerists, they would have been able to adopt a part of them, to vary the comic scenes around the *baquet* [a large wooden tub]" (318). His comments suggest why Amiot's arguments may have generated little interest.

Arguing that Western medicine was enlightened by its anatomical knowledge, Delatour also praised the interchange between the different European countries, and the hospital system as a vehicle for communicating and testing knowledge. Yet even while criticizing Chinese medicine for what he characterized as its practitioners' "ridiculous attachment to astrology" (250), Delatour quoted more laudatory assessments as well. He included Amiot's recommendation that Chinese medical works be translated (although he included the priest's reflections on the related challenges) and Cibot's comments that knowledge of Chinese medicine "would unquestionably be the most useful, because they are the most ancient, and perhaps those of which we have the greatest need . . . Science and knowledge are two very different things: as the first day by day becomes baneful in our Europe, so the other could sweeten the miseries of life" (264). Knowledge—the apparent purview of the Chinese—seemed to trump science.

Yet the more detailed the anatomical knowledge on which Western practitioners depended, the less credible Chinese paradigms seemed. Nor did theories of imponderable fluids bridge the gap, Amiot notwithstanding. Likewise, despite Saillant's insights, the persisting obstacle to acceptance of Chinese pulse taking remained its theoretical grounding. By the time members of the Macartney party got hold of it, the practice embodied "foolishness." Much of the rejection coincided with a general distancing from humoral theory, with which Chinese paradigms had been equated. And yet a single counterexample surfaces, again from Amiot.

Having reiterated his own experience of physician pulse taking,

Amiot repeated his conviction that the "universal Agent" *yin-yang* not only produced, but also modified, all bodies. It was the key that might "open the Sanctuary of nature to us; it is only within it and by it that we can make sense of all the phenomena that are found at each step in the shadowy Regions and that we can succeed in forming a clear idea of the true Theory of the World" (Huard 1978, 77). More importantly, he raised one of the only challenges to Western dismissals of Chinese body theory:

> Let us know, before anything, if those who have advanced what you have just read *have claimed to speak symbolically, and through allegories, or if they have believed due to physical truths.* In the first case, we would have to look for the true meaning of their symbols and of their allegories, and make every effort to find them . . . In the second case . . . if we accept that one should take in a natural sense everything that is said about these particular Agents, it seems to me that we can make use of it for an explanation of the effects produced by the animal Magnetism of Mr. Mesmer. (80; italics added)

Amiot recognized that a different symbolic system was at work, and that it merited investigation on its own terms. This was perhaps one of the only instances in which an observer did not try to draw immediate parallels with Western theories, but instead posited the existence of a truly independent system. Amiot also proposed a vitalist reading of "physical truths," albeit via Mesmer.

It did not help that foreigners had diminishing access to the literati, who might have been able to engage in a comparative discussion, as had Amiot's physician. Delatour, relying primarily on Jesuit accounts, could contextualize the lower strata of practitioners encountered by later observers, noting that street practitioners were no more like elite physicians than were their analogues in Europe. "The small Physicians, runners of the streets of China, true charlatans, ply their trade and do not harm in the smallest fashion the reputation of their wealthier brethren, since the latter have the general esteem for their knowledge and their probity" (Delatour 1803, 321). Post-Jesuit observers, however, at best saw elite physicians in passing, more often encountering marketplace peddler-doctors, who struck them as the epitome of quackery.

The reading of sources on Chinese medicine remained as selective and skewed as it had previously been, even as overall awareness of the constitutive parts grew. Insofar as Chinese theory resisted being grounded in materially discernible physical structures, it was not allowed to stand on its own, but instead was folded into Western formulations to the point of disappearing. Chinese methods were adopted—whether in the bastardized approach to pulse reading, the use of selected herbs, or the application of moxibustion—but divorced from their conceptual frames. It thus became possible both to identify moxa with the Chinese and to decenter moxa's Chinese origins by reclaiming it as one of eternal Europe's practices. The cumulative effect was further consolidation of a Eurocentric frame of reference.

That frame of reference drove increasingly negative assessments of Chinese healing. André Everard van Braam Houckgeest concluded that Chinese medical knowledge had been acquired long before that of the Europeans. But, he added bluntly, in China things had remained in a primitive state, with no apparent drive toward progress. "Regarding all our steps towards perfection as useless and absolutely superfluous, they are quite resolved to attempt nothing to imitate them" (van Braam Houckgeest 1797, 245).[30] Chinese resistance to Western paradigms, and rejection of diplomatic and trade relations, remained incomprehensible to the growing numbers of new observers, who increasingly construed both as indefensible affronts.

CHAPTER 5

Memory, History, and Imagination: 1805–1848

Following American independence, the British reexamined their colonial "responsibility" in India. A growing sense of being destined to rule "lesser" peoples and disseminate British culture, values, and trade merged with missionizing. Simultaneously the Industrial Revolution saw factory building, urbanization, agricultural developments, increased wages, and economic expansion—by midcentury, about a quarter of the world's trade lay in British hands. It also brought economic swings, protests, and riots. By 1843, workhouses held more than two hundred thousand poor. Bad harvests and epidemics struck in 1847. Emigration rose from an annual sixty thousand in the early 1840s to a thousand leaving England daily in 1848.

Napoleon's victories in Europe spurred British efforts to stymie French expansion. Napoleon retaliated, leading to the War of 1812, which involved the United States. Growing nationalism throughout Europe generated discussions of the role of citizens and the individual. In 1820 and 1821, revolts erupted in Italy, Portugal, Spain, and Greece. In 1823 American president James Monroe prohibited further European expansion in the Americas, opening the way for American economic imperialism. The period closed in 1848 with the publishing of the *Communist Manifesto,* revolutions throughout Italy, and uprisings in Paris, Vienna, and Berlin.

In the United States, between 1804 and 1806 Meriwether Lewis (1774–1809) and William Clark (1770–1838) sought an overland route to China. In 1814, Harvard botanist Dr. Jacob Bigelow (1786–

1879) lectured on the elements of technology as reapers, cotton gins, and weaving machines altered production and the factory system spread. By 1821 the country had four thousand miles of turnpikes. During the 1830s, railroad lines outdistanced canals and steamboats traveled the Mississippi. Yet booms collapsed into panics in 1819 and 1837. The brutal expulsion of Native American tribes to lands west of the Mississippi was legalized through the Indian Removal Act of 1830, while the economy became increasingly enmeshed in the international slave trade. Congress outlawed the trade as of 1808, avoiding full-scale abolition, but illegal trafficking persisted up to the Civil War. Artisans, worried by the influx of Irish and German immigrants, promoted unions. A more stratified class system emerged.

Two biblical sources inspired nineteenth-century American visions of change: Calvinism, which cast America as a retelling of Israel in the wilderness—a chosen people founding a Promised Land—and Christian millennialism, with its belief that the end-time was imminent, give or take a century. Missionary societies formed to convert Native Americans and sent missions to China by the late 1820s. Revivalism burned through upstate New York in the 1840s with a heat compared to wildfire. This "burned-over district" saw movements like the Seventh-Day Adventists and the Church of Jesus Christ of Latter-Day Saints (Mormons).

A sense of calling permeated many movements. Newspaperman Horace Greeley was a good example, espousing "socialism, land reform, feminism, abolitionism, temperance, the protective tariff, internal improvements, improved methods of agriculture, vegetarianism, spiritualism, [and] trade unions" (Tindall and Shi 1992, 502). Such commitments included health reform: how to cultivate the body fit to bring about the millennium? Many chose salvation by education, providing individuals with the information to uplift themselves and making the transformation of personal body and social body matters of individual responsibility.

In China, domestic and foreign problems continued to challenge the government's stability. Enough poor men achieved *jinshi* (advanced scholar) degrees through civil service examinations to foment illusions of upward mobility. Yet civil service was also viewed as collaboration with foreign rulers. Chinese were not allowed to rise as quickly or as high as Manchus, which fostered apathy and corruption.

Local officials were held responsible for disturbances in their juris-
dictions but had little authority to effect change, leading many to
underreport unrest. Paid low stipends, they funded administrative
costs through local taxes. Many literati returned to pre-Song Confucian sources, rejecting Buddhist and Daoist "corruptions." This movement, begun during the Ming dynasty, was known as Han Learning.
For example, Ruan Yuan (1764–1849), a leading scholar of his time,
oversaw the compilation and editing of the *Huangqing jingjie,* a collection of classical commentaries, comprising 180 works, in 366 volumes,
produced between 1825 and 1829 (Bruce and Brooks 1993).

Confucian understandings of history construed uprisings as the
weakening of a dynasty's hold on the mandate of Heaven. The White
Lotus Rebellion and the 1813 uprising of the millenarian Eight
Trigrams group seemed to prove the point. By the 1820s and 1830s, rebellions had spread. Part of the dissatisfaction was economic. China's
population in 1741 had been 142 million. A century later, it was 423
million (Fairbank, Reischauer, and Craig 1978). Peasants, although
not entirely isolated from the larger economy, lived with little hope of
better circumstances. No central policy directed the country's economic growth.

The China Trade

Western traders remained restricted to the bounds of the factory
system of Macao and Canton. After the War of 1812 the foreign community was largely English speaking. Friendships emerged between
some British and American traders and *hong* merchants, but foreigners
were still forbidden to study Chinese from locals—missionaries who
did so, like British Robert Morrison (1782–1834) and Prussian Karl
Gutzlaff (1803–1851), risked criminal charges. Perceptions of the Chinese were therefore often limited geographically to a neighborhood
outside of Canton, socially to business encounters, and linguistically to
rudimentary commercial argot.

In 1816 England attempted to renegotiate trade relations. Sir
George Thomas Staunton (1781–1859), who as a child had served as
Lord Macartney's page, assisted Lord William Pitt Amherst (1773–
1857). Fluent in Chinese, Staunton was now president of the Canton
Select Committee of the British East India Company.[1] The mission also

included Morrison. Still, it failed. Sinologist H. Julius von Klaproth (1783–1835) concluded some years later, "The most useless thing that one can do is to send embassies to China, since one is stuck with the results, and [they] only serve to put European governments in humiliating positions" (von Klaproth 1823, 364). In 1834, free-trade advocates overturned the British East India Company's monopoly. The British government sent Lord Napier to end Britain's "tributary" status. Napier, with no experience in Asia, took matters from poor to worse. The *hong* merchants and British traders reached compromises, but the situation deteriorated.

By the mid-1830s, opium was more profitable than other commodities. To the amazement of botanist Robert Fortune (1813–1880), the British and American drug lords were "men of the highest respectability, possessed of immense capital, and who are known and esteemed as merchants of the first class in every part of the civilized world" (Fortune 1848a, 7:290). They systematically ignored Chinese governmental prohibitions. Opium drained the Chinese economy of silver. Two million taels left the country in the 1820s, rising to nine million a decade later. From 1827 to 1828, according to the *Medical Times,* 1,213,832,442 pounds of Bengal opium reached China, increasing in 1833 to 2,883,339,345 pounds (Payen 1843). Efforts by Imperial Commissioner Lin Zexu (1785–1850) to halt the trade in 1839 provided the British with an excuse to launch the first Opium War. The war resulted in the humiliating defeat of the Chinese, the imposition of unequal treaties with England and other nations, the forced opening of five new ports, and subsequent attacks and treaties between 1840 and 1844.

New patterns of emigration arose. Abolition movements in the Americas led some slave owners to seek alternatives through indentured labor. Chinese contractors recruited the financially desperate, particularly from southern China, sending more than five hundred thousand Chinese and South Asian workers to Latin America, the Caribbean, and eventually North America between 1838 and 1870. American shipbuilders and merchants were implicated at each level of the trade. New York merchants, for example, shipped guano fertilizer from South America to southern plantations. Workers, frequently deceived into signing eight-year contracts, were forced into the toxic undertaking of digging and hauling hundred-wheelbarrow loads of droppings day after day. Some committed suicide, so great was their despair (Tchen 1999). The trade instantiated "coolie" labor and marked the beginnings of a traffic that would overshadow earlier forms of social exchange.[2]

Reporters and Reportage

Five genres of reportage and commentary grew from, and generated perceptions of, the Chinese and their practices, the number and kinds of works multiplying exponentially during the period under consideration. The first genre involved reports by foreign observers—diplomats like Sir John Francis Davis (1795–1890), physician-members of diplomatic parties like Clarke Abel (1780–1826) and John McLeod (1777?–1820), or traders like Nathan Dunn (1782–1844). Some naturalists, like Robert Fortune, spent time in China collecting botanical specimens. Most had read at least Barrow (1804) and Staunton (1797) and sometimes le Comte (1698) and Du Halde (1736).[3]

Some were Protestant missionaries, like Robert Morrison, David Abeel (1804–1846), and Karl Gutzlaff (1803–1851), a Lutheran who went to south China in the early 1830s. Becoming fluent in different Chinese dialects, Gutzlaff traveled up the coast disguised in Chinese clothing, proselytizing and dispensing medical care. George Tradescant Lay (ca. 1800–ca. 1845), a British naturalist, was sent as a missionary to China by the British and Foreign Bible Society, later serving as British consul at Canton (Lay 1843n). Samuel Wells Williams (1812–1884) went as a printer for the missionary board. Some of these observers wrote books, Lay also publishing articles on Chinese physiology and surgery for British medical journals. Others, like Thomas Colledge (1797–1879), Elijah Bridgman (1801–1861), William Lockhart (1814–1896), and Peter Parker (1804–1888), were medical missionaries.

Some observers published in the *Canton Register*, founded in 1827 and briefly edited by journalist William Wrightman Wood (fl. 1825–1830), who also wrote a book about his time in China. Missionaries wrote for *The Indo-Chinese Gleaner*, published from 1817 to 1822; for the *Chinese Repository*, from 1832 to 1852; and for the *Chinese Courier*, a monthly periodical. The *Courier*, which was published from 1832 to 1833, was written not only for the foreign community, but also to illustrate "our arts, sciences, and principles . . . There is no more excellent way to show that we are not indeed 'Barbarians;' and the Editor prefers the method of exhibiting facts, to convince the Chinese that they have still very much to learn" (Gutzlaff 1833, 2).

The *Repository*, in particular, reprinted excerpts not only from current observers but also from earlier generations: Louis le Comte (Editor 1832e), Lord Macartney (Editor 1833g), Alvaro Semedo (Editor 1833h), William of Rubruck, Marco Polo, Friar Odoric, Fernão Mendez Pinto (Editor 1834c), and Gabriel de Magalhães (Magaillans) (Editor 1841i). Similarly, John Rhodes Pidding, formerly of the British East India Company, published a newspaper for China-trade merchants—*Captain Pidding's Chinese Olio and Tea Talk*—from 1844 to 1845.[4] He, too, excerpted earlier sources. Although original authors often went unnamed, readers thereby encountered older sources.

Restricted to Canton, foreigners could not speak comprehensively about China—which rarely stopped them from claiming to be qualified to do so. Some missionaries, hoping to raise needed funds, exaggerated Chinese failings, paralleling Jesuit inflation of Chinese virtues. Distorted representations were not conscious lies; generally oblivious to their own biases, observers kept journals and thought the contents worth sharing. For example, C. Toogood Downing of the Royal College of Surgeons was medical officer on a trade ship. The *Chinese Repository* gave his *Fan-Qui in China in 1836–7* (Downing 1838) a critical drubbing, the reviewer characterizing Downing as having "undertaken a task for which he was wholly incompetent" (M. 1838a, 329). Downing's actual sojourn lasted six months, spent mostly on board ship. A better title, added the reviewer, might have been "A Voyage to China made by a literary body-snatcher" (328). Downing compounded the offense by plagiarizing an article by Gutzlaff (1837) on Chinese medicine, printing it under his own name in the *Lancet* (Downing 1842). (The theft went unremarked.) Yet even books like Downing's were read and quoted.

Scholars interested in China formed an academic discipline with related societies and specialized journals, generating a second genre comprising scholarly studies and translations. Some individuals collected Chinese books, which they learned to read. Jean Pierre Abel-Rémusat (1788–1832), for example, while studying Western medicine, learned Chinese from a Chinese herbal owned by the Abbé Tersan.[5] He went on to read Michael Boym and wrote his dissertation on Chi-

nese tongue diagnosis (Abel-Rémusat 1813). Initially serving as a surgeon in military hospitals, he left medicine for sinology, in 1814 becoming the first professor of Chinese at the Collège de France.

Scholars collected Chinese books. H. Julius von Klaproth journeyed
with a Russian embassy to Beijing in 1805 and 1806, assembling a large
collection (Editor 1823f). Robert Morrison built a library of ten thousand volumes, including medical texts. It eventually went to University
College, where a professorship of Chinese language was established
(Editor 1837c). Chinese books even began to be available for general sale (Editor 1843f). George Thomas Staunton donated unnamed
medical treatises, the *Mémoires,* manuscript dictionaries, and works by
Mendoza, Ricci, Martini, Kaempfer, le Comte, Anson, and members of
the Macartney embassy, to the Royal Asiatic Society (Editor 1827d).

Scholars also took up the challenge of translating texts. Abel-
Rémusat's successor Stanislas Julien (1797–1873) translated the *Mengzi*
(Mencius). Such translations appeared to stand apart from the living
culture, particularly when contemporary practices were depicted as
degenerate forms of ancient philosophies (see Christy 1932; Jackson
1981; Versluis 1993). Yet the resulting portrait of China derived not
only from observers and sinologues, but also from Chinese literati. In
particular, the literati*'s* own tradition foregrounded ancient sources as
repositories of the culture's foundational values, leading the literati to
lament what they viewed as the deficiencies of contemporary imple-
mentation (Wright 1992). This construction proved sufficiently com-
pelling to Western scholars that its adequacy went unquestioned. At
the same time, literati critiques were never intended to rationalize the
imposition of Western values and practices.

Translations, in turn, generated commentaries and derivative materials—a third genre—some by American Transcendentalists like Ralph
Waldo Emerson (1803–1882) and Henry David Thoreau (1817–1862).
Such authors posited a universal religion, revealed through the different world religions. Emerson, in this spirit, excerpted from Chinese,
Indian, and other religious texts, ignoring their differences. Mengzi's
assertions of a fundamentally good human nature appealed to Emerson, as did the Confucian ideal of the *junzi*—the profound person
who recognizes his innate nature to be that of Heaven. Emerson and
Thoreau printed selections from Confucius and like authors in the
Transcendentalists' newspaper, the *Dial,* introducing them to a wider

audience. Through the Lyceum lecture series, begun in 1829, Emerson spoke to thousands from all social classes, his reading of Chinese ideas informing his presentations. His approach followed what Arthur Versluis calls intellectual colonizing—a seizing of ideas, like artifacts, and ranging them alongside ideas from disparate settings. Emerson believed he had found something of himself in Oriental literature—in part, after having first projected himself onto it (Versluis 1993). By spiritualizing China and identifying that country with a timeless wisdom, he and his contemporaries could mine Chinese sources for their own purposes. They could even borrow from Confucius while condemning him for the Chinese social order.

Derivative articles also appeared in magazines like the *Edinburgh Review* and the *North American Review,* which reached intellectual audiences, and the *American Magazine of Useful and Entertaining Knowledge,* which appealed to a popular one. Almost every issue of the latter included a China story, and cover illustrations represented Chinese scenes or social roles. One article, "Chinese Small Feet and Long Nails" (W— 1824b), cited Montanus, "Martinus," "Die Halde," Kircher, Trigaut, Polo, De Pauw, De Guigne, Barrow, and "Rubruquis." Some short stories perpetuated idealized stereotypes, as in Priscilla Wakefield's "The Chinese Mandarine" (1811), wherein a devoted son saved his father's honor. Yet within decades, children's books—like the newspapers—transmitted less generous messages. Samuel Goodrich's *Peter Parley's Tales about Asia* (1830), for example, taught children that religion in China was "a system, contrived by cunning priests, to obtain influence over them. Like the religion of Mahomet, it is a false religion" (36; Miller 1969).

Physicians and surgeons who had never been to China, but who had read earlier Western medical works, produced a fourth genre—articles on Chinese healing practices for a Western medical audience. Abel-Rémusat occasionally wrote articles and delivered presentations on Chinese natural history and medicine, including acupuncture (Abel-Rémusat 1825, 1833, 1843). His friend and colleague, surgeon François-Albin Lepage (dates unknown), was a student of the surgeon-librarian Pierre Sue and followed in his professor's footsteps; in his medical thesis he presented an overview of what was known of Chinese medicine (Lepage 1813). He, too, drew on eighteenth-century China narratives, including Jesuit letters. Abel-Rémusat, in turn, reviewed

Lepage's thesis in 1813; the review was later published in 1825. Jonathan Pereira (1804–1853)—son of a Portuguese refugee, reporter for the *Lancet*, apothecary at the Aldersgate General Dispensary, and medical lecturer (Editor 1839d)—wrote about Chinese herbs for *Pharmaceutical Journal and Transactions*, and in his own *Elements of Materia Medica and Therapeutics* (1843).

Some surgeons generated a fifth genre, chronicling experiments and clinical experience with moxibustion and acupuncture in medical and surgical journals both in Europe and the United States. Baron Dominique Jean Larrey (1766–1842), a military surgeon during the Napoleonic wars and chief surgeon at the veteran hospital Hôtel des Invalides, was best known in relation to moxa. Acupuncture research was promoted by French surgeons Louis Berlioz (dates unknown), Pierre Pelletan Jr. (1782–1845), Jean Baptiste Sarlandière (1787–1838), and Jules-Germain Cloquet (1790–1883) and his students. In England it was promoted by James Morss Churchill (d. 1863), surgeon of Thames Ditton, Surrey, England, and London surgeon John Elliotson (1791–1868), who practiced and taught at University College Hospital in London. In the United States, Robley Dunglison (1798–1869)—brought from England by Thomas Jefferson in 1825 as professor of medicine at the University of Virginia—and Franklin Bache (1792–1864), great-grandson of Benjamin Franklin, and later a colleague of Dunglison's at Jefferson Medical College in Philadelphia, experimented with the modality in the United States.[6]

The genres were aimed at different audiences. Foreign observers discussed Chinese healing through missionary, medical, and Asiatic society journals and books. Their audiences included physicians, mission boards, lay supporters, sinologues, and readers of travel narratives. Some articles and papers were reprinted in full or summarized. Such patterns of transmission reveal which content was viewed as significant and by whom. Few readers received every genre, though there was some crossover; a Christian physician might have read medical journals, the *Chinese Repository,* and perhaps China narratives, possibly even encountering Chinese theory indirectly through Emerson.

It remained common for herbs, moxa, and acupuncture to be classified as part of Chinese medicine, and everything else as idolatry and superstition. Unlike earlier periods, however, the disposition to bias interfaced with increasingly negative racial representations of Chineseness, Protestant dismissal of Chinese religious life, and an all but absolute rejection of Chinese medical theory and related practices. As we shall see, during this period the phenomena of racialization, religionization, and medicalization converged most acutely and overtly, making each piece essential to grasping the nuances characterizing the other two.

Of Time, Space, and Humankinds

Eurocentric narratives increasingly represented time as progress, space as expansion and freedom, humanness as whiteness, and religiosity as Christian. It never occurred to most Westerners that their contributions would not benefit the Chinese. To observers viewing China through the miniature world of Canton, the country no longer represented an exemplar of civilization.

Time and Space Revisited

Although efforts to locate the Chinese within biblical chronology persisted, the view of time as a march toward progress reconfigured China as the very antithesis of that progress. The *American Monthly Magazine* castigated the Chinese for adhering to the ways of their ancestors: "It cannot be surprising that no progressive improvement has taken place in the Chinese nation, either as it regards their moral, intellectual, or physical state" (W— 1824b, 9). By the first Opium War, beginning in 1839, newspapers dripped contempt. The *Boston Evening Transcript* wrote, "There is a pompous and pedantic land, which boasts supremacy in wisdom and in science from an epoch anterior to all human record save its own—China, the land of many letters, many lanterns, and few ideas" (Miller 1969, 84).

Goods and objects continued to be imported, but not with the earlier chinoiserie-inspired frenzy. Some objects entered the space of scholars, collectors, and museums. Staunton, for example, donated to the Royal Asiatic Society theater costumes, a mandarin's official robes, other samples of Chinese clothing, and "ornaments of good omen" (Editor 1827d, lxxxvi–lxxxvii). William Bentley, minister of the Second Congregational Church in Salem, Massachusetts, instructed ships' captains on the material culture he wanted for the East India Marine Society and its museum. Society members processed annually through Salem, wearing robes and carrying objects from the collection (Jackson 1981). On a more popular level, inexpensive "album paintings" by Chinese artists, depicting scenes and occupations from Chinese daily life, were widely purchased (see, for example, Figures 22 and 29). Still, earlier fascination often dwindled to comments about Chinese "fondness for tinsel and gilding rather than solidity and grandeur"—for the latter, Samuel Wells Williams (1848, 2:178) added, one had to go to Greece.

Far from providing an inner space of social vision, China was rewritten as the archetype of tyranny. Morrison (1820, 95) thundered, "China does not enjoy *liberty*. Her government is a military despotism. Her virtues and vices are those of slaves." Canton was portrayed as a city whose "dissolute character" was proverbial (Wood 1830, 140). Some writers characterized the Chinese as inherently vicious; others blamed Western traders. Missionary Henrietta Shuck (1817–1844) wrote, "These foreigners are generally mere adventurers, unprincipled, vicious, eager in the pursuit of money, and unscrupulous as to the means of acquiring it" (Shuck 1849, 131). Some observers reminded their readers that Canton—even if corrupted by Europeans—was not all of China; others, however, claimed to have gone "where no European face had ever been seen before" and to have found "the same pilfering predilection" (McLeod 1820, 41–42).

Some foreigners thought the Chinese were justified in calling them *fangui* (often translated as "foreign devils" but more accurately meaning "outsider ghosts"). Yet Chinese merchants sometimes exacerbated matters by telling foreigners that government officials were responsible for every difficulty, while telling those same officials that foreigners "were of so barbarous and fierce a temper, as to be incapable of listening to reason" (Davis 1836a, 1:55). By the end of the period, as foreign accounts had it, the emperor, rather than being the enlightened ruler, was a despot; Chinese education stifled the aggressive inquiry of scientific thinking; and Chinese gentlemen did not play by recognizable social rules. Such polarization rendered Chinese forms of knowledge suspect—a consequence with ongoing repercussions for how Chinese healing practices would be represented and perceived in the West.

Polarized Humankinds

The polarity of blackness and whiteness continued to structure categories of race, along with attributes assigned to them, operating as
organizing principles for European and American political, economic, and social relations. Blumenbach's equation of beauty with
whiteness rarely faced the sort of challenge that appeared in D. B.
Slack's essay on human color in the *Boston Medical and Surgical Journal.* "The mere circumstance of our making the color of the black man
a theme of philosophical speculation," Slack wrote, "confers upon
us no right to make our own color the standard of beauty" (Slack
1844, 518). Noachide racialization continued, albeit inconsistently,
with Shem represented as the forebear of either Caucasians *or* Asians,
while Japheth was also assigned either Caucasians or Mongolians.
Blumenbach's racial typology—Caucasian, Mongolian, Malay, American, and Ethiopian—persisted, as did his subdivisions—"Mongolian"
included "The Mongol-Tartar Family, the Turkish Family, the Chinese
Family, the Indo-Chinese Family, [and] the Polar Family" (Editor
1840a, 40).

The supposed equality of whiteness masked the reality that different
European immigrants did not enter America on equal footing. To become "American" meant assuming "the dominant customs and values
of the white, Protestant, English-speaking, Northern European ethnic
stock" (Schutz 1989, 167–168). Famine in Ireland from the potato
blight in 1845 forced more than one hundred thousand Irish to emigrate to North America; forty thousand died during the crossing.
Protestant Americans quickly identified them as "priest-ridden subjects" whose religion was to blame for their poverty, drinking, disease,
and lack of education. Consequently the Irish were blamed for epidemics like cholera (see Kraut 1995). In turn, the Irish rewrote themselves as Anglo-Saxons to secure the economic and social benefits
of whiteness. Such moves would inform Irish relations not only with
African Americans but also, eventually, with Chinese immigrants.
Phrenology consolidated such racialization. Leading physicians like
Harvard's John Warren collected skulls of different groups for "comparative anthropology." The Boston Phrenological Society collection
included "an English form," a "Jew—tribe of Benjamin," "Negro.

Angelo—remarkable for his knowledge of languages," "Flatheaded Indian," "Hindoo," and "Chinese" (Anonymous 1835a).

The issue of how to explain differences yielded recycled answers: climate, sun and heat, and the influence of civilization (Smith 1814; Harlan 1822). Yet actualities again undermined efforts to stabilize categories, as illustrated by titles like "White Negro" (Fraser 1809c; Editor 1825t). Intermarriage happened more than proponents of absolute difference liked to recognize. The lower wards of Manhattan, for example, brought together free African Americans, Irish immigrants, and Chinese from the China trade (Tchen 1999). Some medical journals reviewed terms for biracial or multiracial persons, to determine which ones functioned as white. One author suggested that in Jamaica persons with no more than one-thirty-second African ancestry were both free and "rank[ed] as white persons to all intents and purposes" (Lewis 1839, 735). Slack (1844) countered that, whether a biracial individual and his or her descendants married whites or blacks, persistence in one form of intermarriage or the other would erase one set of physical differences. Such debate surrounded reflections on meanings assigned to Chineseness.

Race and the Chinese

James Cowles Prichard (1786–1848) noted that although Linnaeus had defined the Chinese as "Homo monstruosis," the description was exaggerated: "The Chinese, in general, are of a middle stature . . . their complexion yellowish or brownish, according to the places which they inhabit, and their mode of living. Those of the northern provinces are much taller and fairer . . . The coolies or porters, being continually exposed to the air, are more tanned than the Konang or Mandarins, and much browner than the women, who live shut up in the harems" (Prichard 1844, 521). Downing compared Chinese with Spanish women, suggesting that some of the former appeared European. Peter Parker observed a child and her mother with "their faces highly painted, to increase the fairness of the complexion, although they would be considered white persons anywhere" (Editor 1843c, 419).

Years earlier, le Comte (1698) had admonished his readers not to be misled by figures on China trade ware, for "they are not so ill-favored as they make themselves" (124). One missionary now commented,

"They are not facsimiles of the farsical caricatures which we are accustomed to see delineated, but powerful and well-shaped men" (S. 1837, 520). He may have meant insulting caricatures that circulated after failed British embassy expeditions. By the first Opium War, the *Boston Evening Transcript* had turned virulent: "Peopled by the long eared, elliptic-eyed, flat-nosed, olive colored Mongolian race, [China] offers a population singularly deficient in intellectual physiognomy; though to its absurd ugliness, the women of the higher classes occasionally offer striking exceptions" (Miller 1969, 84).

Nevertheless, the bias was not fully entrenched as of 1841. "Libertas"—Washington correspondent for the *Colored American*—attended a lecture by Peter Parker, facing whom "sat a colored man, in the most conspicuous part of the Hall, among the finely dressed ladies. And how some of them did shake hands with him after meeting. And all this in a slave city. This colored man was darker than many a mulatto, whom their ladyships would not think of noticing at all. This can only be explained by the fact, that mulattoes are Americans, and the colored man under consideration is a Chinese! . . . Isn't Chinese color better than American color? Who can but admire the discrimination of their ladyships?" (Libertas 1841). Here sat Parker's Chinese teacher. Exoticism trumped color within circumscribed settings, although fascination did not necessarily equal acceptance. Class differences played a part as well. Given competing variables of assessment, the Chinese both had, and had not yet, fully registered within racialized typologies, revealing the fundamentally arbitrary nature of the classifications.

An Imagined Chinese Character

Racialized physiology blurred with moral assessment. German physician, botanist, and historian of medicine Kurt Sprengel (1766–1833) now wrote, "We learn about how the perfecting of social institutions may operate among a nation of Mongol origin, whose physique alone seems already to indicate the false direction that ideas have taken among them" (Sprengel 1815, 192). For some, the Chinese could not be moral, "for true morality resides in the heart or understanding, and must be reared upon a right knowledge of our Creator in all his ways and works" (Lay 1841a, 21). Others differentiated, favoring individuals whose social positions resembled their own. Samuel Shaw (1847), for example, observed: "The merchants of the co-hoang are as respectable a set of men as are commonly found in other parts of the world . . . They are intelligent, exact accountants, punctual to their engagements, and, though not the worse for being well looked after, value themselves much upon maintaining a fair character" (183). Some friendships lasted for years. *Co-hong* Howqua (1769–1843), for example, invested through Boston merchant families, arranging for his estate to be managed by Russell & Co. Until it failed in 1890, the company paid his family up to $45,000 a year (Downs 1997).

In contrast, small shopkeepers and itinerant vendors on New China Street, Old China Street, and Hog Lane met with disdain. John McLeod (1820, 158) wrote, "They are a people, who, by early education and constant habit, are *manoeuvrers,* and always enjoy a much higher satisfaction in obtaining any purpose by fraud, trick, and overreaching, than by the most direct, candid, or honorable means." Such opinions entered children's books—"From the Emperor to the beggar, through every rank of society, through every grade of office, there is a system of cheating and hypocrisy, practiced without scruple, and without remorse" (Goodrich 1830, 36)—contaminating the perceptions held by upcoming generations.

The smearing of Chinese character merged with descriptions of the urban poor. Wood (1830), for example, described a beggar who roamed the streets with a dead cat tied to a stick, entering one shop after another. People gave him money to leave. Blind mendicants might or might not be blind. The poor were judged for eating "rice or millet, seasoned with a preparation of putrid fish that sent forth a stench quite intolerable to European organs," due, Clarke Abel insisted, to their being "utterly insensible to bad smells" (Abel 1818a, 246).[7] Markers of race, character, and poverty intertwined. Such character assassination was exacerbated by descriptions of physical punishments imposed by the legal system, loosely referred to as "torture." Chinese documents and prints illustrate that some of these punishments did occur, but Western writers also embroidered their accounts, presented as evidence that the Chinese lacked human feeling.

Chinese men's masculinity continued to be interrogated. Although European Romanticism favored certain "feminine" qualities in a man, the point was to show his moral attunement to the suffering of the oppressed. No such ambiguity characterized a fabricated description of mandarins pursuing foreigners passing overhead in a hot-air balloon: "We launched into the air . . . while the panting Mandarians ascended with as much rapidity as their corpulent bodies and their petticoats, would permit" (W— 1824a, 441). Some observers, noting the absence of dueling, questioned Chinese honor. Downing (1838) suggested that Western contempt was "founded almost entirely upon [the Chinese] unwarlike, cowardly character" (3:324). Yet identical behavior just as readily supported opposing conclusions. Morrison (1817) wrote, "They have no conception of that sullen notion of honor, that would lead a man to prefer being shot, or shooting somebody else, rather than explain and prove the truth and reasonableness of his words and actions" (122).

Some observers, of course, still pointed to Chinese virtues. Abel (1818a), having read about infanticide, sought instances of "a lower degree of parental affection." Instead, he repeatedly witnessed impoverished parents "expose themselves to the lashes and insults of the soldiers in defending their children from the pressure of the crowd" (235). (Meanwhile 4,323 individuals were implicated in infanticide in France between 1830 and 1839; Bayard 1841, 407). Parker and other physicians provided similar details: One father was so affected by watching surgery performed on his daughter that he left the room in tears, only to return when she cried out. On the other hand, children were also described as undergoing operations impassively (Wakley 1837a, 481). Gutzlaff (1837, 156) wrote that the Chinese "can take the most nauseous drugs with stoical indifference, and have generally a very strong constitution; even when afflicted with the most painful malady, they still move about, and are able to support the most excruciating pains." Such portraits reinforced stereotypes that Chinese lacked human feeling. Given British privileging of stoicism, undemonstrativeness, and a newly coined image of the stiff upper lip (Reinders 2004), such conclusions can only be read as ironic.

Chinese Abroad

Encounters with Chinese in the West remain difficult to enumerate. In England, for example, some Chinese sailors adopted Anglo-Christian names; some servants assumed employers' surnames. References to London's "Chinese poor" surfaced early in the century. In 1808, Chinese and Lascars rumbled in the East End (Myers 1996). In 1824 the *Times* reported the "Death of a Chinese Lady." Yhou-Fung-Queou, who had accompanied her husband and brother to London, was "beautiful." Her countenance was "pleasing, and bespoke gentleness and courtesy" (Anonymous 1824a, 3; H. 1824). The couple contracted a pulmonary illness, the husband dying first. Yhou, treated by a Dr. Webster, awoke one morning after dreaming of her husband, "and therefore she knew she must die" (Anonymous 1824a, 3). The *Times* lamented her passing. As the only Chinese woman known to have visited England, she had seemed an insightful observer.

In France, although various publications recalled earlier Chinese visitors (Breton 1811; Editor 1823i; A-Z. 1824), attitudes were changing. A Mme. Celliez—hired to teach one man French—represented him as a potentially valuable resource (Philibert and Celliez 1823). A reviewer disagreed, citing counterexamples: Tschoung-ya-san, a young trader captured from an English ship, had arrived in Paris as a prisoner. In 1819 seventeen-year-old Tchang-ya-kin had come as a servant. The third, Kiang-hiao—Celliez's student—was a merchant's son who had left China at fifteen. The reviewer concluded, "There is not a scholar of the *collège royal* who, at the end of six month's study, would not be able to derive a hundred times more from Chinese works" than from such sojourners (A-Z. 1824, 242).[8] Texts again overshadowed persons, given the knowledge sought and the social class of the visitors.

In 1829 four young Chinese men arrived in Paris to study theology with the Lazaristes. Some newspapers questioned whether they were, indeed, Chinese. The *Universel* reported a meeting between the young men and Abel-Rémusat and some of his friends and students. The purpose was to authenticate the visitors and to show that the professor did know Chinese, never having previously heard it spoken. Because of variations in dialect, members of the group used a blackboard to communicate, surprising the Chinese visitors (Lundbaek 1995).

In Berlin, the *Litterarisches Conversationsblatt* reported the presence of "Assing" and "Hass." Both met Blumenbach—who pronounced them "veritable Chinese"—and Johann Wolfgang von Goethe (1749–1832). Assing, using gestures and words from different European languages, explained Chinese legends and ordinary subjects. After a year, both visitors spoke enough German to converse in greater detail. Assing could play an air from German opera on an instrument called an *erhu,* "a type of violin with two strings" (Editor 1823i).

Italy had the Chinese College in Naples. M. Viesseaux, a visitor, described the main hall, hung with portraits of students. Instructed in Latin and learning Italian through daily conversations with teachers and servants, students eventually returned to China as missionaries. "Those who have suffered martyrdom are represented with the instruments of their death," Viesseaux commented, "others have chains round their necks, as a sign of their having suffered imprisonment" (Viesseaux 1824, 266).

Evidence of Chinese presence in the United States is fragmented. The Eighth Census of 1860 recorded that, from 1820 to 1830, three entered the country; from 1831 to 1840, eight more; and from 1840 to 1848, an additional three. However, as we have seen, direct and indirect evidence indicates earlier and more extensive arrivals. When President Jefferson declared an embargo in 1808 to prevent ships from being captured as war with England loomed, thousands of sailors, including Chinese, were stranded. Some entered North America through the West Coast, like the cabin boy on the *Bolivar* who arrived in San Francisco in 1838. Some married and had children, not uncommonly with Irish women, some couples running boardinghouses for Chinese ships-cooks, stewards, and sailors. A sailor named Appo went first to Boston and from there to New Haven where he married a Catherine Fitzpatrick. The two then went to New York, where he worked in a tea store (Tchen 1999). China trade merchant John Cushing brought a retinue of servants to Boston. "Marie Seise"—a Chinese woman—served an American family in the Sandwich Islands (Hawaii), returning to China six years later. She found work with the Charles Gillespie family, whom she accompanied to San Francisco in 1848.

In 1817 a John Nitchie wrote to Robert Morrison about a twenty-six-year-old Chinese man whom his mother had met in New York. She arranged for "Tschin-San-Chai" to attend Sunday school and learn to read. He had come to the United States as a waiter to a James Milnor, stayed for eighteen months, went back to China, and then returned to America in 1812, hoping to develop sufficient fluency in English to work as an interpreter. While attending school, he worked as a porter in "a China-ware store," again lodging with Mr. Milnor, "who always had a great regard for him, considering him as a very trusty man, of very good morals, and superior to any of his countrymen, in the same rank in society, in intelligence and behaviour" (Nitchie 1818, 79). Tschin had converted to Christianity and hoped to assist Morrison.

The goal of educating young Chinese as missionaries led the Foreign Mission School in Cornwall, Connecticut, to bring five boys from Canton between 1818 and 1825. Two—Ah Lan and Ah Lum—and possibly a third student, were expelled. Of the fourth, Chop Ah See, little is recorded. The fifth, Lieaou Ah See—"William Botelho"—later returned to China to missionize. The Monson Academy in Monson, Massachusetts, was another such venture. In 1847, Rev. Samuel R. Brown of Yale brought three students to the United States from the Morrison Educational Society in Macao (Chu 1987). The academy closed in 1827. It is not clear where the students went.

Chinese merchants occasionally visited. During the 1808 embargo, John Jacob Astor petitioned Jefferson for permission to provide passage for merchant Punqua Wingchong. New York senator Samuel Latham Mitchell argued that Punqua had come to collect money owed to his family and needed to return home for his grandfather's funeral. Newspapers suspected Astor of bypassing the embargo, suggesting that his "mandarin was 'a Chinaman picked up in the Park,' 'a common Chinese dock loafer,' a Lascar, and even an American Indian 'dressed in Astor's China silks and coached to play his not-too-difficult part" (Bonner 1997, 1). Jefferson granted permission. Punqua reappeared in Canton, where he owned a silk and fancy goods shop.

In 1847 merchant Chum Ming visited San Francisco with colleagues to negotiate trade arrangements (see Chu 1987; China Institute in America 1983; Yung 1986). Other individuals referred to fleetingly include a Chinese man from the vessel *Sally,* dressed in "full Mandarin costume," at church services in Plymouth, Massachusetts, in 1813 (Morison 1921, 203). By 1845 "Atit" from Canton had lived in Boston for eight years, becoming an American citizen. In 1848 an etching commemorating the piping of water to Boston from Lake Cochituate included a Chinese man, wearing a queue, in the crowd (Chu 1987).

Chinese entertainers also came. In 1808 New York's *Commercial Advertiser* announced a circus newly arrived from Boston and Spain. "The Young Chinese" would "display a variety of Comic attitudes and Vaultings, over his Horse in full speed." In 1841 juggler Yan Zoo performed in New York, as did juggler Ah Fong in 1842. New York stages also presented a "Tartar Cavalry," "Chinese necromancers," and "tumblers and combatants" (Tchen 1999, 97).

Collections of objects, like that in Salem, attracted visitors, one explaning that it allowed him to escape New England's mundane realities. The "arcade of sitting and standing figures became real friends of mine. Mr. Blue Gown and Mr. Queer Cap must be greeted whenever I went to the Museum" (Goldstein 1984, 257). In 1838 merchant Nathan Dunn organized a Chinese Exhibition in Philadelphia (after first building a Chinese-inspired mansion of his own). More than a hundred thousand visitors viewed its 1,341 items, collected by Dunn and his friend William Wood, a journalist. The collection included a summer pavilion, manufactures, religious iconography, models of junks, and oil paintings of *hong* merchants, along with life-size wax figures of mandarins, priests, shopkeepers, literati, servants, actors, and ladies. Chinese artisans had used individual models. Parker's Chinese teacher, taken to the exhibition by his student, "was so overcome by the extraordinary verisimilitude exhibited, that he burst into tears" (Editor 1841f, 536). Dunn sold fifty thousand copies of his *Descriptive Catalogue* (Dunn 1839) during the first months of the exhibit (Goldstein 1978).

E. C. Wines, reviewing the exhibition in the *Chinese Repository,* enthused over a twofold wonder: the speed with which travelers could now reach distant countries, and "the still greater convenience and safety, with which those who quietly remain at home may form the most accurate conceptions of places they never expect to visit." The reduction in travel time had annihilated distance; the presentation of "exact resemblances" could now "approximate places" (Wines 1840, 581–582). Time, space, and humankinds had entered a new relationship, older barriers collapsing. So faithful a representation was Dunn's "peep at China," Wines argued, "that China can be studied to more advantage in Philadelphia than in Canton or Macao" (584), given the logistical restrictions placed on foreigners. It was the effect of a *"tout ensemble"* (585)—an entirety claiming to present a whole.

After keeping the exhibition open from 1839 to 1842, and encouraged by friends, reviews, and the Royal Asiatic Society, Dunn shipped the exhibition to England. Madame Tussaud positioned figures of a young Chinese man and an English gentleman to look like spectators, and a wax Chinese couple, the woman moving her head as she spoke to her husband (Altick 1978). A British reviewer rhapsodized, "There is nothing wanting to give the visitor a complete idea of what the Chinese really are, and the result will be to raise them to a much higher degree in the estimation of Europeans than our prejudices have hitherto permitted them to attain" (Editor 1842a, 341–342; see also Editor 1843h). One function of the exhibit—coming in the years after the first Opium War—was to rehabilitate the Chinese in foreign opinion.

In 1841 the Boston Museum opened, initially displaying more than a hundred cabinets of Chinese "curiosities"; by early 1842 it provided entertainment, including juggler Yan Zoo, who was admired for balancing seven plates on seven sticks (McGlinchee 1940). A few years later, John R. Peters Jr., a member of Caleb Cushing's 1844 China mission, opened another China museum above Boston's Marlboro Chapel. The glass cases—many displaying mannequins representing different social roles—corresponded to the detailed catalog, whose cover stated, "Words may deceive, but the eye cannot play the rogue" (see Figure 19). To enhance the supposed realism, Peters hired two Chinese guides: T'sow Chaoong, who spoke English, and Le Kaw-hing, a music teacher who had left China to overcome opium addiction "and

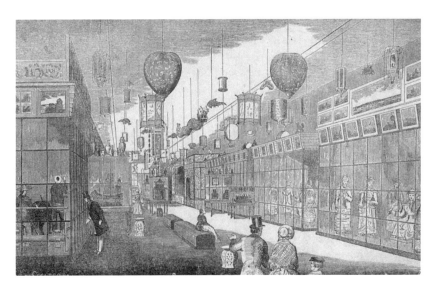

Figure 19. View of the interior of the Chinese museum. John Peters, *Ten Thousand Things on China and the Chinese,* 1850. Widener Library of the Harvard College Library.

who will occasionally favor visitors with a Chinese song, accompanying himself on some of his original and curious instruments" (Peters 1846, 7).[9] In 1848 Phineas T. Barnum bought the exhibit, incorporating it into his own in New York (see Zboray and Zboray 2004).

Individuals viewed as racially or sexually exotic drew audiences in Europe and the United States. Those displayed were sometimes represented as "monsters." Medical journals published typologies of the monstrous, organized by a "redundancy of parts," a "deficiency," or the "unnatural formation or position of organs" (Pendleton 1827, 291). The brothers Chang and Eng, billed as the Siamese Twins, found themselves so categorized, leading to a stage career for which they wore Chinese clothing and queues and performed acrobatics. Medical literature contributed to voyeurism. Dr. John K. Mitchell published "An Account of a Monster," describing a sixteen-year-old Chinese boy in Canton named Aké, from whose belly grew "the form of a headless child, more than thirty inches long" (Mitchell 1821, 78). Mitchell's article included a drawing. Exhibited by his uncle, Aké was examined by Western doctors.[10] In 1825 the *Boston Medical Intelligencer* reported on a Mitchillian Museum's having received a cast, "done from the life, of Akee, the double-man of China," who was "in the enjoyment of pretty good health" (Editor 1825r, 148).

The *Medico-Chirurgical Review* described a London man who planned to "make a fortune by exhibiting two poor Chinese damsels in the modern Babylon. They were accordingly incarcerated for a season in a little room in Pall-Mall and astonished a few of the British belles" (Cooper 1830, 494; Cooper 1829). Barnum followed suit, by 1834 featuring Afong Moy in traditional dress and advertising her four-inch, "monstrous small" feet. She eventually became so well known that newspapers simply announced "the Chinese lady." In 1847 she was billed to appear with Tom Thumb, after which she left for Boston. Barnum then recruited another woman, Pwan-ye-koo. The *New York Times* described her as "a genuine Chinese lady . . . prepared to exhibit her charming self, her curious retinue, and her fairy feet (only two and a half inches long), to an admiring and novelty-loving public." Both women were presented as specimens of exotica (Yung 1986, 14; see also China Institute in America 1983; Bonner 1997), relocated in constructions of monstrosity no longer represented as geographically distant.

Foot binding was increasingly represented as "barbarous" and "a cruel and revolting practice" (Lay 1841a, 32). The *Boston Medical and Surgical Journal* reported the case of a foot-bound seven-year-old who developed gangrene and lost both feet (Editor 1848f). Medical missionaries increasingly disparaged Chinese women's inability to walk without shoes and support (Editor 1848f), although some observers still drew comparisons with corseting. Davis, for example, wrote, "Quite as absurd, and still more mischievous, is the infatuation which, among some Europeans, attaches beauty to that modification of the human figure which resembles the wasp" (Davis 1836a, 1:254). Indeed, Western health reformers targeted corseting.

Physicians viewed the bound foot as an artificially induced deformity, a quasi monstrosity, and medicalized its physical details. Blake Cooper (1829, 1830) described a specimen taken from the body of a drowning victim, comparing it with a clubfoot. A Dr. Simpson (1845), after describing the physiological effects and providing precise measurements, lamented fashion's influence. The *London Lancet* called it "pedal mutilation" (Editor 1846g, 251). Missionaries speaking to women's groups suggested that the practice was perpetuated to please men, thereby further challenging Chinese manhood. Such polemics buttressed the argument that the Gospels "civilized" men toward women. By targeting "heathen" women as "ignorant—degraded—oppressed—enslaved," Western men represented their own women as enjoying relative freedom and respect (Drucker 1981). Even so, the displays continued to fascinate, permeated by the lure of the sensational.

In 1847 Captain Kellett sailed a Chinese junk, the *Ke Ying*, from Canton to New York, exhibiting it in New York, Newport, Providence, and Boston before departing for London. The performance opened on Thanksgiving, with crew members performing martial arts exercises on deck with pikes and shields, the junk becoming the stage on which they played themselves. In Boston alone, more than four thousand people attended (Chapin 1934; Bonner 1997; Tchen 1999).

By 1848 the Chinese had entered at least eleven East Coast cities, along with Mexico, California, and the Northwest.[11] They came, and sometimes stayed, as sailors, servants, merchants, students, performers, and stage exhibits. Most other Americans would have seen them in these roles only at a distance, minimizing true familiarity or equality. Moreover, Chinese travelers and immigrants did not generally publish travel narratives. One exception—a travelogue narrated by Xie Qinggao (1765–1822), an illiterate native of Guangdong—described succinct impressions of Portugal, England, and the United States. Unlike Western observers in China, Xie restricted himself to the descriptive narrative style used by gazetteers in geographical writing, avoiding assessments of what he saw (Ch'en 1942). He did not discuss Western healing.

The State of Western Medicine

These different perceptions of the Chinese, along with knowledge involving Chinese healing, entered a medical world characterized by a mélange of self-styled practitioners, often in competition. Reflecting such flux, Thomas Wakley (1795–1862) founded the *Lancet* in 1823 to circulate medical lectures that were otherwise unavailable to a broader medical audience, and to promote or denounce some of the competing practices and theories. Medical exchange increased. Between 1830 and 1840, 222 American doctors went to Paris. While in Europe, they visited teaching hospitals, attended courses with famous physicians, purchased books, specimens, and instruments, and subscribed to European medical journals (Warren 1978; Packard 1932). This international circulation of ideas contributed to the dissemination of medical journal articles related to Chinese practices.

Illnesses of the time could be ferocious and fatal. The standard therapeutic responses provided by "regular" physicians were equally fierce. In addition to bloodletting, calomel—a poisonous salt of mercury used to the "point of salivation"—produced a laxative effect, interpreted as the expulsion of depleted humors. (It actually indicated the body's attempts to eliminate a toxin.) Many of these therapies reflected the persistence of humoral underpinnings, even though humoral theory itself increasingly held less sway. Physicians generated blisters, infecting them to expel "laudable pus," followed by tonics such as whiskey or brandy. Likewise, popular medicine relied on emetics, cathartics, diuretics, and bleeding—all therapies that "exhibited" visible responses. Physician-authored domestic medical books instructed families to keep opium, mercury, tartar emetic, and ipecac on hand.

Some reformers proposed alternatives. Sylvester Graham's version of vegetarianism, Thomsonian herbalism, the eclectic medical schools, hydropathy or water cure, homeopathy, "Physical Education" for both men and women, and less restrictive women's clothing all emerged in the process. Arguments for more accessible medical language persisted—as, in the United States, did the nationalistic emphasis on developing medicine particular to American climates, illnesses, and botanicals. Hence, some reformers promoted American drugs over imports. Reformers favored what was "natural," with "Nature" functioning as both a scientific and a religious construct.

The dominant dynamic was one of movements and countermovements. As Paul Starr (1982) notes in relation to the United States, "Sectarianism intensified not only because American society was open, but also because it was closed" (95; see also Warner 1987; Cassedy 1977; Malmsheimer 1988; and Rothstein 1972). Confronted by challenges from sectarian groups—particularly the homeopathic practitioners, who founded a national organization in 1847—the regulars countered with the American Medical Association in 1848. Ironically, as John Harley Warner (1987) argues, the presence of the new movements pressed the regulars to adopt harder definitional lines than they otherwise might have done. The real issues were power, legitimacy, and who had the authority to define what constituted legitimate medicine. Medical journals targeted everyone from the makers of patent medicines (G— 1806), Thomsonian practitioners (Editor 1837e), "root doctors" (Editor 1843g), hydropaths, homeopaths, and Mesmerists (Editor 1845b) to "doctress-botanists" (Editor 1846a). Even the clergy were chastised for their testimonials used to advertise various nostrums (Roberts 1848).

Little consensus prevailed regarding what "science" meant. In Europe some suspicion lingered toward potential connections between science, technology, and radicalism. In the United States, science was expected to further democracy, and popular wisdom charged that science, too, should be democratic. Insofar as progress, the movement toward perfection, and scientific improvement were conflated, both science and medicine were to be set within the purview of the ordinary person. Various nineteenth-century medical groups wanted to be thought of as scientific, as becomes apparent in reading their debates. The term *scientific* would also be employed when assessing the Chinese.

Appraisals of Chinese Medicine and Its Practitioners

In *Recherches historiques sur la médecine des Chinois* (Historical Research on the Medicine of the Chinese, 1813), a thesis presented to Paris's Faculty of Medicine, François-Albin Lepage advocated understanding the state of the medical sciences among other peoples. He proposed the long-range task of studying Asian systems and the more immediate one of reviewing those of the Chinese.

The Medical Art among the Chinese

Speculating as to why science, as known in Europe, had not developed in China, Lepage (1813) posited three reasons. Longtime China observers could attest "that the Chinese had carried certain arts to the highest degree, and are thus strong friends of the sciences, since their emperors themselves did not disdain to be instructed in astronomy, jurisprudence, and medicine by our missionaries" (9). But, he added, the missionaries' expulsion from China had truncated the exchange's scientific potential. Second, China's isolation prevented communication with neighbors. If the Chinese were "strangers to the sciences cultivated in Europe, it is less their genius that one must accuse than the political circumstances in which they find themselves" (10). Third, China's written language had proved a hindrance.

Abel-Rémusat, in reviewing Lepage's thesis, commended his friend for avoiding prejudices toward China to which even the most educated men sometimes succumbed (apparently not counting Lepage's reiterated rejection of Chinese medical theory). He agreed that Chinese medicine had declined, but he challenged the argument about written Chinese. In a subsequent presentation delivered in 1828, he developed his own view (later published in 1843). Pointing to the visual structure of Chinese characters, he argued that early characters were pictorial representations that became stylized over time. Nevertheless, they still prompted the imagination. The paradoxical advantage of imagistic writing arose from the impossibility of creating as many images as there were things to name. The Chinese had, however, addressed this problem. Each character consisted of a visual classificatory component, plus a second visual component that specified the partic-

ular thing *within* the category: "In that way, they have established ge-
nuses, families, they have traced the outline of a natural classification.
They have placed in the family of the dog, the wolf, the fox, the cat,
the lion, and other carnivores; in that of the pig, the elephant and
rhinocerous; in that of the ox, all the large ruminants; in that of
the sheep, all the smaller ruminants; in that of the rat, all the rodents.
Following this arrangement, each natural being has received a sign
formed from two parts of which one is the type to which this being is
related, and the other an accessory [part] to distinguish the species"
(Abel-Rémusat 1843, 213). The organization of the Chinese language,
he concluded, was inherently scientific.[12] In China, to study words was
to study the classification of things.

Even so, physician Robley Dunglison (1833) concluded that medicine had "long but most imperfectly been practiced by the Chinese"
(1:184). Gutzlaff delivered a paper—published by the Royal Asiatic Society and reviewed in the American *Asiatic Journal* (Editor 1837c)—titled "The Medical Art amongst the Chinese" (Gutzlaff 1837).[13]
Praising the sophistication of pulse taking and herbal knowledge, he
added that the Chinese were "ignorant of anatomy, helpless as surgeons, and in time of sudden danger next to useless" (155). Missionary Walter Henry Medhurst (1796–1857) suggested that the Chinese
had received more praise for their medical knowledge in the past, perhaps reflecting the passing of Jesuit influence (Medhurst 1838). The
Chinese Repository put things still more bluntly: "There is so much error
mixed up with the little that is correct and true in the medical books of
the Chinese—so much that is manifestly either of no utility, or posi-
tively injurious, connected with this little that is worthy of commenda-
tion—that it becomes highly desirable and very important to ascertain
. . . what they actually do know, and how and with what effect they employ their knowledge" (Editor 1840c, 488).

Similar opinions filtered into Western medical journals. The *Boston
Medical and Surgical Journal* observed, "The Chinese are more ignorant
of medicine and surgery than of most other things which confer direct
physical benefit on the race, and will not be questioned by those who
have the leisure to investigate the present condition of either, as practiced by them" (Editor 1841e, 176). Peters's museum catalog critiqued
the "low state of medical science in China, which, in its connection
with astrology, closely resembles the practice of the healing arts in Eu-

rope, less than two centuries since" (Peters 1845, 87). Samuel Wells Williams (1848) concluded, "In all departments of learning, the Chinese are unscientific . . . they have never pursued a single subject in a way calculated to lead them to a right understanding of it" (2:192). Little seemed to redeem Chinese medical knowledge. Nevertheless, Lockhart (1841) advocated greater openness: "It is not to be supposed that all the opinions they entertain on medical subjects are mere nonsense, for some of their works have evidently been written by men possessed of considerable talent, and who have carefully examined into the nature and causes of disease; and the rules and precepts given for the management of some affections are by no means to be despised" (307). Few followed his advice. Wilson's condemnation reiterated a broader racialized judgment of Chinese civilization as a whole: "In medicine . . . the Chinese appear to have remained for centuries . . . in a state of 'petrified fixedness,' which nothing has moved" (Editor 1846g, 251–252). Medicine, that is, was construed as mirroring the state of Chinese culture as a whole.

Education and Sources

Western authors recognized the broad strokes of Chinese medical training. Sprengel (1815) quoted Martini: the most prestigious physicians learned medicine from their fathers, passing it on to their sons. The journal of an anonymous observer added, "Instruction in medicine does not appear to be at all an object, any further than it is to be gained by practice,—the practitioners not being brought up in the institution, but being received into it after having previously acquired some knowledge of their profession" (Editor 1835b, 184). In contrast, Wakley (1826a) drew on other sources to commend training involving acupuncture figurines, adding: "If our examiners at Lincoln's Inn would give every candidate for their diploma a sharp examination upon a *Tsöe-bosi,* not made of wood, but of other materials . . . they would do more to make men good surgeons, than all the little narrow-minded by-laws they have ever framed. We hope the good example of the Chinese examiners will not be lost upon them" (794). Yet apprenticeship was increasingly rejected in the West. As "Aliquis" (1830–1831) wrote in the *Lancet,* "In a profession so highly scientific, it is useless as a means of education" (44). The absence of teaching hos-

pitals in China seemed a shortcoming, although benevolent institutions and government-sponsored foundling hospitals were occasionally acknowledged (Williams 1848). Only Lockhart (1841) pointed to
"a great medical college" in Beijing, where "persons most thoroughly
acquainted with medicine, and possessing an unblemished character,
are after examination selected to enter the college, to fill its offices,
and to practice therein" (305). Such training, however, was not the
norm.

How aware of Chinese sources were Western physicians? Lepage not
only noted the number of Chinese medicine texts, but also quoted earlier Jesuit authors like Fr. Cibot: "As to the Chinese books on medicine, we have remarked that most of the great compilations were made
with much order and method." Alluding to the translations of European anatomical works commissioned by the Kangxi emperor, Lepage
argued that these made it "difficult to distinguish what belongs exclusively to [the Chinese], and what they have borrowed from the Europeans" (Lepage 1813, 35). Further complicating this, he added,
most travelers writing on the topic could do so but imperfectly. He lamented the absence of more physician observers: "What precious exchanges of knowledge could one not then make with Asia! Things
would be immediately appreciated at their true worth, and physicians
would know much better how to distinguish between that which could
enrich the domain of medicine, or that which one should leave under
the name of useless or ridiculous things" (102). Abel-Rémusat (1825)
asked whether any of his contemporaries was sufficiently familiar with
Chinese scientific works even to pronounce on their value. "Almost
none of these books have yet been translated," he wrote, "and almost
all those who reproach the Chinese for their ignorance, are outside of
the state [of being able to] judge them, since they don't know the language" (242–243). Two imperatives pertained: to learn to read Chinese, or turn to those who could. The first would be more certain; the
other a briefer undertaking. After all, sources were available.[14]

Missionary journals sometimes alluded to Chinese medical works
without explaining their contents, as when the *Chinese Repository* first
acknowledged the thousands of such books, while recommending "the
Golden Mirror" as "the best work of the kind we have yet seen in this
language" (Editor 1840c, 488). The editor meant the *Yizuan yizong*

jinjian (the Imperially Commissioned Golden Mirror of the Orthodox Lineage of Medicine, 1742).

Physician Edward Sutleffe alerted readers to the *Golden Mirror* and to the "E-shoo-hwuy-tsan" *(Yishu huican)*, "a comparative compendium of medical books" (Sutleffe 1820–1821, 2[14]:425), while also sketching the history of Chinese medicine.[15] Sutleffe purchased "all the books on medicine which were to be found in the populous and opulent city of Canton: they amounted to 892 volumes" (Wakley 1826b, 107; Medhurst [1838, 112] also alluded to this purchase, adding, "If the Chinese know little of the science in question, it is not for want of books or theories.") Sutleffe anticipated deriving little benefit, however, arguing that since Bacon had introduced experimental science, European knowledge had outdistanced everything else in both degree and accuracy. Sutleffe later appended his overview of Chinese medical history to a collection of his own cases (1825), but he gave no indication of having incorporated Chinese practices, only making a case for training missionaries to provide medical care (1825, vol. 2). Wakley (1826b, 102) criticized the work "as worthless as the letter-press is excellent" due to its mix of "christian humility, sectarian rancour, and gross and stupid vulgarity."

Occasionally authors exhibited familiarity with developments in Chinese medical history, as when physician Alex Pearson (1780–1874) described the Qianlong emperor's order to revise the *Shanghanlun*— "to arrange each disease under its proper head; to exclude what is contradictory, to retain what is perspicuous and practical, and to add the discoveries of modern practice" (Pearson 1826a, 126). Other observers drew sweepingly negative conclusions: journalist William Wood (1830) commented that, although Chinese medical works were numerous, "those which are justly celebrated are small in proportion to the many indifferent treatises" (154). He cited no specifics.

In 1836 a Dr. Lumqua donated 352 Chinese books to the Asiatic Society of Bengal, among them five volumes "on Anatomy and Surgery, with prescriptions," seven on pediatrics, six on medicaments and ailments, eight on prescriptions, four on the moral preservation of life, and six on horoscopy (Princept 1836, 247). It is not clear whether they reached Europe. Gutzlaff, in his paper for the Royal Asiatic Society, reviewed the "Ching che chun ching, i.e., Approved Marking-line of

Medical Practice, a very celebrated work in forty volumes" (Wang Kentang's *Zhengzhi zhunsheng,* 1602). Yet even he found "the advantage derived from their perusal so trifling" as not to recommend them (Gutzlaff 1837, 156–157). When asked about the best Chinese medical books, Lockhart commented that this was a difficult question, as each branch of practice had its authorities. "But for matter and method," he added, "none equal the 'Golden Mirror of Eminent Authors,' and the 'Comparative Compendium of Medical Writers.'" He also noted the *Bencao gangmu* (Lockhart 1841, 306–307).

Doctors, Quacks, and Mountebanks

Occasional portraits of Chinese physicians surfaced. Drawing on "notes of conversation with a Taou priest" recorded by "doctor Yellow" in 1832, the *Chinese Repository* reported on "the fashionable Doctor in Canton," *Chin Shetih,* who had risen to his present position from an earlier career of peddling drugs. Preserving simple habits, "early in the morning [his house] is open for patients, who, as they come in, are conducted to a room adjoining the doctor's, where they wait for him in silence. Patients who wish him to call at their houses enter their names and places of abode with his door-keeper. About 9 o'clock he sallies forth, committing himself entirely to his faithful servant and chair-bearers, who carry him round to the patients in the order of time as reported at his gate . . . without reference to their condition, whether poor or rich. He makes no charges" (Editor 1832d, 343). Patients paid what they could, although payment was not required. The description corresponded closely with one produced years earlier by Lepage, of chests brought on house calls, divided into "[more than] forty small compartments full of roots and plants of different properties, which they administer according to the needs of the patients" (Lepage 1813, 20). Physicians who chose not to bring medicines with them wrote out prescriptions much as European doctors did, for their patients to fill with pharmacists. Risen from a lower social order, Dr. Chin spoke a heavily accented mandarin, "as a Scotchman speaks English," and would not discuss the strengths of the medicines he prescribed, "which," commented the editor, "it is said, are very few" (Editor 1832d, 66–67). The doctor relied on some two dozen medicines, unlike a predecessor who had been known as "the rhubarb doctor." He was popular among the wealthy. "They say that, although he does not speak good mandarin, and is not able to explain the properties of his prescriptions, yet people very generally get well under his care" (67).

The *Repository* described members of "the *medical community*" as commanding respect when skilled, some becoming quite able, "but as a community they are anything, rather than masters of 'the healing art.' They are very numerous, amounting, probably, to not less than two thousand" (Editor 1833f, 306). A discussion of the structure of the government included the *Tae E yuen (Taiyiyuan)* or "grand medical hall." Its officers' duties included overseeing medical practice in relation to "the nine classes of diseases," directing subordinates, and providing medical care to the imperial family (Editor 1835b, 184). The *Repository* also explained penal law regulating practice:

> All persons rearing *venomous animals,* preparing poisonous drugs, or using magical writings and imprecations with a view to occasion the death of any person therewith . . . shall suffer death.—An unskillful practitioner of medicine, who administers drugs, or performs operations with the puncturing needle, contrary to the established rules and practice, and thereby, though without any design to injure, kills the patient, shall be allowed to redeem himself from the punishment of homicide, but shall be obliged to quit his profession for ever. If it shall appear, however, that he intentionally deviates from the established rules and practice, and aggravates the complaint in order to extort more money for its cure, and the patient dies, the money shall then be considered as stolen, and the medical practitioner shall be decapitated. (Editor 1833c, 104)

Insofar as laws reflect abuses recognized as requiring regulation, one can cautiously read backward from the penalties described. The link between individuals bent on harm and incompetent physicians appears to have been whether or not their actions resulted in death.

Gutzlaff (1837) characterized physicians as scholars who had failed the civil service examinations or poor scholars who needed to earn a living. Medhurst (1838) warned against assessing Chinese medicine's efficacy "by the number of doctors' shops throughout the country: for though the celestial empire literally swarms with medical works and apothecaries' shops, yet the number of successful practitioners we believe to be small" (112). Such statements prepared readers for descriptions like one from George Smith, who described having observed a patient grossly swollen from edema. Local practitioners "had been pursuing their irrational mode of treatment, on the supposition that it was a little globule of coagulated blood which was circulating in the body, and must be expelled before any hope of recovery could be cherished. For this purpose, among other specifics, toads had been prescribed for the patient" (Smith 1847b, 168). The patient died. Western readers were thus given little general reason to associate Chinese physicians with medical skill and sophistication.

Chinese patients were also described as resorting to multiple doctors. An elderly man with a chest complaint sought medicine from Downing, who gave him a box of pills. Some time later the patient requested another box, saying the first was helping. Downing chided him for not finishing it sooner. The patient showed him "a small bottle half-filled with black, dirty-looking balls, which he told me were the medicines prescribed for him by his native doctor. He said that he had a great deal of faith in us both, and therefore thought that he could not do better than follow both prescriptions . . . he took a dose of each of the pills alternately; two or three of mine one day, and half a teaspoonful of his fellow-countryman's the next" (Downing 1838, 2:150–151). Downing acknowledged that the man had improved. Unable to ascertain the precise source of efficacy, he concluded, "I was content to divide the credit of the cure with my unknown brother of the Central Empire" (2:151). Williams wrote that patients received remedies in amounts more suitable for horses, "for the doctor reasons that out of a great number it is more likely that some will prove efficacious, and the more he gets paid for, the more he ought to administer." The patient who did not recover as expected scolded "his physician for an ignorant charlatan who cheats him out of his money, and seeks another, with whom he makes a similar bargain, and probably with similar results" (Williams 1848, 2:186). Wood (1830) believed that most remedies provided permanent relief by sending the patient to his ancestors.

Public places thronged with "conjurers, quack doctors, and innumerable vagrants" (Wood 1830, 77). The *Asiatic Journal* detailed Cantonese magistrates' struggles to prevent "quack-doctors" from advertising aphrodisiacs. Police whitewashed over signs; vendors posted new ones "describing the properties and the mode of using their aphrodisiacs, in language which . . . makes Canton look like one vast public brothel" (Editor 1831a, 139). Wood (1830) described street practitioners "surrounded by a chaos of medicinal herbs and simples, with a small cabinet of preparations, and a granite mortar before them" (107–108). George Smith (1847) observed, "In every little open space there are crowds of travelling doctors, haranguing the multitude on the wonderful powers and healing virtues of the medicines which they expose for sale. Close by, some cunning fortune-teller may be seen, with crafty look, explaining to some awe-stricken simpleton his future destiny in life" (22). The parallel structure of the description suggested an indirect equation of duplicities. Robert Fortune (1848), commenting on the Temple of Confucius in one city, wrote, "In front of the principal tea-houses, are the tents of astrologers, doctors, dentists, necromancers, booksellers, almost all itinerant trades, peepshows, dancers on the tight-ropes, and Punch" (16).

One itinerant doctor displayed a snake (Lay thought it a cobra), bringing it to his face. When it tried to bite him, he jerked it away. Having attracted a crowd, he rubbed a ball of medicine on his face. The

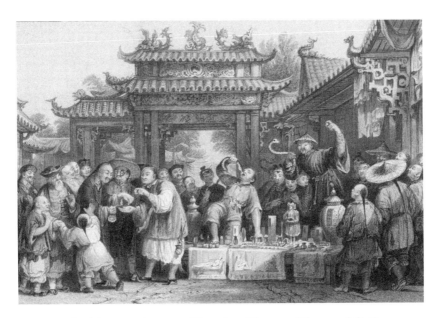

Figure 20. An itinerant doctor at Tien-sing. Thomas Allom and G. N. Wright, *China: Scenery, Architecture, Social Habits, Etc.*, 1843. Widener Library of the Harvard College Library.

snake pulled away. (See Figure 20.) Several displays of this test sold the audience on the repellant. Another practitioner had to hire a young man as a clown to help attract a crowd (Lay 1841a). In Peters's museum, the ninth display case included a street doctor. The catalog explained:

> Some are surrounded with roots and herbs, some have long strings of teeth which they have extracted, in front of them, and others, like our Esculapius, have their medicines exposed in small jars for sale, with printed advertisements of their virtues, and directions for use. Occasionally one may be seen with some large bones, or thick skin, such as that of the rhinoceros and elephant, disposing of them in small pieces to the passers-by, who suppose them to possess eminent strengthening properties. One of this last-mentioned class of Chinese M.D.'s might be seen at the entrance of the American grounds . . . with the skeleton of an ourang-outang, which he was disposing of . . . and as an evidence of the virtues of the medicine, an unhappy-looking chicken stood upon one leg, beside the skeleton, with a duck's foot and leg banded to the other. (Peters 1845, 93)

Such images, coupled with faint praise for literati clinicians, conflated the two in foreign imagination. The realism of the museum display also lent veracity to the China narratives—upon which the display was based.

An 1837 critique of animal magnetism suggested that humans had long succumbed to quackery: "In medicine, from Hoangti to Hahnemann, have we not had a succession of absurd doctrines?" (Editor 1837h, 268). The emperor—who apparently was assumed to be known by name to readers of the *American Journal of Medical Sciences*— was relegated to the ranks of the detested homeopaths. In 1802 the British *Medical and Physical Journal* had published a letter from "Medicus" on patent medicines, singling out the "Chinese apostate Ching-si, so celebrated of late for his brown and yellow lozenges, [who] vends at an enormous price jalap and calomel" (Medicus 1802, 396). The description suggests an immigrant practitioner in England. Two years later, "Aminicus" submitted a handbill circulated by a father whose daughter had died from the mercury in Ching's lozenges. Mr. Ching declined to comment—probably, as Aminicus noted, because he had died some time prior to the case. "He was a regular country practitioner of some celebrity, and from the successful exhibition of his lozenges in private practice, was induced to advertise them" (Aminicus 1804, 173–174). Someone continued to sell the pills. An 1843 article in the *Medical Times* exposed the ingredients of selected patented medicines, including Ching's brown and yellow Worm Lozenges. The author warned that many nostrums for curing worms contained calomel—and then provided instructions for making both brown and the yellow sorts (Paris 1843). The cumulative effect of such characterizations and calumnies was a far cry from observations generated by earlier writers like Frs. Amiot and Cibot.

Readings of the Body

Western focus on the dissected body gained further ground. An American physician wrote, "With a view to enlarge our knowledge of the nature of diseases, we ought to open dead bodies as often as it may be convenient" (Passamaquaddy 1807, 327).

The Body Anatomical

By the 1820s, dissectors required thousands of bodies each year. Besides the corpses of criminals and Resurrection Men, there were no sources. In 1830 the Massachusetts legislature legalized anatomical study, authorizing overseers of poorhouses, boards of health, and town selectmen to dispense unclaimed bodies to surgeons (Editor 1831d). Two years later the English Anatomy Act made similar provisions. Both extended the stigma of dissection from the criminal to the poor. Race entered the picture in the United States, where grave robbers shipped corpses of blacks to northern medical schools. Southern medical schools secured black bodies from hospitals and the cemeteries of poorhouses, slave owners, and black communities (Jackson 1997).

Advocates of anatomical dissection not only composed apologetics (Editor 1832a); they promoted the practice to a general readership. Ten thousand copies of Edward Jarvis's *Primary Physiology for Schools,* for example, were printed between 1848 and 1853, filtering a medicalized understanding of the body into a popular worldview. The privileging of the anatomical body continued, therefore, to inform perceptions of Chinese anatomical models. Lepage (1813) wrote,

"One feels in effect how imperfect must be the knowledge that the [Chinese] anatomy provides, if one limits oneself to it alone, and into how many errors one must find oneself led, when one wishes next to apply it to the sick person" (13). The question proved tautological: if structure and function constituted essential knowledge, then knowledge from which they were absent could only be imperfect.

Lepage acknowledged the Confucian premise informing the Chinese position and, like earlier Jesuit writers, pointed to forensic medicine as a source of anatomical knowledge. He cited the *Neijing* as including discussions of anatomy, and reminded his readers that the Kangxi emperor had commissioned a translation of "the anatomy of *Dionis* into Tartar Manchu, which Fr. Parennin sent to Mr. De Fontenelle in 1723, with a body of medicine" (14). It was, he thought, sometimes considered permissible to open bodies. Abel-Rémusat (1825) probed this comparative question, challenging its Eurocentric premises. First, China's anatomical treatises did, in fact, provide a general idea regarding the parts of the body. The system was comparable to that of the early Greeks. There could be no more reason to criticize the Chinese than "the prince of European medicine" (245). While not accepting the Chinese physiological system *per se,* he interrogated Lepage's analysis: "One would have to conclude that [the Chinese] are either really bad physicians, if they conduct themselves according to their principles, or really bad reasoners, if in starting from similar principles, they never arrive at curing their patients. In truth, in the sciences of observation, experience and theory are never so intimately connected that the progress of the one is always in proportion to the perfecting of the other, and Chinese physicians would not be the only ones who support a reasonable practice on absurd reasoning and ridiculous explanations" (246). Although no pure endorsement, it urged recognition of observation and experience. Equally important, as one of the few scholars in Europe who labored to learn to read Chinese and Manchu, Abel-Rémusat commented on the limitations of the translated sources, applying to Boym's work cautions raised earlier by Amiot. "In China, as in Europe, science has a technical language—expressions and twists—of which a knowledge, albeit extensive, of the general language does not give a perfect understanding. Boym, a stranger to the art of healing, has followed the literal sense of the words in translating books of medicine . . . he at most often translated without understanding, and I ask which of our theoretical works would not run the risk of being disfigured in passing through the hands of a similar interpreter" (247).

The admonition appears not to have unseated Western confidence that China was being correctly read—as wrong. An 1840 discussion of the *Golden Mirror* in the *Chinese Repository*, for example, discussed several "anatomical terms"—selecting the terms *arms, clavicle,* and *fontanelle* as evidence that "though brief and more or less erroneous . . . the Chinese, albeit they so much dread the knife, are yet not wholly ignorant of human anatomy" (Editor 1840c, 488). Lay, however, was less accepting: "The Chinese meddle not with dead corpses except it be to give them a decent burial, and therefore we need not marvel that their notions of human anatomy are very wide of the truth" (Lay 1841a, 238). Downing (1838, vol. 2) credited them with knowing skeletal structures due to disinterring the dead and cleaning the bones to rebury them in more favorable locations. Williams (1848) disagreed: the skeleton represented "a kind of internal framework, on and in which the necessary fleshy parts are upheld, but with which they have not much more connexion by muscles and ligaments than the post has with the pile of mud it upholds" (2:182).

One must locate such critiques among disputes between "regular" physicians and other groups. In defending the legitimacy of their own practice, regulars asked how "quacks," knowing "nothing of the structure of the human body, or the laws by which it is governed, should be more successful, when the method of cure is either the impulse of the moment or the effect of credulity?" (G— 1806, 70). Not to know anatomy, that is, was tantamount to quackery. Three decades later, the *Boston Medical and Surgical Journal* charged Thomsonians with knowing nothing of anatomy, adding that "any system of practice resting upon any other basis than that of a thorough knowledge of Anatomy, Physiology and Pathology, can never be productive of any great benefit to the community" (Editor 1837e, 400). Such judgments contextualize the rejection of Chinese readings of the body.

Moreover, Western writers did not know that views within China itself were not uniform, or that some Chinese physicians contested Chinese anatomical representations. In 1830, for example, the author of *Yilin gaicuo* (Correcting the Errors of Physicians) generated controversy in China and Japan by arguing that the drawings were wrong.

The earlier work of Wang Qingren (1768–1831), who had introduced revisions into Chinese medical knowledge based on his observations of the bodies of epidemic victims, continued to provoke concerns related to anatomy's moral dimensions. Physician Lu Maoxiu (1818–1886) noted, "This teaches people to study the way of medicine from rotting corpses in burial grounds and on execution grounds" (Andrews n.d., 10). Once life had ceased, how could one learn anything significant?

Body as Process

Dismissive critiques from Western observers did not go unnoted by the Chinese. In 1820 "Son of Han" published "Man as Microcosm" in the *Indo-Chinese Gleaner.* Just as a person breathed, he observed, so did nature, as witnessed in the tides, which corresponded to human "k'e hoo keih," or "expiring and inspiring" (Son of Han 1820, 373). According to Western philosophers, he said, "Man was by the Greeks termed the Little World, being supposed by some, an epitome of the universe, a great world." He added caustically, "Greek perversions of Asiatic History, are believed in Europe much more readily than the accounts which Asians give of themselves." Therefore it should not prove difficult to accept a Chinese theory corresponding to that of the Greeks. The point? "'Man is a little universe,' or as we Chinese express it, 'a little heaven and earth'—for with us the phrase Heaven and Earth means much the same as your European terms, 'Universe, nature, &c.'" (372). It was, he suggested, gratifying to see Western theory catching up with the Chinese understanding of Man as "an Epitome of the Universe" (373; see also Editor 1820c).

Still, Western writers rarely revised their generally critical stance. Even Abel-Rémusat (1843), commenting on Chinese theories of change, critiqued their "mendacious physics" predicated on processes of "spontaneous development," wherein one substance could transform into any other. "Following these principles, there is nothing astonishing in seeing the fluid of lightening and the stars themselves convert into stones, like that taking place in meteorites. Sentient beings become insensate, witness fossils and petrifactions . . . The tone with which these marvels are recounted by authors is certainly somewhat equivocal; but there is room to believe that they admit at least a certain number as proven, and that they see nothing truly impossible in the others" (216). He meant the varieties of change designated by terms like *hua* and *bian,* that allowed a piece of jade to become a boy, as with the character Baoyu in the novel *Hongloumeng* (Dream of the Red Chamber) by Cao Xueqin (ca. 1717–1763).

Elisabeth Hsu notes that in classical Chinese the observer's perception of change plays a role in its specific conceptualization. This subjective dimension means that although terms like *hua* and *bian* are not strictly synonymous with "change," they may at times be used as equivalents. "*Hua* designates a change within one mass and *bian* a transition from one state of the mass to another one. The question then arises what such a mass is. Is, for instance, the change from a frog into a quail a change within one mass or a transition from one state of the mass into another one? Both views are possible. *Hua* would emphasize that a 'mass' is being transformed and *bian* would emphasize that a transition from the frog-state into the quail-state is taking place while simultaneously indicating a connectedness between these two states" (Hsu 1994, 51). In a universe of *qi,* the subtle typologizing of change becomes not merely possible, but fundamental. Yet even for sympathetic observers like Abel-Rémusat, the very idea that such changes could occur was so implausible—"mendacious"—as to prevent his accepting core concepts in texts like the *Huangdi neijing suwen* or intuiting the aspect of reality they signaled.

Various authors revisited the challenge of explaining *qi.* Morrison posited that it corresponded to the "'materia subtilis' of the Cartesians; and to the 'subtile spirit'—the subtile and etherial medium' of Newton's Principia." He quickly acknowledged that they were not synonymous; his aim was to suggest correspondences. In turn, *qi,* aggregated, produced "Chîh" *(zhi)*—matter or substance. "The Ke [*qi*] and Chîh taken together make Sing [*shen*], the nature and property of bodies. Ke and Hing [*xing*] are the Primary Matter and Form. Ke and Sin [*xin*] are Matter and Mind" (Morrison 1819a, 147).

Qi, that is, along with its denser forms *(zhi),* constituted *xing*—the inherent characteristics and properties of a thing, its innate propensities. (Note the transformative implications.) The term was also applied to "human nature." *Qi* functioned as the essential vital stuff, while "Hing" could refer to the form it assumed. *Xin* (heart-mind) lay at the core of Confucian thinking about human nature. When Morrison differentiated between *qi* and *xin,* calling the one matter and the other mind, he transposed a Cartesian distinction where it did not entirely apply, insofar as both were *qi*. Years later, Medhurst (1838) would rehearse a similar explanation, differentiating between "chîh, which is the gross and sensible part of things" and "ke, primary matter, or the substratum on which figure, and other qualities of bodies, are reared" (190).

In relation to medicine, Gutzlaff (1837) explained, "throughout the human body a vivifying ethereal fluid is transfused, which is called Ke, and resembles the ether of nature" (160). *Ke* made fifty full cycles in twenty-four hours. Lay linked *qi* to Galenic theory, even as he validated limited aspects of it by referring to Western experiments:

> The Chinese hold the opinion once so prevalent in the West, that air circulates in the human body; and they caution the operator against letting it out, by the unguarded use of his instrument. They seem to speak as if they could see the steam issue from a puncture made into the vessels which contain it. Whether they were really sharp-sighted enough to see the *ke,* or air, as it escaped from a wounded artery, it might be presumptuous perhaps to decide; but that the body of man is bathed internally with some ethereal fluid, as well as with blood, seems to have been proved by some recent experiments upon the horse; and . . . the fact that air is secreted from blood to fill the air-vessels in birds and fish, would lead us, I think, to conjecture that this is the case. The Chinese are right then in the main, though in details we find them at their old work of blundering. (Lay 1841a, 242)

The critical factor resided in being able to connect the theory with a scientific experiment grounded in a Western paradigm, and to speculate that they dealt with the same phenomena. Even so, Lay could not altogether move beyond condemnation.

In a different literature, Emerson also wrote about *qi*. Ironically, he characterized Chinese religions as the worship of "crockery Gods which in Europe & America our babies are wise enough to put in baby houses" (Jackson 1981, 55). (Presumably, he read Confucius and Mencius as philosophers and not as religious thinkers.) Every reader of "Experience" was unwittingly exposed to Mencius's understanding of *qi*. Referring to Mencius (1970, II.A.2.76–78), Emerson equated *qi* with a pervasive reality [represented in] Thales by water, Anaximenes by air, Anaxagoras by (Nous) thought, Zoroaster by fire, Jesus and the moderns by love; and the metaphor of each has become a national religion. The Chinese Mencius has not been the least successful in his generalization. "I fully understand language," he said, "and nourish well my vast-flowing vigor [*qi*]."—"I beg to ask what you call vast flowing vigor?" said his companion. "The explanation," replied Mencius, "is difficult. The vigor is supremely great, and in the highest degree unbending. Nourish it correctly and do it no injury, and it will fill up the vacancy between heaven and earth. (Emerson 1903–1912, 72–73)

Perhaps because Mencius was not a medical text, Emerson did not link *qi* to vitalist vocabularies.

Both Morrison and Medhurst, like Amiot before them, added to the mix "Le" (*li*). "An immaterial and incorporeal principle, it has no figure. It is a kind of Principle of organization; answering to the internal and essential forms of Europeans" (Morrison 1819a, 147). Medhurst (1838) characterized it as "an universal principle, which is present with every existence, inhering or adhering to it . . . inherent in material bodies, and considered as their root and origin" (190). *Li* had long fascinated Confucian thinkers. Where Mencius had argued that to know one's own heart is to know the heart of Heaven, because both involve *qi*, later teachers proposed that *li,* too, inheres in both. Morrison's editor parodied the argument, writing, "They also invert the order and say—Le is heaven, and Le is the heart; or, in other words, heaven is Le, and Le is heaven; the heart is Le, and Le is the heart!" (Morrison 1819a, 150). Yet when one assumes a pervasive dynamic reality, that is, indeed, what they were saying.

Commentaries on the *Yijing* (Classic of Change) characterized sages as teaching the imperative to "investigate principle (*li*) to the utmost and fully develop one's nature until destiny is fulfilled" (Chan 1963, 269). Medhurst wrongly concluded that because *li* was conceptualized as impersonal, and because it was linked to the material dimensions of reality, Chinese cosmogony was by definition rooted in materialism. He did not understand that the privileged element in the paradigm was not matter. Rather, it was the workings of the *Dao* in its many expressions—substance, vital force, and ordering principle—that mattered.

Such discussions flowed into considerations of *yin* and *yang.* Humoral comparisons persisted for some writers, such as Lepage. Others sought additional metaphors. Morrison (1819a) resorted to Linnaeus's botanical model, particularly what he called "a sexual system of the universe," in which *yin* was female and *yang* male. "This notion," he added, "pervades every department of knowledge in China. It is the foundation of their theory of anatomy, and of medicine" (145). The journal's editor agreed, suggesting that "no definition suits the Chinese Yin and Yang so well as that of a Physical Hermaphrodite" (149). Shifting to the language of optics, Morrison saw little promise in attempting "to introduce these technical terms into the cosmogony of Moses; for it appears to me that the Chinese Yin and Yang mean many things not included in the 'Light' and 'Darkness' of the Book of Genesis" (146). Both sets of meanings were inherent in *yin* and *yang;* the fragmented analogies, both scientific and religious, illustrate how ill-fitted Western classificatory systems were to effect a translation.

Sutleffe (1820–1821) began by discussing "the one eternal principle"—"Tae-keih" *(taiji)*—which subdivided into "a dual power"; this he translated as "Vis Inertia" and "Vis Mobile," a rendering that exaggerated the static and dynamic dimensions of *yin* and *yang.* Yet he also recognized their interdependence, and that excess or deficiency in either one generated disorder in human, natural, and social systems. Moreover, "in each animal body, whether male or female, the Dual Powers exist; and every part of the body is ascertained to belong either to the Vis Inertia, or the Vis Mobile" (3:2). He understood that therapeutic interventions entailed preserving and restoring balance between them.

Gutzlaff (1838) recognized that "the Yang and Yin principle is as prevalent in medicine as in the whole of nature" (176). The human body was, indeed, a microcosm. Lockhart (1841) remained unsympathetic: the Chinese were familiar with basics of anatomy, "though many of their ideas are so much obscured by what is frivolous and absurd, as to be almost entirely undeserving of attention. This is strikingly exemplified in their endless disquisitions on the *yin* and *yang*" (308). Still, Lay (1841a) counseled readers not to "despise the poor Chinaman's spiral" (149)—the *yin-yang* diagram, drawing analogies with the nervous system:

If we look at the nervous activity and nervous rest as the inverse of each other, I think we shall come nearer to the ideas of the Chinese. Both of them are necessary to life: if the nervous system is too much excited, the mind and body are injured; if too little, disease and bodily inaptitude are the results. Let us call the nervous activity *yang*, and the quiescence, or rest of that system *yin*, and we have two quantities which are the inverse of each other, but both alike necessary to life and health. Then let us consider the former as denoted by the bright part of our figure, and the latter by the dark, and we have a graphic or pictorial representation of a well-understood phenomenon in the human constitution. (148–149)

Such attempts to introduce alternative comparisons notwithstanding, the lingering power of Galenic metaphors is striking. In a British medical meeting, Mr. Streeter, a surgeon, "perceived in some of the Chinese doctrines a resemblance to the humoral pathology" (Bird 1842b, 805). Sinologists, too, perpetuated the paradigm, one editor writing, "They give the name of *yang* to the vital heat, and that of *yin* to the radical moisture" (Editor 1844d, 27).

Gutzlaff (1838) also explained the Five Phases, "which revolve in [man] as well as in other parts of the universe" (178). But Lay, again, proffered the most insightful reading, rejecting the materialist interpretation that gave Chinese philosophy "a most whimsical and absurd appearance." Instead, "The word rendered material in dictionaries has an abstract sense, and refers to the essential characteristic of an object, and not merely to the stuff or substance of which a thing is made" (Lay 1839, 382–383; see also Lay 1841a). One sinologist editor explained that each "element" predominated in, and governed, specific parts of the body. "Thus, fire rules the heart and first intestines, air the liver and gall-bladder, water the reins [kidneys], metals the lungs and great intestines, earth the spleen and stomach, &c." (Editor 1844d, 28). Lay (1841c) later explained Chinese understandings of anatomy in the *Lancet*, accompanied by an annotated traditional drawing. (See Figure 21.)

Such drawings failed to impress Lockhart (1841), who commented that they looked "as if some person had seen an imperfect dissection of the interior of the body, and then had sketched from memory a representation of the organs, filling up parts that were obscure out of his own imagination, and portraying what, according to his opinion, the parts ought to be, rather than what they in reality are" (308). Still, he glossed the parts. For example, *Tan,* the gallbladder, "is placed below the liver, and projects upwards into it; it has the office of judge; determination and decision proceed from it; when people are angry, it ascends or expands" (309). A Mr. Liautaud purchased an anatomical plate dating from 1576, accompanied by a description, which Stanislas Julien translated. Liautaud presented both to the French Academy. Multiple medical journals reproduced his review, although none in-

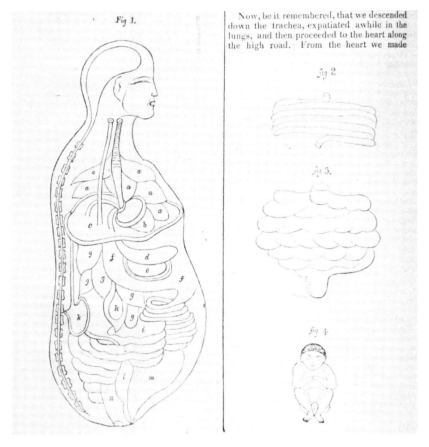

Figure 21. Chinese physiological drawing. George Tradescant Lay, *London Medical Gazette,* 1839. Francis A. Countway Library of Medicine.

cluded the plate (Liautaud, 1844a, 1844b, 1844c).[16] In contrast, Williams (1848) published a diagram that named each of the details.

Western authors registered mixed understandings of the *jingluo,* or meridians. Sprengel (1815) recycled Du Halde's description of the "twelve gates." Downing (1838, 2:158) accepted that the Chinese had long ago discovered the blood's circulatory system, but believed them to have recognized only veins and arteries, and not the blood's passage to and from the lungs. "As yet," wrote Thomas Colledge, "we are not aware that any correct knowledge regarding the circulation of the blood obtains in China." Medical missionaries rejected using *jîn (jing)* to designate "veins, arteries, nerves, and tendons." As a term referring to anything resembling a vein, including the vein of a leaf, they found it maddeningly imprecise, instead of metaphorically exact (Colledge, Parker, and Bridgman 1838, 41–42).

Medhurst (1838) alluded indirectly to the *Huangdi neijing* and the *Nanjing,* wherein the circulatory movement of the blood was recognized. "It must not be imagined from this, however, that the Chinese understand the circulation of the blood, as the phrase is used in Europe; or know anything distinctly about the veins and arteries through which it flows. Not having practiced anatomy, they are unacquainted with the internal structure of the human frame, and remain satisfied with the fact of the blood's circulation, without attempting to explain it" (110).[17] The description avoided dismissing the Chinese model; it was simply different.

Lay described the meridians as "the circulation, or the apparatus for irrigating the rest of the body with the vital streams" (Lay 1841a, 238–239; Lay 1841c). Each "viscera" connected to a "duct" connecting hands and feet to the head or other parts of the trunk. "It is not easy," he grumbled, "to translate fiction into the language of truth without some abuse of terms or something that looks like ambiguity or equivocation" (Lay 1839, 753). Lockhart (1841) struggled less, simply suggesting that the Chinese divided the channels into two categories, *jing* and *luo*—the *"king"* referring to the straight vessels, and the *"lo"* to the lateral branches. "For in the *Nan King* it is said, '*king chih hing chay,* the *king* are the vessels that follow a straight course; and *lo pang hing chay,* the *lo* are those that have a lateral direction" (308).[18]

Multiple journals reprinted Wilson's explanation of organs, vessels, and the "sexual system"—the "male" and "female" aspects of the twelve "arteries," discussing their positions and citing Wilson's description of the heart as "the ruler, from which the spirits proceed; it is also held to be the receptacle of the marrow, which comes from the brain, and goes to the reproductive organs" (Wilson 1846a, 1847a, 1847b).[19] Williams (1848) settled for a Daoist explanation, in which "the brain is the abode of the *yin* principle in its perfection, and at its base, where there is a reservoir of the marrow, communicates through the spine with the whole body" (2:180). He bypassed the alchemical roots of the image.

Pulses and Balances

It remained a commonplace that Chinese doctors based "their science in a profound knowledge of the pulse and all its modifications" (Lepage 1813, 15). Boym, Cleyer, Hervieu (as reprinted in Du Halde), and sometimes members of the Macartney party continued to serve as primary sources. Through them, Western readers became aware, to limited degrees, of Wang Shuhe. Abel-Rémusat (1825) even challenged earlier judgments, suggesting that missionary translations, albeit inadequate, would have rendered pulse theory "absolutely intelligible, if a French physician, the celebrated Bordeu, had not judged it otherwise" (248). He did not elaborate on the problem of conflicting paradigms, the fundamental sticking point.

   D. B. de Malpière's illustrated collection of Chinese social roles included a discussion of pulse reading in relation to the Chinese doctor (de Malpière 1825, vol. 2), while Wood—citing Du Halde—noted that "the success of an examination of a candidate for a medical degree depends principally on the state of his knowledge on this point" (Wood 1830, 154). Medical missionaries characterized Chinese diagnosis as "minute descriptions of the pulse, which they classify and connect with the five metals, the five planets, the five daemons" (S. 1837, 520). According to the *Medical Times,* "The patient must . . . have his arm resting on a cushion . . . both [the physician] and the patient are to remain calm, silent, and collected. The fingers are now applied in due *succession,* in order to judge of the compressibility of the artery" (Editor 1841c, 215). Physicians compared pulses with the intervals of a patient's breathing. The pulses—"the superficial, the profound, the quick, and the slow"—were equated with "the choleric, the sanguine, the phlegmatic, and the melancholy" (215). Such lingering humoral comparisons continued to bias the assessment of Chinese practice. Sprengel (1815) rehashed Cleyer, le Comte, Du Halde, and Staunton, but called Chinese pulses "puerile and absurd" (1:199–200). In 1823 Johan L. Formey rejected Chinese theory as sophistry (Kuriyama 1999). Citing the *Doctrine of the Pulse,* Davis (1836a) derided "the prejudice which distorts some portions, and the nonsense which encumbers others" (1:2). The *Boston Medical and Surgical Journal* described the practice as feeling the "length of the arm, and minutely recogniz[ing] the variations for every half inch, if such exist, which is indeed problematical" (Editor 1841e, 177).

John Peters's museum catalog proved equally damning: "As an evidence of their ignorance of the circulation of the blood, they distinguish twenty-four different and distinct pulsations in the body, and twenty-four different diseases at each of three pulses in each arm" (Peters 1845, 94). Dr. Samuel Jackson (1830a) concurred, adding that "the Chinese . . . possess a doctrine of the pulse which is artificial and complicated in proportion to their ignorance of the circulation" (104). British surgeon Golding Bird (1842b) dismissed a colleague as having "perpetrated quite as many absurdities concerning the pulse as the Chinese" (805–806).

Medhurst (1838) appeared initially more forgiving, describing Chinese doctors as able to detect pulse variations "with a nicety and precision, scarcely equaled by European physicians" (110). Such skill enabled the Chinese to discern twenty-four pulse types and to prescribe without needing to ask the patient any questions. Nevertheless, even Medhurst ultimately called the system "more the result of fancy than experience; and the connection they pretend to trace between the five points at which the pulse may be felt, the five viscera, the five planets, and the five elements, is the fruitful source of innumerable mistakes in their practice" (110–111). Still, he added, European doctors until Bacon's day had linked medicine and astrology, suggesting that the West remained close to practices equally subject to censure. Gutzlaff alone, for reasons that are not entirely clear, appeared to take the topic seriously, even though he, too, dismissed the core Chinese paradigm. "The science of the secret of the pulse is perhaps one of the most intricate in existence, and requires long practice before it can be well understood. There are twenty-four different kinds of pulses, with their sub-divisions; as for instance, a quick, a slippery, a rough, a deep, a slow one . . . It would require a whole volume to describe all the peculiarities of the pulse, and how every disease can thus be prognosticated" (Gutzlaff 1838, 179). Skilled physicians not only understood the course of an illness, but also detected the phase currently affecting the patient.

Lepage (1813) characterized pulses as "susceptible to an infinity of variations, following the differences of the seasons, gender, age, and stature" (25) (he rejected seasonal influences). He noted the sense of touch through which Chinese physicians detected subtle distinctions, articulated as images, capturing nuances unknown to most European clinicians. "The Chinese author explains the nature of each type of pulse by comparisons that seem quite strange: he says, for example, that slippery pulses feel like when one moves pearls under one's fingers; that the superficial pulse produces a sensation similar to that which one feels in touching the skin of a small onion; that the sharp pulse causes one to feel a sensation like that of a knife that scrapes bamboo; that the mobile pulse produces the same effect as stones that one touches in water, etc." (29).

As Shigehisa Kuriyama observes, the challenge for European commentators lay in determining whether the apparent obscurity of such descriptions was due to real differences between the systems, to mere variations in terminology, or to flaws in available translations. The problem resided in the nature of the pulses being taken. The *mo* system emphasized flow; the Greek-based, rhythms related to a pulsating artery. Such differences both reflected and generated corresponding differences in feeling, knowing, and speaking in relation to the body (see Kuriyama 1999, 61–108). Judgments reached by some observers proved equally contradictory, blurring affirmation and rejection, as when Lepage (1813) concluded, "But to recognize a particular sagacity among them in pulse examination is hardly to grant them the truth of all the false applications which they make in it, in their practice" (27). Moreover, Lepage complained, symptoms became secondary, leading Chinese diagnosticians to "occupy themselves only very superficially with what should be made the principle object of their study" (36). It was a semiotic issue, the debate involving not only the nature of pulses, but also the signs considered most significant in reading an illness.

A British author calling himself "Dion" merely submitted an outline to the *Indo-Chinese Gleaner,* explaining points on the wrist where pulses were felt: "the space below the wrist bone, between that and the root of the thumb, which, from its shortness, they call 'the inch' [*cun*]; Secondly, That immediately opposite the wrist bone, which they call 'the bar' [*guan,* to bar the door; frontier gate]; and Thirdly, That above the wrist bone to the elbow, which, from its length, they call 'the Foot (measure)' [*chi*]" (Dion 1821, 129). He spelled out twenty-four kinds of pulse—floating, deep, slow, quick, slippery, rough, substantial, empty, vibrating, failing, rapid, moderate, large or broad, small or minute, long or protracted, short, impeded, sudden or throbbing, hidden, moving, strong, weak, hard, and contracted—adding that only practitioners with extensive practice could differentiate between them. The practitioner, he added, learned a table linking pulses to disorders. For example:

5. A slippery pulse, if in the
    Right and left "inch," is indicative of asthma, and a fulness in
        the breast
    Right and left "bar," [ditto]. heat in the stomach, difficulty of
        breathing, and loss of appetite
    Right and left "foot," [ditto]. retention of urine, or dysentery; in
        males, an haemorrhage, and in females, a stoppage of the
        menses. (130)

The journal's editors confessed their own limitations in the "technological phraseology of this most excellent science," excusing themselves for possible mistakes or awkwardness related to the translation (Dion 1821, 129).

Occasional writers recognized other Chinese diagnostic methods. Abel-Rémusat's thesis (1813), written in Latin, reviewed tongue diagnosis. Lepage (1813) commented that it illuminated what one might draw "from the translation of the best works of Chinese medicine" along with "the abuse in relying on everything that has been written on this subject by people who were barely versed in medicine" (104). De Malpière (1825) noted "the color of [the patient's] face and his eyes, the sound of his voice, the inspection of his tongue, his nostrils, [and] his ears" (2:n.p.). Wakley quoted Sutleffe, who also reviewed directives to "first *look* at the patient's countenance; next mark the *tone* of his *voice;* then ask him all about his Ping-yuen [*bingyuan*], the probable *source* or *origin* of his malady; and finally, feel his pulse" (Wakley 1826b; see also Sutleffe 1825, Rehmann 1838).

Few Western authors discussed Chinese etiological theories. Pearson (1826a) listed cold, referring to cold-damage disorders. Gutzlaff explained that because *yin* blood was in the veins, "a hundred various diseases arise from the bad state of the blood." Phlegm generated different kinds of cough, sometimes due to a deficiency in stomach *qi*. Pain was often related to "fire," but the accompanying swelling, to moisture. "Both owe their origin to wind and cold" (Gutzlaff 1837, 158–161). Surgeon T. M. Dantu (1826), following ten Rhijne and Kaempfer, characterized the primary factor as wind. Pearson (1826a) posited that the concept of harmful winds resembled Western ideas about the effects of congested or seeping blood.

Pearson, Gutzlaff, and Lockhart understood the role of the Five Phases *(wuxing)* in illness, "morbid phenomena resulting from their . . . deficiency, preponderancy, or distribution" (Pearson 1826a, 129). The physician's task was to determine which phase had gained ascendancy and to counter its effects. For example: "During the spring the wood of the liver is invigorated, in autumn metal predominates, and affects the wood; in summer fire is the most powerful. Metal having lost its power, wood and fire predominate, and injure the earth of the stomach, the body becomes heated, the pulse very full; thus the aliment cannot be digested, and dysentery naturally ensues" (Gutzlaff 1837, 162). Such ideas occasionally filtered into medical literature, as when the *Boston Medical and Surgical Journal* explained Chinese theory: "All diseases arise from disturbing the equilibrium of these constituent parts, and the art of healing consists in restoring their mutual relations" (Editor 1839a, 194).

Only Gutzlaff included worms, reviewing an author who discussed eighteen types, some resembling imps, lobsters, serpents, or frogs. He also provided a theoretical overview. "The external causes of sickness are wind, cold, dryness, and moisture; the internal, the seven passions (anger, pleasure, sorrow, fear, love, hatred, and desire,) and the six affections, (the temper, disposition, natural feelings, natural affection, animal passion, and sexual desire)" (Gutzlaff 1837, 164). Similarly, few Western medical writers discussed Chinese illness classifications. Again Gutzlaff (1837) listed fourteen from his Chinese source, the "Approved Marking-Line," subdivided into nine categories organized by cause. There were fevers and agues; respiratory problems—suffocation, short breath, dropsy, or cough; the vomiting of phlegm, pus, green and sour water, or obstructions in the throat. The list covered diseases accompanied by loss of blood, different kinds of pain and paralysis, and diseases of the viscera. Mental disorders unfolded into madness, immoderate laughing, fits of rage, and fear and trembling. Forty-one eye diseases concluded the schema. "His remedies would astonish the medical faculties in Europe," added Gutzlaff; they were, however, too many and too complicated to detail (162).

Western authors acknowledged Chinese smallpox vaccination, but they privileged their own methods.[20] The *Medical and Physical Journal* lauded Staunton for translating Pearson's treatise on cowpox vaccine (Editor 1806), while Downing credited Pearson with introducing the approach to Canton in 1820. In actuality, Pearson reported in 1816 that the king of Portugal had arranged for vaccine to be brought from South America to the Philippines. From there, Portuguese subject "Mr. Hewit," a Macao merchant, brought it to Macao in 1805. Both Pearson and Portuguese practitioners provided the inoculations (Wu 1931, 9–10). Abel observed Chinese assistants working under Pearson's direction. One, Yao Hochun—called "A Hequa" by foreigners—vaccinated more than a million people, over a period of thirty years. Abel observed hundreds of parents bringing children to a temple near the British factory for vaccination (in Downing 1838, vol. 2). Pearson's final report characterized A Hequa as "a man remarkably qualified for the business, by his accuracy of judgment, method and perseverance" (Wu 1931, 11).

In 1840 Dr. W. Beck Diver sent Dunglison a history of vaccination in China—beginning it, however, with the work of Western doctors and suggesting that the spread of the practice derived from Pearson's wisdom in training assistants. Opposition, he added, arose from Chinese practitioners who specialized in treating smallpox, and from Buddhist monks who provided the older Chinese method and "were well paid for certain ministrations with their deities to avert or mitigate the scourge" (Diver 1840, 211). Such practitioners gained no credence through Lockhart's translation of a treatise on infant inoculation. It ended by explaining these practitioners' emphasis on choosing lucky days for the operation. For example, "the eleventh day of the moon ought to be avoided, for at that time a person's spirit is in the pillar or septum of the nose" (Lockhart 1843, 560–561). Wilson simply limited his report to the Chinese method without editorializing, a detail his many reviewers reiterated.

Gardens, Dispensatories, and Sovereign Remedies

The collecting of Chinese plants continued. Lepage alluded to large numbers of Chinese plants in the hands of a Mr. De Jussieu, originally sent by Fr. d'Incarville to his uncle, Bernard De Jussieu. "It is most remarkable that these plants are almost all the same as those in the environs of Paris" (Lepage 1813, 103). Interest in Chinese flora inspired Abel (1818a) to stroll the hills surrounding the monastery housing the Amherst embassy party. He observed *Smilax China*—China root—and ferns steeped and used medicinally. Botanist John Russell Reeves (1804–1877), employed by the British East India Company, lived in Canton for thirty years. He sent lists of Chinese *materia medica* to the Royal Medico-Botanical Society of London in 1827, along with plates from the *Bencao gangmu*. He also trained local painters to produce botanical illustrations in a style more familiar to Western botanists (see Fan 2004). Some plants Reeves identified with "Chinese travelling doctors," who pounded them "into a pulpy mass, and applied [them], poultice-like, to wounds, bruises, swellings, and sprains" for "the poorer classes of people" (Reeves 1828, 24–25). American doctor Benjamin Ellis recognized some herbs on Reeves's longer list: "such as datura stramonium; ficus, or fig; plantago or plantain; ricinus communis, young shoots, unripe capsules, and also the ripe seeds; young shoots of two or three species of croton; croton tiglium; seeds which have been long known among the Chinese as a drastic purgative; some species of euphorbia, and taraxacum" (Ellis 1830, 150–151).

The *Chinese Repository*, commenting that few foreigners had "pushed their botanical researches into the interior of this country" and that the field had no Thunbergs or Kaempfers, listed Reeves as an exception (Editor 1833i, 225). A subsequent review of extant research began by critiquing the Jesuits for having produced little more than translations of Chinese sources, which mixed "dissertations on plants of all kinds and qualities, chiefly those used in medicines" with "accounts of tiger-elephants, dragons, and other similar fantasies." Ironically, the *Chinese Repository* itself published a series on Chinese natural history, by missionary Samuel Wells Williams (1838), none based on direct observation, but also taken directly "from Chinese authors," with Chinese illustrations. The primary source was the *Bencao gangmu*. Williams's objective was "to show what has been done, in this department by this people, and how it has been done" (1838, 45). Despite earlier collecting carried out by chaplain Peter Osbeck in 1750, or by Abel, William Kerr (a gardener sent by the Horticultural Society of London in 1819), and Reeves, Chinese natural history required "thorough investigation, for what has been done needs to be done again" (Editor 1834e, 85).[21]

The Botanical Gardens

Nineteenth-century botanical gardens experienced uneven fates. From 1846 to 1848, Robert Fortune curated the Physic Garden at Chelsea, having previously traveled to China for the London Horticultural Society. To venture outside the thirty-mile radius to which foreigners had been confined in the area around Amoy, Fuzhou, Ningpo, and Shanghai, he donned Chinese robes and wig; he succeeded in gathering specimens and observing gardening and agricultural practices. Multiple pharmaceutical journals reviewed and excerpted his book (Fortune [1847]1979, 1848a, 1848b, 1848c). At Chelsea, Fortune did what he could to restore the garden, which had deteriorated due to lack of funding, but finally he abandoned the task and returned to China in 1848, commissioned by the British East India Company to collect tea plants for cultivation in northern India. The House of Commons deliberated over whether to remove the garden to Kew, consulting with physician-herbalist Jonathan Pereira. They eventually decided to support another collection at Kew. According to a "Provincial Surgeon" (1848), conditions at Chelsea worsened. He observed jumbled plants lacking labels, and walkways of carelessly scattered gravel. In contrast, Kew—which remained a leading repository for Chinese specimens—organized its plants with students in mind. Visits rose from 9,174 in 1841, to 46,573 by 1846 (Bell 1848).

In the United States, Dr. David Hosack bought twenty acres from the City of New York in 1801, establishing a botanical garden for instructing medical students. Located at Elgin, three and a half miles from the city, it eventually housed some three thousand species (Editor 1810, 1811). The collection focused on native plants and included American ginseng (Hosack 1806).

On Chinese Pharmacy

The social standing of apothecaries was more clearly established in Europe than in the United States. Facing challenges from other herbal practitioners—"the whole vast tribe of Thompsonian, Botanical, Indian, and other vegetable *doctors*" (Davis 1848, 342)—by the 1830s American pharmacists struggled to elevate their status as "scientific apothecaries" (Fisher 1837, 274). The one regularly reprinted article on Chinese pharmacy involved a brief description of imperial efforts to regulate Chinese practice. Chinese apothecaries had to have a license, keep specific medicines in stock, sell certain drugs only with a prescription, and have "a sufficient supply of *Ginseng root,* and to superintend the growth of the plant furnishing this very costly, but favourite Chinese Remedy" (Editor 1847h, 176).[22]

Foreign observers recognized various kinds of herbal practitioners in China. De Malpière (1825, 2:n.p.), for example, included drawings of both an itinerant pharmacist and a scholar-physician. On China Street, wrote Dr. William Ruschenberger (1838, 2:231), street herbalists "are usually seated in the midst of little baskets of dry herbs, which they are always compounding in a rude mortar, when not engaged with the complainings of a patient." Some displayed "small jars, packets neatly folded up, and a store of pitch plasters" (Lay 1841a, 204). Williams (1848, 2:186–187) described a vendor who attracted clients by pounding his chest with a brick, turning it red, and then applying a remedy that immediately healed it. The more learned simply set up a pavilion, awning, or flag on a pole, quietly awaiting patients.

One anonymous author, recording his observations while walking through the foreigners' district of Canton, described a great hornet's nest hanging outside of an apothecary's shop. He entered to investigate: "After the usual civilities, taking a cup of tea, wishing health, wealth, &c., [I] began to inquire of the principal person . . . concerning the properties of various medicines then before us; at length the hornet's nest came to be noticed: 'it was brought from a great distance,' said the old gentleman, 'it grew on a very high tree, its cruel and poisonous inmates had all been driven out' . . . The conclusion of the whole matter was, that his medicines would cure all kinds of diseases, and the hornet's nest was a proof of it!" (Anonymous 1835c, 244). One suspects the author of ignoring the power of metaphor.

Abel (1818a, 116–117) compared pharmacies in Dongzhou, Beijing suburb, with those of Europe, noting similar neatness and "the arrangement of their various drawers and jars." Davis's description of shops on "Apothecary street"—their drawers "neatly arranged and lettered, but filled principally with simples"—migrated into the *American Magazine of Useful and Entertaining Knowledge* (Davis 1836b, 241). Williams (1848) wrote that, instead of "huge glass jars at the windows filled with bright colored liquids, and long rows of vials and decanters in glass cases, three or four branching deer's horns are suspended from the walls, and lines of white and black gallipots [small earthenware jars] cover the shelves" (2:185–86).

John Wilson's description circulated the most widely, under "pharmacy in China": "The drug shops of China are large, and are commodiously fitted up. They have a great array of drawers and jars, arranged much in the same way as in England; glass vessels are very rare. Different departments are allotted to separate classes of medicaments; care is taken to keep things in order; and there is a degree of neatness and meth,od in their appearance which would not be discreditable to a London laboratory. They do not seek notice by partly-coloured bottles and cabalistic signs, which make so great a figure in the windows of some English medicine vendors, but are rigorously plain" (Wilson 1846b, 567; see Editor 1847h, 1847i, 1848c). Abel (1818a) observed formulas dispensed in small paper packets with directions written on the outside. Lay (1841a) elaborated: "Everything indicates care and importance;—the prescription is laid upon the counter, the different medicaments are taken from the drawer or the jar and weighed in the order set forth in the formula, and not a single circumstance omitted to make you feel that the doctors of the East and the West, with their faithful helper, the apothecary, have, either from instinct or instruction, followed the same model" (230). A written prescription, wrote Wilson (1847c), occupied "a large sheet of paper, . . . often diversified by red, added to the ordinary black characters," and rarely involved fewer than nine or ten substances. Ordinary ingredients were wrapped in white paper, more esteemed ones, like ginseng, in red (130). (See Figure 22.)

Gutzlaff (1837) and de Chavannes (1845) commented on correlations drawn between parts of the body and of medicinal plants. The tops of plants treated diseases in the head, both partaking of the nature of Heaven; middle parts treated the trunk; and roots, the lower parts of the body. Some substances could only be used alone; others, in compounds or as vehicles for still other drugs. Pharmaceutical preparations included "decoctions, to purge and to promote the circulation of the blood; others made up into pills, to expel the wind and open the bowels; others are mixed with liquor, vinegar, and other strong essences; to augment their effect, others are ground to powder, or fried in fat to absorb the bad humours" (Gutzlaff 1837, 167; see also Lockhart 1841). Williams (1848, 2:185–186) added details: hartshorn was filed to a dust, roots like rhubarb and gentian were sliced thin, and others were powdered with a mortar and pestle. Vegetable substances were usually taken as pills or in decoction.

Doses sometimes occasioned skepticism. Gutzlaff (1837) pointed to the difficulty some patients had swallowing decoctions and pills, faint-

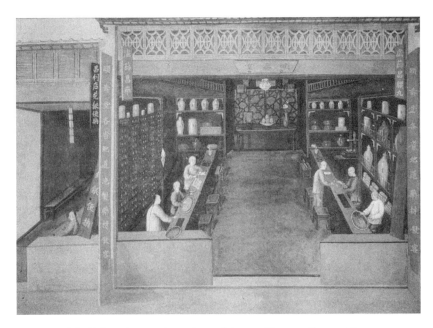

Figure 22. Medicine shop—view along thirteen Factory Street, Canton. Gouache ca. 1830. (E82.547.) Such drawings were produced by Chinese artists and purchased by foreign visitors. They were also bought by a wide clientele in the West (see Huang and Sargent 1999; Goldstein 1978). Photograph courtesy of the Peabody Essex Museum.

ing and being revived when warm animal's blood was poured down their throats. Death, he added dryly, was not infrequent but, resulting from an ancient system, it aroused little comment. Ruschenberger (1838) suggested that doses sometimes resembled mash for a horse. Wilson commented on a bowel remedy entailing five large pills: "How the patient, without the assistance of a probang, contrived to gorge them was the wonder. Men who should order or issue such perilous looking pellets in England, would be considered fit to deal with the diseases of horses only" (Wilson 1847c, 131).[23] Nothing underwent "adulteration"—chemical processing—a point that Gutzlaff (1837) questioned, as few natural substances were "fit for exhibition in medicine without a previous preparation." Still, he characterized Chinese pharmacopoeia as "richer than that of any other nation" (164).

Resemblance between Western and Chinese versions of pharmacy did not prevent some observers from rejecting the latter. The issue was not individual drugs but rather the physiological model upon which prescriptions were based. Lay (1838, 202), for example, concluded that "the mistaken ideas entertained by their doctors about the parts and their respective functions in the human system, utterly disqualify them for undertaking a case of any importance," including the prescribing of medicine. It was the routine sticking point. Even when translations were accurate, like some intangible weight the immateriality of Chinese models repeatedly pulled observers and readers alike away from engaging with Chinese paradigms in their own right.

Botanicals, Dispensatories, and Pharmaceutical Literature

Accompanying the interest in collecting plant specimens from around the world, new botanical works achieved acclaim. In 1827 John Stephenson's and James Morss Churchill's *Medical Botany* was commended for reconnecting with ancient works like Dioscorides. It also culled from the London, Edinburgh, and Dublin pharmacopoeias, providing local and foreign names of plants, detailed descriptions, properties and uses, and colored lithographs. Medical students were urged to study it, given the difficulties of learning about plants in their countries of origin (Editor 1827h). John Lindley's *Flora Medica* (1838) made another case for an international perspective. Lindley, who had assisted Fortune at Chelsea, observed that many young men, when overseas, could not obtain Western drugs. But reviewers characterized Pereira's *Elements of Materia Medica and Therapeutics* as "the best English text-book on the subject" (Cormack 1841a). It was Pereira who demonstrated the greatest knowledge of some Chinese *materia medica*.

Family herbal books remained popular, American authors often adopting a nationalistic tone, as when John Gunn (1834) advised his readers to use only American plants. Others described themselves as "Indian doctors" (Henry 1814; Anonymous 1836; Foster 1838; Mahoney 1846), claiming direct links to authentic American herbal knowledge. American physicians, however, found the country's *materia medica* largely a *terra incognita* (L. 1839). Titles emerged like the *American Dispensatory* (Coxe 1806), *Vegetable Materia Medica of the United States, or Medical Botany* (Barton 1817–1818), *American Medical Botany* (Bigelow 1817), the *Pharmacopoeia of the United States* (National Medical Convention 1831), and the *Dispensatory of the United States* (Wood and Bache 1834). The last underwent successive reprintings. Each publication was intended to function as a comprehensive reference work for American practice. As we shall see, some discussed medicinal plants that were also identified with China.

Paul Unschuld (1986a) reminds us that the term *pharmacopoeia* did not correspond to the variety of herbals produced in China. Any private citizen could assemble family recipes, travel observations, textual criticism of older works, or other materials. Eclectic works, being shorter, were often more popular than encyclopedias, being easier to use. Still, when Western authors referred to Chinese *materia medica* by name, they usually cited only the *Bencao gangmu* (Schott 1843; see also Fan 2004). Occasionally some writers exhibited grosser ignorance, as in this comment: "The vegetable kingdom, rich as it certainly is in this country, has never been an object of much attention among the Chinese" (Editor 1833i, 225).

Even Abel-Rémusat, who was more familiar than most with Chinese sources, foregrounded the *Bencao gangmu* in a piece on Chinese natural history (Abel-Rémusat 1833), reviewing its classificatory scheme in detail. So did Medhurst (1838), more briefly, concluding with less than faint praise. "This arrangement will be seen to be far from scientific," he wrote, "but that they should have examined the vegetable kingdom at all, and made any sort of classification, shews that they are by no means an unthinking or an uncivilized people" (109). In contrast, the

Boston Medical and Surgical Journal simultaneously commended and derided Chinese botanical knowledge for its careful observation of facts, methodical organization, and "no want of information upon a variety of subjects of which they are too generally thought to be profoundly ignorant" (Editor 1841b). Where or how the impression of ignorance arose is not clear, apart from the fact that it was allowed to stand for more pervasive and unexamined forms of bias.

Classifying Drugs

Lepage (1813) and Gutzlaff (1837) explained that Chinese drugs were categorized by taste, and by whether they were warming or cooling, Lepage adding that the Chinese had also studied the exact times when plants should be collected, and whether they should be dried in sun or shade, according to their nature. Gutzlaff summarized the *Bencao gangmu*'s classificatory system and metaphoric ranking—one group was called "sovereign remedies," another was likened to ordinary government ministers, and a third to extraordinary ministers. Prescriptions marshaled a "sovereign" with "servants" of different ranks (Gutzlaff 1838, 174–177). Illness categories provided the basis for other classifications. Pearson (1826a) reviewed an unnamed work with prescriptions for "diseases of a cold nature" and fevers. An author reviewed by Gutzlaff (1838) organized remedies by disease, and then by each phase, showing how to modulate therapies accordingly. Gutzlaff (1837) wrote, "Maladies accompanied by cold, require warm remedies, and vice versa; indigestion may be relieved by emetics; worms, and humours of the abdomen, give way only to poisonous drugs; and bad humours may be expelled by moist medicines" (167).

Despite awareness of these systems, Western sources discussed a relatively small number of specific drugs, generally independent of Chinese classifications. Lepage (1813) noted the difficulty of commenting on *materia medica* known only by Chinese names. One could determine neither their Latin names nor whether they also grew in the West. He and other commentators generally limited themselves to substances known both in Europe and Asia, only occasionally including those that "however particular they may be to China, are so in use in the country that one could hardly pass over them in silence" (69). Such herbs were listed under romanizations of their Chinese names and discussed as exotica, drawing mostly on earlier Jesuit sources. Abel-Rémusat (1825), commenting on Lepage, observed: "He gives a list of some medicines equally known in Europe and Asia, and informs his readers that the rest of the medical substances indicated by Cleyer, that is, by Boym, and by Du Halde, being designated only by their Chinese names, it is not possible to recognize them, nor to appreciate the use made of them by the Chinese.[24] It is an inconvenience which will continue as long as one does not have a synonymic nomenclature of the plants of China, related to the places they should occupy in our European systems" (250). Of this second group, Lepage listed only *Lin-tchi*, a type of agaric reduced to ashes and used to arrest hemorrhages (lime, reduced to a powder, was also used). *Ou-poey-tse* had been known to botanist Étienne-François Geoffroy (1672–1731), who believed it analogous to an excrescence on elm leaves. The Chinese explained it as shells formed by small worms, mixing it with other drugs to produce tablets called "violet-colored precious nails." (See Figure 23.) "These tablets are so precious that the emperor has them made in his palace, and offers them to the grandees of his court and to European foreigners as a mark of distinction" (Lepage 1813, 73). *San-tsi* was the plant most valued after ginseng. It was the same color as a gray goat, leading the Chinese to think that gray goats' blood also had medicinal properties. (Indeed, the missionaries reported surprising results in cases of falls and contusions.) Chinese doctors used it to treat female ills, especially blood loss. Rare and costly, it was used against smallpox as well.

Lepage also included *Okiao,* the glue made from the skin of an ass (see Chapter 4). There was *Tsée-jen-toung* (demi-metal), a substance from copper mines. A cube, attached to a silk thread and steeped in wine, water, or tea, communicated to these liquids the virtue of reanimating circulation and strengthening the nerves. Roasted, reduced to a powder, and given in doses of three *fen*—around three gross in a half-glass of wine, or approximately 1500 milligrams—it helped bone fractures knit. Patients were also kept absolutely still for one hundred days. "One easily guesses," Lepage commented, "to which of these two means one should attribute the healing" (75). *Hiung-hoang* was a reddish-yellow soft stone marked with small black spots, used as a sovereign remedy against malignant fevers. Other small blue stones, taken powdered, prolonged life. Finally, an author writing for *The Chinese*

Courier described bear paws as a delicacy "prized by the Chinese as restoratives, and . . . administered to aged people to give them strength and prolong life: they are also used as aphrodisiac" (Anonymous 1833, 3).

A second group of *materia medica* consisted of those so common to both Europe and China that no one felt a need to introduce them into the China trade. Lepage (1813) reviewed several of them—sulfuric acid, borax, cicadas, coral, deer's blood, nitre, raisins, and sal ammoniac. What he knew, he had gotten from Du Halde. Mugwort was another. Although some discussions related it to moxibustion (see

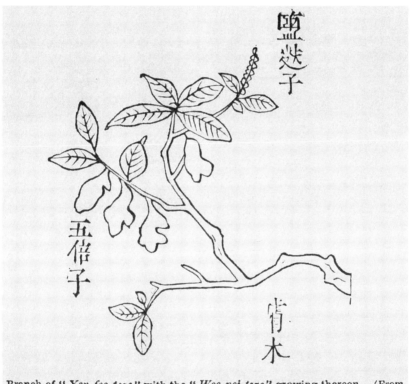

Branch of "*Yen-foo-tsze*" with the "*Woo-pei-tsze*" growing thereon. (From the Pun-Tsaou).

Figure 23. Branch of *"Yen-foo-tsze"* with the *"Woo-pei-tsze"* growing thereon, from the *Bencao gangmu.* Jonathan Pereira, *Pharmaceutical Journal,* vol. 3, 1844. Godfrey Lowell Cabot Science Library of the Harvard College Library.

below), the herb also appeared in other connections. One "Gentleman in the Course of His Travels" (1807) described mugwort growing in "fields, hedges, and waste places" in Scotland and England. A "uterine and anti-hysteric," its aromatic, bitter leaves—infused either alone or with other substances—suppressed menses (117). Somewhat confusingly, another author claimed that the ancients considered it an *emmenagogue*—a medicine for inducing menstruation. In China, he added, women made poultices of the leaves, mixed with rice and sugar, for amenorrhea and hysteria, and applied the fresh plant, bruised, to wounds (Withering 1808; see Hill 1812). Lepage (1813), too, wrote that it grew in all the provinces of China and was frequently used by the Chinese, who recognized in it the same properties as did Europeans. Samuel Henry (1814) described the leaves as "deobstruent, laxative, diaphoretic, diuretic, emmenagogic, anti-hysteric, anti-spasmodic, anthelmatic, and corroborant" (497).[25] German Dr. Hufeland (1824a) used mugwort for epilepsy, gathering the root in mid-October, shade-drying it, powdering it, and administering it in warm beer half an hour before an oncoming seizure. His report enjoyed multiple reviews and reprintings, although Dunglison (1846a) eventually cautioned that mugwort's anti-seizure benefits were exaggerated.[26]

Drugs Shipped to China

The largest group of drugs discussed involved those commodified through the China trade. Lists of imports and exports published in 1834 (Editor 1834d) and 1843 (Editor 1843i) show substantial congruence both with each other and with an earlier list in Lepage (1813). Of those shipped into China through Hong Kong, the first was asafoetida. "The vessels employed to carry this drug are so scented with the odor, that they spoil most other goods. Considerable quantities of it are brought to this market; and it ranks high in the materia medica of the Chinese physician" (Editor 1834d, 449). Bird's nests were considered "a great stimulant and tonic, but their best quality, perhaps, is their being perfectly harmless" (453). Bezoar—the "concretion found in the stomachs of a goat in Persia"—was once valued as a medicine, until its actual ingredients had been determined. Cow bezoar continued to be "used by the Chinese solely as a medicine" (452). "Dragon's blood," a resinous gum, was used by alchemists. Putchuck *(Aplotaxis auriculata)* came from India and Persia "and appears to be the roots of a plant which grows in those countries. The color and smell are similar to that of rhubarb, and when chewed, it becomes mucilaginous in the mouth" (468). It was also used in joss (incense) sticks.

Lepage (1813) wrote that cinnabar was used to strengthen and open the viscera, reanimating weakened pulses, relieving oppression, resisting the malignity of smallpox, and promoting sweat in fevers. "One takes the water in which cinnabar has boiled for a long time. Mixed with sulfur and thinned with a woman's milk, it serves against skin illnesses" (75–76). In turn, women's milk was used as an eyewash for ophthalmia, although "the eyes of elephants which one soaked it in gave this remedy an air of charlatanism" (78).

Quicksilver entered China from Europe and sometimes America (Editor 1834d). It was used to treat worms, scabies and other skin conditions, and venereal disease (Lepage 1813). Abel, Reeves, and Peters commented on Chinese uses, although Abel (1818a) criticized mercury's not being administered to salivation. Gutzlaff (1837) wrote that quacks in China used it for venereal disease—Downing (1838, vol. 2), that Canton's apothecaries treasured it. Bell (1844) discussed its importation from China.

Europeans had introduced quinine to China when the emperor had fallen ill of a fever in 1692, and Frs. Fontaney and Visdelou had offered it to him. "The emperor, encouraged further by the example of several nobles in his court, took it in turn, and was also cured of his fever" (Lepage 1813, 74). In gratitude, he had given them accommodations at one of his palaces.

Cooked shark's fins were valued as a tonic and stimulant (Editor 1834d); sea horses had only to be put in the hands of a woman in labor to help her deliver with greater ease (Lepage 1813). Trade lists also included the teeth of elephants, and "Horns, Unicorn's or Rhinoceros," without specifying their uses (Editor 1843i, 2).

An Excellent Restorative

Two drugs—ginseng and opium—dominated the drug trade into China. Regarding ginseng, Mérat and de Lens's medical dictionary noted, "Its name, which is written still as *gin-seng, gin-chen, jin-chen* in China, *nindsin, ninzi* in Japon, [and] *orheto* in Manchu, signifies the first of plants, marvel of the universe, etc., as if to paint the sublime qualities that the peoples of these countries accord it" (Mérat and de Lens 1831, 356). Western sources described ginseng as a perennial from "Tartary" and North America (Coxe 1806), although one author argued, using specious etymology, that it was Homer's "enigmatical" root "Moly" (Deverell 1805, 131). One botanical source reported it growing in desert regions (Burnett 1835), while Downing (1838) located it in Tartary, Shandong, and "Liaudong"; Fr. Calau (1843c) added Korea, speculating that it also grew in Russian territories. N. Wallich (1829) reported locating another species in Nepal.

In the United States, ginseng grew in Florida, South Carolina, and New Jersey (Henry 1814). Barton located it farther west "both on the high rocky banks of the Wissahickon creek, under deep shade, and in the umbrageous woods above the falls of Schuylkill" in Pennsylvania (Barton 1817–1818, 194–195). The *Indian Vegetable Family Instructor* (Anonymous 1836) claimed it abounded in Vermont. Indeed, the *Boston Medical and Surgical Journal* commented that Vermont and New Hampshire ginseng had "laid the foundation of some large fortunes in New England" (Editor 1839a, 194).

It became clear that such geographic variety corresponded to multiple strains of the root. Mérat and de Lens (1831) consulted with Abel-Rémusat, who showed them Chinese botanical books and manuscripts from the king's library, containing different figures of the "true" ginseng—each of them distinct. "We thus see," they concluded, "that the name gen-seng cannot belong to a single plant, since the Chinese have so many species, that for them it is a complex name, and that they are always able to designate as *true* the rarest among them, and as a consequence the most expensive; it is, for this people, a collective appellation" (359). It was therefore wrong to think there was only one ginseng.

Chinese regard for ginseng—whichever one was meant—was well known.[27] "The missionaries and other Chinese travelers have told the most marvelous stories," noted Ellis (1830, 153), while Wilson (1846b, 131) characterized the admiration as "bordering on religious adoration." The *Dispensatory of the United States* (Griffith 1833) suggested that the Chinese generally used American *panax quinquefolium* only as a substitute for Asian ginseng—which Reeves (1828) witnessed "at one of the shops in Doctor-Street, carefully shut out from profane eyes, and excluded from the air in two or three canisters one within the other" (27). Ironically, Mérat and de Lens (1831) hypothesized that ginseng was no longer used in China: despite the number of species available, Western travelers were not mentioning it. They wrongly concluded, "It seems that it is no longer any more than a historic object . . . For Europe, it has never been but an object of curiosity, and soon gen-seng will be nearly relegated among the fabulous medicines, with *hippomane, nepenthes, connamomun,* etc., of the ancients" (360).

American ginseng trade gradually diminished. Barton had heard of cargo shipped to Canton and then jettisoned, to evade duties exceeding its value. By 1821 the United States still shipped more than 1,000 tons a year; in 1824 exports dropped to 375 tons. In 1825 Samuel Thomson called ginseng trade a thing of the past. He was partly right. Ginseng still came through Knoxville daily, but prices had fallen (Gunn 1834). The *Chinese Repository* agreed that profits had initially run at 500 to 600 percent but had dropped to the point of hardly being worth the investment. Clarified ginseng—skinned and boiled roots—sold at $60 to $65 a picul (about 133.33 pounds); raw, they went for $35 to $40 (Editor 1834d). Although ginseng was still gathered in Ohio and West Virginia, and exported through Philadelphia and port cities (Wood and Bache 1847), the *Western Journal* reported that in 1847, American shipments totaled only 2,796 piculs—somewhat over 186 tons (Editor 1848b).

Barton (1817–1818) explained that the Chinese used ginseng to treat fatigue, facilitate respiration, invigorate digestion, cure nervous conditions, reinforce the healthy system, and recover powers lost to aging. According to Downing (1838), it was used to alleviate fatigue and "render man immortal"—adding, "If anything on earth can do so" (2:146). It offset "habitual consumption of tea and opium" (2:149). Calau (1843c) described its tonic properties for tuberculosis and debility, and its stimulative effects against depression.

Barton (1817) wondered whether Chinese regard for ginseng resulted from "the imagination of a people remarkable for their prejudices, civil, moral and religious" (1:200; see Wood and Bache 1847). Western practitioners rarely thought it warranted such encomiums (Edwards and Vavasseur 1829). Only John Lindley (1838) called for further investigation, as few Western doctors had used actual Chinese ginseng. J. W. Cooper (1833, 97–98) instructed readers to gather roots in the fall, and cut them lengthwise into thin pieces: "The bark of small roots should be beaten or scraped off while green, as it would be difficult to get it off after it is dry; besides, it will dry the better after it is off." Generally, however, American traders failed to duplicate Chinese methods of drying it.

Western physicians made modest claims. Coxe (1806, 493) thought ginseng "a gentle and agreeable stimulant"; Samuel Henry (1814, 139), that it stimulates appetite, "invigorates the system, and is an excellent restorative to those fatigued by traveling." Barton (1817) considered it a stimulant, a stomachic, and a "masticatory" (1:201; see Edwards and Vavasseur 1829). Wood and Bache (1847, 531) wrote, "Some persons . . . are in the habit of chewing it, having acquired a relish for its taste; and it is chiefly to supply the wants of these that it is kept in the shops." Thomson (1825) recommended it for "nervous affections." Brooks (1833, 22) compared it with licorice, used "in asthmas, pleurisies, coughs and all foulness of the lungs," while Cooper (1833) suggested it for stomach gout and indigestion. Gunn (1834) used it for "nervous debility, weak digestion, and feeble appetite, and as a stomachic and restorative." It was, he said, good for children, and for "asthma, palsy, and nervous affections" (428).

The Shakers, famous for herbal medicines, promoted ginseng for lost appetite, nervous debility, weak stomach, asthma, and gravel (Miller 1998, 151), selling it at $1.25 a pound.[28] They may have known about Chinese uses, but many Shaker communities also sustained cordial relationships with local Native Americans; it is unclear how much they learned from the tribes or from American herbals. Robert Foster (1838), a "North American Indian doctor," characterized ginseng as a tonic against epidemic fevers and chest pains, and for cleansing the blood (152). Lindley (1838, 59) classified it as a "demulcent," a soothing substance for easing pain, while Mahoney (1846)—calling it "O-taj-le-gah-le"—recommended it for "weakness of the womb, and nervous affections, convulsions, palsy, vertige and dysentery" (376).

Some writers provided recipes. Henry steeped chopped ginseng in Jamaican rum for two weeks. The patient drank a wineglass three times a day for excessive "venery, pain in the bones from colds, and gravelly complaints." He described a New Jersey man "so debilitated and afflicted with pains in his bones, that he expected nothing but death every day, who by taking ginseng in rum was able to follow his business on the farm, and his pains entirely removed in a few days" (Henry 1814, 139; see also Gunn 1834, Foster 1838). Thomson (1825) counseled a teaspoon of powdered ginseng in sweetened hot water; the *Indian Vegetable Family Instructor* (Anonymous 1836) likewise recommended treating children for stomach and bowel pains with dried grated root in hot water, sweetened with sugar. Cooper's strengthening bitters included goldenseal, ginseng, chamomile, and lemon peel steeped in wine or whiskey (Cooper 1833).

Nationalist sentiment prompted botanical doctor Samuel Emmons's preference for ginseng as an American drug over "deadly foreign minerals" (Emmons 1836, i). He treated Saint Vitus's dance by pulverizing and mixing lady's slipper, ginseng, and nutmeg with alcohol, setting the bottle in the sun for ten days, straining the contents, adding anise, and administering doses of up to a tablespoonful, several times a day (99–100). His restorative bitters contained unicorn root, bloodroot, ginseng, tamarisk bark, nanny bush bark, devil's bit, rue, seneca snakeroot, sassafras bark, and goldenseal (113–114).

Still, the 1842 National Medical Convention in the United States relegated ginseng to its "secondary list"—medicines "little employed or of doubtful value"—a position from which a drug could be elevated, but from which it was more likely to be dropped (National Medical Convention 1842, xviii–xix). Although ginseng continued to be included in American sources, increasingly the articles went unrevised, indicating that the publishers thought no new material merited addition.

Opium Eating, Opium Smoking

Opium, by contrast, was accepted in Western medicine. In 1812, Moses Dennison of Shirley, Massachusetts, cultivated white poppies, decocting an extract favorably compared with Turkish opium (Editor 1812). Dr. G. G. Sigmond (1837a, 1837b, 1837c) lectured on opium's properties. Yet it was also recognized that opium consumption could result in addiction. The most widely recognized habit involved eating it; the country most associated with the practice was Turkey. In 1829, for example, a Dr. Madden described Turkish men high from opium in a coffee shop. (He also detailed his own experiments.)

Debates concerning the impact of laudanum (an opium derivative) on longevity surrounded an insurance company's refusal to pay on a policy for a Lord Mar, due to his overindulgence. Some Western physicians equated opium with excessive drinking (Christison 1832a, 1832b). "Opium eaters" were generally viewed as individuals who used opium for some "nervous affection," inadvertently becoming addicted (Editor 1833b). It was recognized that closet addicts "in the United States are vastly more numerous than is suspected," particularly among the affluent (Editor 1839g, 18–19). Doctors published articles on how to help them (Seeger 1833).

The Chinese were rarely represented as opium eaters. Abel (1818a) noted that although opium was not displayed in pharmacies—"probably because it is a contraband article"—it was frequently mixed with tobacco (214). Reeves (1828) described it as a luxury used by government officials—a point repeated by Ellis (1830), who noted that consumption drained "the country of eight millions of dollars" (151–152). Indian opium sold at $600 to $700 a chest; the Turkish sort, from $620 to $680 a picul (Editor 1834d). Gutzlaff (1837) explained medicinal uses for pain and dysentery, but moved quickly to the miseries of addiction. Some missionaries pointed to "nominal christians"—Western merchants—"deeply implicated in this crime of freighting a poison, which leads to certain moral infatuation, degradation and death" (Johnson 1837, 193–194). Lay (1838, 194) urged "non-participation in the sale of opium," arguing that a valuable medication had become "a bane that destroys both body and soul."

Articles detailed the practice in China (for example, Bird 1842a; Smith 1842a), explaining how opium was prepared and smoked, and its effects on users. Smith described the interior of a smoking shop—an emerging trope—adding that many officials supposedly blocking the trade were themselves users who turned a blind eye. Even so, some physicians discussed the potential benefits of replacing laudanum with Chinese methods of smoking opium for "painful diseases that defy the power of opium taken in the common way" (Johnson 1837, 710).

Public representations increasingly linked the Chinese with widespread addiction. Said an article in *Dwight's American Penny Magazine,* "In the city of Amoy alone there are as many as one thousand opium shops" (Polhman 1846, 731). Smith described men waiting for a proprietor to measure out their doses. They told him there were nearly a thousand such establishments in the city (Beck 1848, 302; see also

Smith 1847a, 1847b). Robert Fortune's travelogue included sections on opium smuggling and smoking, although Fortune insisted that the number of addicts in China was exaggerated (Fortune 1979; 1848a, 1848b, 1848c).

Some Chinese physicians offered drug treatment programs. The *Chinese Repository* described one placard advertising "an angelic remedy for opium smoking"—a prescription received through spirit writing upon sand on a table, whose secret ingredients, coupled with daily reduction in one's opium consumption, eventually enabled the addict to quit even the substitute (Editor 1832c). On rare occasions the American public read Chinese objections to the drug trade. A former *hong* merchant, Tang Shin, author of moral treatises, was made an honorary member of the Historical Society of New York. In his acceptance letter, he expressed his certainty that American literati were dedicated to righteous deeds. They should therefore, he said, labor to abolish the slave trade *and* oppose opium trafficking—"to eternity," he wrote, "let opium be prohibited" (Thonching 1845, 718–719). Indeed, Smith (1847b) recorded a conversation wherein Tang characterized the opium traffic as even worse than the slave trade.

The Drug Trade to the West

An 1843 tariff list on goods exported to the West included and described multiple drugs. Alum *(pé-fan),* for example, was used by the Chinese "to moderate the heat of fever, to stop stomach flux" (Editor 1843i). The powder treated rectal prolapse. Tea, mixed with alum in equal quantities and taken with cold water, countered poison (Lepage 1813, 75).

The Chinese used "aniseed stars" (star anise) mostly for cooking, exporting them at $11 or $12 per picul, and the oil at $2 a catty, both for medical purposes (Editor 1834d). Camphor, more valuable, was a "bitter and hot remedy, to dissolve and dissipate the humors in the treatment of scurf and scabies" (Lepage 1813, 74). Among the gums displayed in one Chinese pharmacy, Abel (1818a) recognized only camphor, used to eliminate vermin and to treat many diseases. Reeves (1828) belittled Chinese distinctions between types, which to Europeans appeared identical. Nor were the Chinese impressed by "specimens of the finest refined camphor from England" (26). William

Procter Jr. (1839) reviewed Chinese, Japanese, and Borneoan varieties, while G. G. Sigmond (1839) discussed camphor's mind-altering effects and its uses for fever and mania in the West.

Camphor shipped to Europe and the United States came from *Laurus camphora,* a tree growing in China, Japan, and Taiwan—the Japanese was viewed as the best, followed by the Taiwanese. Prices ranged from $20 or $30 a picul to $1,000 to $2,000 for "the Baroos" sort (Editor 1834d, 454). E. O'Reiley of Amherst, Massachusetts, sent samples from the Tenaserim Coast to assistant surgeon John McClelland in Calcutta. He had learned to evaporate camphor granules and wanted to compare their chemical properties with Chinese camphor for potential commercially viability (O'Reiley 1845).

Cardamom came in several varieties, the "lesser" being more pungent and flavorful when used in cooking by the Chinese. Europeans imported them "for medicinal and other uses" (Editor 1834d, 455). Cassia tree—differentiated from "the true cinnamon tree"—provided wood, bark, buds, pods, and oil for the China trade, all sought "for various purposes in carpentry, medicine and cookery" (456). Wood and Bache (1847) discussed Western uses of cinnamon as an aromatic often added to less pleasant-tasting medicines; it was "warm and cordial to the stomach" (249–250).

China root still figured. Lepage (1813) identified it as the fungus *fuling,* used as a sudorific and purgative. However, the list of exports from China described it as "the root of the *Smilax China,* a climbing plant. The roots are jointed, knobbed, thick, of a brown color, and break short; when cut, the surface is smooth, close, and glossy; but if old and wormy, dust flies from it when broken" (Editor 1834d, 456). Clearly the confusing application of the same name to two distinct drugs persisted. Lindley's *Flora medica* described China root as hard, knotty, dark externally, and whitish within. An emetic, it caused nausea and vomiting and could substitute for sarsaparilla. "The Chinese," he added, "eat it under the idea that it invigorates them" (Lindley 1838, 599). Pereira (1843a, 134) identified it as *Smilax China,* also comparing it with sarsaparilla, and decocting it for venereal disease, rheumatism, gout, and skin diseases. According to Wood and Bache (1847), sarsaparilla—like *Smilax China*—had been used in Europe for venereal disease. Over time it had fallen from favor, until restored through use as an additive to mercury.

"Gamboge"—so called because of its origins in "Camboja"—also came from China. Sun-dried sap was made into rolls used "as a beautiful pigment and as a medicine; and it is carried in considerable quantities from China and India to the west" (Editor 1834d, 461). Musk, deriving from an antelope found in Tibet, Siberia, and China, was costly and often adulterated. "When good musk is rubbed on paper," advised the *Chinese Repository*, "the trace is of a bright yellow color, and free from any grittiness" (Editor 1834d, 465). It was used in the West for both perfume and medicine.

The literature on rhubarb was the most extensive. Most writers recognized China and Turkey as points of origin; some added Asia, "Tartary," Russia, and occasionally Native Americans. Identifying varieties proved more complicated. Stephenson and Churchill (1834) located palmated rhubarb in Russia and several other species in the mountains between China and Tibet. Another author concluded that commercial rhubarb was neither *Rheum palmatum* nor *undulatum* (Paravey 1837). Pereira detailed six types: Russian, Dutch-trimmed, Chinese, Himalayan, English, and French (Pereira 1845; see also Pereira 1847). The best was Russian, although the drug known in England as "Russian rhubarb" was, in St. Petersburg, called "Chinese rhubarb"—which in turn differed from rhubarb from Canton, with which the Russians were unfamiliar. Most rhubarb used in the United States came through Canton, leading one entrepreneur to send a shipment of European rhubarb to Canton, where he repacked it in half-picul cases to sell as Chinese.

Some authors detailed how rhubarb was gathered and prepared. Stephenson and Churchill (1834), for example, compared "Tartar" and Chinese methods. The former involved cleaning and slicing the plants, laying the pieces on long boards and turning them multiple times a day, fixing a thick yellow juice with the root. Four or five days later, the pieces were pierced and hung to shade-dry for two months. Seven loads of green roots yielded "one small horse-load" of dried. The Chinese skinned and sliced the roots, drying them on stone slabs heated over fires. When mostly dried, they were hung on cords, producing round or flattened pieces, smooth as though scraped, with residual bits of cord (Dunglison 1846a, 1:166). As Calau (1843a, 1843b) explained, traditions governed the choice of plants from which one selected pieces, and how one pared, examined, dried, and packed them.

Pharmacy journals reported chemical tests—soaking rhubarb in different substances, burning it in different kinds of vessels, and trying to determine its active ingredients (Brugnatelli 1812; see also Schlossberger and Doepping 1845). Some tried to determine under what conditions it lost its properties, and formulas that enhanced its effects (Henry 1814). Using ioduretted hydriodic acid in decoction, for example, one could differentiate, by color, between the Russian, Chinese, English, or French (Birbeck 1835).

Rhubarb had a "peculiar somewhat aromatic smell, and a bitter astringent taste, is gritty when chewed, imparts a yellow colour to the saliva, and affords a yellowish powder with a reddish-brown tinge" (Wood and Bache 1847, 591–592). A mild purgative, its astringent qualities tonified the stomach and intestines (Gentleman in the Course of His Travels 1807). "There is scarce any chronic disease in which rhubarb is not serviceable," enthused Hill (1812, 291). So well known were its properties, wrote Stephenson and Churchill (1834), that it bordered on supererogation to list them. In small doses, it was a tonic; in larger doses, a purgative. When nursing mothers took rhubarb, their milk turned purgative (Pereira 1843a). Only one source mentioned Chinese use, M. Paravey (1837) wrongly claiming that Chinese herbal books represented it as a tonic, not a purgative.

Patients with hemorrhoids and "costiveness" (constipation) could chew the root nightly for fifteen to twenty minutes, and then swallow it; this was an acquired taste (Jackson 1830b). Tincture of rhubarb made "an excellent stomachic, given with some bitter infusion" (Stephenson and Churchill 1834, 3:n.p.), or one could make a liquid extract (Procter 1847). M. Chevallier (1835, 258–259) published his recipe for syrup—"clear, and of a fine amber color." One could even make rhubarb wine (Dunglison 1846a). *Carpenter's Annual Medical Advertiser* recommended that new druggists stock the extract, whereas new country storekeepers should stock the root (Carpenter 1844). (Reasons for the distinction were not provided.)

Tea still received credit for the low incidence of "stone" and gout in China (de Chavannes 1845). Dublin doctor Edward Percival (1818) suggested that, in excess, green tea's stimulant effects damaged the heart, but that nevertheless it alleviated some fevers and regularized certain pulses. A later author argued that it could harm an already weakened constitution (Cole 1840). Medical and pharmacy journals reviewed reports, from Mr. Warrington of London's Apothecaries' Hall, accusing the Chinese of adulterating tea shipments with other leaves (Pigou 1836; Warrington 1844a, 1844b; see also Dunn 1835). The *American Magazine* repeated the charge (Dwight 1835c). Pharmacists wondered how many species there actually were, and to what the varieties (detailed in the *Journal Asiatique* by von Klaproth [1824]) owed their distinctive flavors. Commissioned by the British East India Company, Mr. F. Pigou (1836) dispatched agents, including a certain Chou-qua, to investigate. They attributed differences to soil and preparation.

Westerners' dependence on rhubarb and tea was apparent to the Chinese. A memorial submitted to the emperor recommended strategies for using both to restore China's wealth: "The foreigners, if deprived for several days of the tea and rhubarb of China, are afflicted with dimness of sight and constipation of the bowels, to such a degree that life is endangered. How trifling, in comparison with tea, then, are the medicinal benefits derivable from opium, and its power of keeping off what is hurtful!—Opium is not smoked by every one in China; while tea and rhubarb are necessaries of life to each individual foreigner" (M. 1838b, 311). The memorial's author proposed fixing tea and rhubarb prices, not allowing foreigners to exchange opium for them, and requiring payment in silver alone.

The Hubbling, Bubbling Caldron

Unfamiliar ingredients in China's pharmacopoeia alternately fascinated and repulsed observers. Pearson (1826a, 146) recorded "bat dung, viper's flesh, scorpions, and larvae of silkworms." Wood (1830, 154) listed rhinoceros horns, elephant parts, dried insects, wild cat bones, and "plants peculiar to the country." Comparing decoctions to the "hubbling, bubbling caldron of Macbeth's witches," Williams (1848, vol. 2) argued that the stranger the ingredient, the more potent the Chinese believed it to be.

Accounts were mixed. Gutzlaff (1837) demystified elephant parts— the eye, "burnt to powder, and mixed with human milk," cured eye inflammations. Pulverized bones in liquor helped digestion; the ivory, similarly prepared, treated diabetes; elephant teeth, epilepsy (167; see also Lepage 1813). One author reported Chinese ink used for coughs, chest conditions, sore throats, fluxes, and spitting blood (Editor 1816). De Malpière (1825, vol. 1) cited serpents, adding that ancient European physicians had prescribed grilled snake meat or snake wine for elephantiasis and leprosy. Parker observed "a man with his whitlowed [inflamed with pus] finger thrust into the abdomen of a frog—the poor writhing reptile being tied on to cure the disease" (Editor 1841e, 176). Ellis (1830) described deer horns sliced thin, boiled in restorative soups, and pharmacy employees preparing bird's nests. Montgomery Martin (1847, 2:278) wrote harshly that pills of pounded tiger bone confirmed "the defective state of medical knowledge in China." Revisiting Du Halde, Pereira (1843b) discussed the "summer-plant-winter-worm," a caterpillar from whose neck grew a fungus (actually a plant, *cordyceps sinensis*).

Lines between *materia medica* and food blurred; the perception of some ingredients as alien led to scurrilous accounts of Chinese diet. *Dwight's American Magazine* published the supposed menu for a Chinese banquet: bird's nest soup, pork fat fried with potatoes, hogs' hoofs, stewed mushrooms, kitten hash, fried Irish potatoes, rat hash, shark's fins, fried ducks, dog stew, pork stew, fried cucumbers, paté of rats, sucking pig, snail paté, and snail soup (Dwight 1846b, 619). Stereotypes of the Chinese as consumers of rats, cats, and dogs gained currency, particularly given the custom of serving exotic meats at banquets.

Some accounts reported on "medicine" that intersected with murder. In 1830 the *Asiatic Journal* reprinted an article from the *Canton Register* on "Medical Anthropophy in China"—a boy supposedly killed in Macao for a piece of his flesh, to restore a dying man; human gallbladder on sale; a man who killed eleven girls to drink "certain fluids to add vigour to his constitution" (Editor 1830c, 254; see Cooper and Sivin 1973). The *Albany Farmer's, Mechanic's, and Workingman's Advocate* reprinted segments (Miller 1969). It was a short step to speculations of cannibalism, returning full circle to medieval narratives. D. McPherson, for example, wrote that when the Manchus evacuated Canton in the 1840s, witnesses claimed "that the Tartar troops ate the flesh of the Chinese that were slain" (McPherson 1842, 150).

No one flagged discussions about equally suspect Western practices. Yet the *Medical News-Paper* printed a piece on "The Gastric Juice of Dead Bodies used by Physicians as a remedy for Diseases of the Living." Revolted, Elias Smith (1824) described proponents' claims to cure dyspepsia and intermittent fever when the juice was taken internally, and putrid and scrofulous ulcers when applied topically. He added caustically that it would make a useful emetic, if one informed the patient of its origin. "If this would not cause the person to puke, antimonials and epecac would be unavailing" (95).

A Nation Stationary

Western observers and writers concluded that Chinese pharmacology represented the virtues of antiquity *sans* science. Ellis (1830) charged that the Chinese blended "correct views of practice" with "the most childish prejudices and puerile conceits" (150). At issue were both processes and content. Gutzlaff (1838, 172) wrote, "They do not spend their time in making chemical experiments, but follow their ancestors." Downing (1838) compared an older Western "doctrine of signatures" (the idea that a plant's appearance indicated its properties) with the Chinese idea that the upper half of a root had ascending properties; the lower half, descending; branches, extending properties analogous to the limbs; the peel, an influence over the flesh and skin; and the pith of the growth above ground, the viscera (2:171). Arguing that Chinese doctors, "without a ray of science to illumine them . . . have yet stumbled upon useful and valuable remedies," he nevertheless relegated the bulk of Chinese medical successes to luck, trial, and error (2:170).

   Wilson (1846b) found preparations designed "to arrest cholera instantly, to communicate strength directly, to infuse courage, to excite love, and to confer the faculty of being loved" no more absurd than compounds sold in England "under the names of antibilious, antidyspeptic, antinervous, *antiomnia mala* medicines" (568). Ultimately, however, it was often a comparison of apples and oranges. The spurious in Chinese practice—nostrums that would have been ridiculed by Chinese literati as well—were taken as evidence by many Westerners that the system itself had little evidentiary basis and less merit.

Western Doctors in China

Where the Jesuits had concentrated on scholar-officials, the Protestants focused on merchants and the lower classes, translating the Bible into the vernacular (leading the literati to perceive them as writing like peasants). East India companies employed surgeons, but they usually provided care to the Chinese only when they had been wounded by Europeans or Americans; this was to avoid penalties for causing a death. Eventually, however, medicine also appeared to provide additional venues for proselytizing.

The Medical Missionaries

In 1827, Thomas R. Colledge, a British East India Company surgeon, established an eye infirmary in Macao. Gutzlaff, although not a physician, treated boat captains and pilots along the riverbanks, gradually expanding his medical work in his forays into the countryside and coastal areas. Despite understanding Chinese medical theory, he appears to have routinely challenged the Chinese practitioners he encountered. Not concealing his triumphalism, he wrote, "To stand against men of this description, who are so very wise in their own imagination, was not an easy task; but I always convinced them, by facts, that our theories, when reduced to practice, would have the most salutary effect" (Gutzlaff 1832, 182; see Hamilton [1833]1834).

Parker, who trained in theology and medicine at Yale and was the first American medical missionary, opened the Canton Ophthalmic Hospital in 1835, treating 1,912 patients during the first year (Editor 1837a). The hospital was located in Factory No. 7, a building belonging to merchant Howqua, who waived the rent. Parker reported the hospital's efforts to European and American medical journals; his dispatches were listed under works received for review and sometimes were published.[29] An 1839 report recorded that the hospital treated not only eyes, but also "abdominal organs," generative and pelvic organs, skin, and bones, "general and constitutional diseases," "preternatural and diseased growths," and injuries (Cormack 1841b).

Between 1841 and 1842, Parker visited Europe and the United States to raise funds. The yield proved uneven. In Philadelphia he got one $50 subscription; in Boston he raised $5,550 (Editor 1844a). While in the States, he married Daniel Webster's niece, taking her to Canton in 1842, despite regulations prohibiting women in the factories. Customs collided, as evidenced in a memorial to the throne by Imperial Commissioner Koying, one of Parker's patients, describing his reactions to the Western practice of having a wife receive a guest as a mark of respect: "Your slave was confounded and ill at ease, while they, on the contrary, were greatly delighted at the honour done them. The truth is, as this shows, that it is not possible to regulate the customs of the Western States by the ceremonial of China, and to break out in rebuke, while it would do nothing toward their enlightenment, might chance to give rise to suspicion and ill-feeling" (Wu 1931, 20). Comments would indeed probably have been folded into negatively gendered perceptions of the Chinese. Parker also trained four Chinese students in surgical techniques for removing cataracts and tumors. One of them, Kwah Ato, was the nephew of Lamqua (fl. 1830–1850), a Chinese artist who may have studied with George Chinnery. Kwah performed many operations.

In 1838 Colledge, Parker, Rev. Elijah Bridgman, and Rev. David Abeel organized the Medical Missionary Society in China, to bring to the Chinese "some of those benefits, which science, patient investigation, and the ever-kindling light of discovery, have conferred upon ourselves" (Colledge, Parker, and Bridgman 1838, 37). They hoped to gain entry into more of China, and to gather information valuable to Western merchants—reflecting the ongoing close connection between religious and commercial objectives—"for a sick man will often deal frankly with his physician, however he may be disposed to conceal facts" (Editor 1844c, 404–405; Editor 1844d).

The *Lancet* announced the medical missionary society's founding with some ambivalence, writing, "Many good and conscientious men . . . regard the proposed means for 'entrapping the Chinese' as perfectly justified by the object" (Editor 1837f, 784). The *Boston Medical Intelligencer* wrote, "China . . . may yet be distinguished for her advancement in science and in practical Christianity" (Editor 1841e, 432). Some medical missionaries viewed it as their mandate to challenge the resistance to anatomical dissection. With that goal in mind, the society proposed to establish an anatomical museum "of natural and morbid anatomy, paintings of extraordinary diseases, &c." (Slade 1843, 85).

The London Missionary Society sent William Lockhart to Macao. He arrived in 1839 and took up Parker's work, but had to leave later that year due to growing tensions between the Chinese government and the British. He went to Batavia to practice medicine and study Chinese with Medhurst. In 1840 he reopened the Macao hospital, but soon he left for Chusan. British doctor Benjamin Hobson (1816–1873) stepped in. Lockhart returned, remaining until the end of the war. By 1841 more than thirty-five hundred patients had received treatment. In 1843 Lockhart went to Hong Kong, where he oversaw the building of the Medical Missionary Society's hospital, which was then put under Hobson's direction. In 1844 he extended the Society's work to Shanghai (Wu 1831). During later rebellions, the hospital was untouched, and the sick and wounded from both sides received care there.

Dr. D. J. McGowan, affiliated with the Medical Mission of the Baptist Convention in America, taught Western medicine "by the employment of anatomical preparations and plates, and more particularly by the use of a model contrived by an ingenious Parisian physician, Dr. Azoux" (Anonymous 1844b, 172). The model showed muscles, tendons, bones, nerves, and arteries in correct proportion and relation to one another. The parts could be disassembled and reassembled, with additional models of the eye and ear. Nevertheless, missionaries also described being pelted with mud and stones. Downing (1838, 3:94) wrote, "the common people really considered us something superhuman, as ghosts and demons." The missionaries were not deterred.

Treaty agreements imposed after the first Opium War included "toleration clauses," permitting foreigners to build not only schools and churches in the treaty ports, but also hospitals. Traders supported the endeavor. As Captain Pidding observed, "Many of the commercial transactions with China have had, it is well known, a very injurious influence on the people, and the consideration of this circumstance has induced some of the principal European and American merchants in China to support very freely the medical missions" (Anonymous 1844c). In 1845, Western physicians in Hong Kong organized a China Medico-Chirurgical Society, and Baptist missionaries in Canton opened a Medical Dispensary near the factories. "The Dispensary is always opened with prayer in Chinese," wrote a reporter, "and each patient receives a tract and Christian teaching" (Friend of China 1845, 543). The "English lady" Miss Aldersey—one of the early women medical missionaries—joined the Medhurst family, learned Chinese, and went to Chusan. She lived with "a good Chinese family," treating patients twice a week until retiring to Ningpo to live with "several Chinese ladies of pleasing manners" (Martin 1847, 493). No other women were reported as being involved in medical missionary work, reflecting gendered practice in the West.

Treating Chinese Bodies

Themes of monstrosity shaped the medicalizing of Chinese bodies, particularly in relation to tumors—defined as any unusual growth or swelling and characterized already in the medical literature as "monstrous productions" (Roper 1817, 74). Physician writers pointed to the prevalence of tumors in China, particularly among the poor, in whom "every form of disease which can render man miserable, or loathsome, prevails unchecked," perhaps due to a vegetable diet and lack of salt (Lay 1840b, 214).

Parker commissioned Lamqua to paint tumor patients. Larissa Heinrich (1999) argues that such images contributed to stereotypes of the "Sick Man of Asia," corresponding to case notes that pathologized a racialized Chinese identity seen as both cause and source of illness. Likewise, these images insinuated the "curability" of China and the Chinese through missionary efforts. Dr. Robert W. Hooper donated twenty-eight such paintings to the Anatomical Museum of the Boston Society for Medical Improvement in 1845 (Jackson 1847), where physician Oliver Wendell Holmes reviewed them: "It is really an instructive sight to see what a bad business Chinese Grahamism and the *vis medicatrix* together make of it with these poor creatures. And it is truly gratifying to know that after Nature has deformed them with such hideous additions, making *China monsters* of them, sure enough, a kind and skilful hand has reached them in their misery, and divorced them from these horrible encumbrances" (Holmes 1845, 318). The paintings persuaded viewers that missionary accounts were accurate, and that removal of monster status required Western intervention.

Accounts of Chinese tumors came home on April 5, 1831. The London *Times* reported that thirty-two-year-old "Hoo-loo" from Canton was admitted to Guy's Hospital for removal of a tumor that weighed seventy to eighty pounds from his lower abdomen (Anonymous 1831a). Thanks to the article, the operating theater was packed, leading surgeon Sir Astley Cooper to relocate everyone to a larger theater that would hold eleven hundred (it was still packed). Aston Key operated, assisted by Cooper and other surgeons from Guy's. A reporter observed, "During the whole of the operation, the patient appeared to be unusually affected by the loss of blood," sixteen ounces altogether. Brandy was administered, fresh air allowed to blow over him, and "warm applications were applied to his feet and chest." He still felt faint; the surgeon injected brandy into his stomach. When his heart stopped, a medical student donated blood, to no avail. The observer concluded that Hoo-loo had died from blood loss and shock. His tumor measured four feet around (Anonymous 1831b, 2). (See Figure 24.)

The *Lancet* condemned performing surgery so soon after Hoo-Loo's arrival in England, in a theater rendered airless by the crowd. The operation had lasted too long: "The vital energy is unable to contend against the long continuance of such unusually severe pain" (Wakley

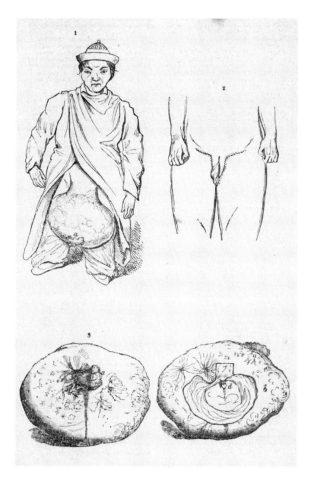

Figure 24. "Poor Hoo-Loo." *Lancet,* April 16, 1831. Francis A. Countway Library of Medicine.

1831b, 83–84). People of different ranks had visited Hoo-loo in the hospital; they found him to be in good spirits, anticipating the operation "with satisfaction." His death led his nurses—among whom he had become "a great favorite"—to shed tears (Wakley 1831c). A month later, the *Asiatic Journal* elaborated: Hoo-loo had been a laborer at the Canton factory. A student of Cooper's had encouraged his trip. The author criticized the failure to provide an interpreter, including "Ho-Lô's" cries recorded by a spectator, who knew some Chinese: "'Unloose me! unloose me!'—'Water! help! water! let me go!' The last articulate sounds he was heard to utter were, 'Let it be! let it remain! I can bear no more! unloose me!'" (Editor 1831b). The representation of Chinese stoicism dissolves, replaced by an image of intolerable suffering. Years later, we are left wondering about the supposed silence with which the missionaries' Chinese patients bore their operations.

Such events did not prevent Western physicians from believing that their practice was superior or lead them to refrain from treating Chinese patients. The *Chinese Repository* reported on Case No. 6565, involving "Lin Tsihseu" (Lin Zixu), the commissioner who had attempted to block the opium trade. The inspector never came in person, sending messages instead through a local magistrate and through *co-hong* Howqua, requesting medicine for a hernia. In return, he was sent an explanation in Chinese of his condition, as well as an anatomical diagram and a recommendation for a surgically designed instrument. Reluctant to allow a foreigner such intimate contact, he was reassured by a colleague who had used such a truss, and one was sent to him. Other symptoms suggested he also suffered from asthma (Editor 1840b).

Another official, Judicial Commissioner Wang, suffered from a paralysis on the left side and from dropsical swelling (edema) in his legs. He was treated with bleeding, blisters, and strychnine, as well as electricity. Although the paralysis persisted, his health otherwise improved. "He is an amusing, talkative, old gentleman," wrote the anonymous author, "and is very fond of dwelling on the circumstances of his father being one of the legates attending lord Macartney's embassy." He still inquired after Macartney, and the Stauntons, continuing to wear a pair of spectacles given to his father by Staunton senior. The hospital regularly sent medicines to members of the commissioner's family, based on "his minute explanations" of their cases (Editor 1840b, 638).

Lay adopted Blumenbach's typology to contrast Chinese bodies with Caucasian, attributing to the latter "a geometry of beauty" and intellectual superiority. Calling on phrenology, he argued, "Of our superiority over the Chinese, the Ethiop, or the Indian, we are not the owners but the stewards only, and consequently are bound to use it for their benefit." He believed the Chinese would accept this "superiority" if it were exhibited through acts of goodness (Lay 1841a, 14). Dr. John Wilson's *Medical Notes on China*—widely reviewed in medical journals—reported that the Chinese suffered from "scrofulous affections, ophthalmia and its results, and cutaneous affections, including elephantiasis" (Editor 1846e, 375). Some observers related these problems to hygiene. In contrast, Dr. William Lockhart (1841) suggested that the Chinese understanding of preventive medicine *was* hygiene. Wilson's influence prevailed, however: a review in the *Dublin Medical Press* concluded, "The inhabitants are essentially a filthy race." Through reprints and reviews, such attitudes resurfaced as far away as Cincinnati, Ohio (Editor 1848d).

Over time, Chinese bodies suffered increased targeting as sites of a supposed convergence of vice and disease. Rev. G. A. Smith (1847a) charged the Chinese with "all the vices charged by the apostle Paul upon the ancient heathen world." Resorting to a hydraulic metaphor, he described a "free, unchecked torrent of human depravity borne along in its tempestuous channel, and inundating the social system with the overflowings of ungodliness" (385). Such metaphors would gradually infuse anti-Chinese rhetoric.

Medical Exchanges

Occasional accounts surfaced of Chinese practitioners treating Western patients. Dr. John McLeod, traveling with HMS *Alceste,* described how the ship's captain broke his arm and dislocated a forefinger. A local doctor encased the injury in a dough, wrapping it in the skin of a fowl. His medicine chest contained some 180 materials—"wood-shavings, roots, seeds, and dried flowers"—along with ginseng. He was delighted to hear the following day that the patient was doing well, although in fact the remedies were never taken. "A new application was now brought for the finger, termed a fish-poultice; so composed as to look, and indeed to smell, something like currant-jelly . . . The physician, more especially, seemed to be a very respectable man, and was treated as such by those about him" (McLeod 1820, 121–122).

John Frances Davis (1836a) cited two other cases. One failed to impress him. The other involved a well-known physician who had risen "from hawking herbs" and successfully treated an Englishman. The paucity of such narratives does not mean such encounters were rare. De Chavannes (1845, 292–293) commented, "Many of the European residents in Canton really find themselves abandoning the English doctors for the Chinese physicians, when it is a matter of intermittent fevers and rebellious dysenteries."

A few observers actually endeavored to learn Chinese medicine. In 1819 physician John Livingstone (d. 1829?) wrote to Morrison about an Anglo-Chinese college being established in Malacca.[30] He anticipated botany being included in the curriculum, with translations of Chinese botanical books to follow.[31] He had encouraged the London Horticultural Society to send a gardener who, with assistance, could collect plants (Livingstone 1819b). Morrison agreed to supply the books and recruit a local assistant, once the gardener arrived. Morrison also purchased a medical library of eight hundred volumes, hired a Chinese physician and an herbalist, and bought out the latter's stock to establish a clinic for the poor, where he spent mornings. Livingstone observed ten to fifteen cases daily. Some patients received Western treatments, but the Chinese physician treated most of them. Dr. M., reported Livingstone, was an intelligent and amiable man. Both missionaries recognized the difficulties in understanding what Chinese patients meant in explaining their afflictions, and the importance of understanding Chinese systems before they could assess or explain Chinese practice (Livingstone 1819a; Morrison 1819b).

Roughly half the cases involved chronic stomach, pectoral, and bowel complaints, and a few, chronic rheumatism. For more acute cases, Dr. M. applied diagnostics for cold-damage disorders—"all the diseases which originate in checked perspiration, whether by exposure to March miasmatic cold, damp air, &c. Its species varies with the season of the year." Impressed by the system's complexity, Livingstone confessed he could still only "enumerate the fever from cold, conjective fevers, dysentery, intermittent and remittent fevers, and rheumatism" (Morrison 1839, 2:23). From herbalist Le Seen-sang he discovered that even though apothecary shops in Canton commonly contained some three hundred medicines, only some thirty were routinely employed.

Pearson, often identified with smallpox vaccination, sought prescriptions related to paralysis. He recruited a Roman Catholic missionary to approach local practitioners and present them with "cases or conditions of diseases," requesting observations and prescriptions. The priest recorded the responses in Chinese, then translated them into Latin, the medium of his communication with Pearson. Pearson then collected the related medicines, which were explained to him by "a respectable and intelligent Chinese apothecary, from whom I procured them." He forwarded the whole to England, but the intended recipient had passed away in the interim and the herbs presumably were lost (Pearson 1826b, 2:138–140).[32]

Medical Missionary Society members recognized correspondences between local illnesses and remedies discovered in the area, and proposed enhancing their own dispensaries with such remedies. Likewise, they expected that familiarity with Chinese illness models would round out their own conceptual frameworks. Such understanding, they argued, would also allow them to correct Chinese "errors." Downing, for example, befriended a local pharmacist, "my professional brother," to answer his questions. "A very grave, respectable-looking personage," he expressed similar interest in knowing how illnesses were treated in Europe. On one occasion, when he fell ill, he asked Downing to prescribe for him. Downing (1838) went through the pharmacy pots and drawers, and the older man "pulled out his most valuable panaceas from secret and unthought-of nooks and corners," allowing Downing to view Chinese *materia medica* firsthand (143–144).

Lay hired a physician tutor, hoping to visit patients together and to pay for their prescriptions in exchange for instruction. His second agenda was to meet local people and proselytize. He wrote, "In this way a man, being crafty, may catch a people with guile, and yet not deceive them, as Lucretius says, because he sought their health, and not their harm" (Lay 1841a, 232–233). His stay in China proved shorter than expected, however, ending his project.

The Remedy Par Excellence: Moxibustion

Among the observers, Abel detailed how one prepared cones of artemesia fiber in China, placed them on afflicted points, and lit them. He believed moxa was used for other internal diseases when these expressed as "external uneasiness," and in "affections of the head," having observed individuals with scarred foreheads (Abel 1818a, 217–

218). His informant assured him the process was not painful. Lay (1841a) was less sanguine, insisting that even amputation, with its "glittering display of knives, saws, forceps, and so forward," was nothing in comparison with "a Chinese physician, [who] with a handful of dirt and as much tinder, is able to inflict more torture than an amputation usually occasions" (234). Williams (1848) described cases at missionary hospitals, where what had begun as small sores from moxa had spread, "until a large part of the tissue, and even important organs have been destroyed, the charlatan amusing his suffering patient by promises of ultimate cure" (2:183–184). "Mugwort also grows in China," wrote a Fr. Dubois (1848, 190), where "they make moxas with the pounded and crushed leaves. Ansiaux, professor of clinical surgery on the faculty of Liege, sometimes uses moxa."

Moxa Revived

Moxibustion as promoted by Pierre-François Percy and Claude Pouteau continued to find favor in Europe, particularly in France. All agreed that when it had verged on falling into oblivion, Pouteau had restored it to favor (Morel 1813). L. M. Lecointe, Dominique Jean Larrey, Louis Benoit Guersent, Claude Jean Baptiste Cothenet, Antoine Jacques Louis Jourdan (1788–1848), Jean Morel, J. V. F. Vaidy, Jean Baptiste Sarlandière, and Alphonse Tavernier (d. 1850) reported their experiences with moxa in medical journals and textbooks.[33] European application of moxa was so identified with the French that in 1821 Franklin James Didier (1821) wrote, "The horrid resources of cautery, moxa, &c. are much resorted to by the French practitioners. Baron Larrey, in particular, is too fond of these extreme means" (481). Still, many of these men were surgeons on leading French medical faculties; their students included other Europeans and Americans.

While emphasizing progress as the hallmark of science, medical writers still substantiated their knowledge by discussing a topic's origins. Some authors looked to "the father of medicine," Hippocrates. Poets like Damophanes, Virgil, and Quintus Serenus Sammonicus were said to have celebrated moxa. Cothenet and Lecointe recognized Arabic and Egyptian origins, as did Jourdan, who referred to Albucasis and Rhazes. Both Percy and Jourdan also cited Prosper Alpini. Sometimes Native Americans, Africans (Ethiopians and Libyans), Indians (the Brahmins in particular), the Lapps, the Turks, and the Armenians were listed as practitioners.[34] The pervasive use of moxa in China and Japan was also recognized (Cothenet 1808; Morel 1813; Percy 1826), Jourdan quoting Kaempfer and ten Rhijne. Sarlandière (1825) believed it was reserved primarily for chronic conditions, although also used at the commencement of certain illnesses, and when a deep effect was needed.

Many authors—having located the modality historically—produced a string of European authors: Pouteau, Alpini, Matthias Glandorp, Fabricius of Aquapendente, and Percy. By 1816 Jourdan could construct an entire European genealogy of therapeutic fire. A bibliography of twenty-one annotated citations from Western literature supported his discussion.

Only Robley Dunglison's introduction to Larrey's work (1822) referred to nonmedical sources, suggesting a familiarity with broader representations of China. His footnotes included Grosier, the Jesuit *Mémoires,* Buschof, Temple, Barrow, Abel, Kaempfer, ten Rhijne, and Cleyer. He even mentioned Benjamin Rush's *Medical Inquiries and Observations* for its discussion of Native American uses of "punk," potentially an analogue to moxa. Dunglison's familiarity with literature both medical and nonmedical exposed him to accounts of Chinese practices of all kinds. In contrast, William Wallace (1827) cited only French surgeons, which suggests that he presumed the sufficiency of their interpretation of the practice.

Pyrotechnical Surgery

Moxibustion was categorized as "pyrotechnical surgery." Some authors classified it with agents that were allowed to burn down and produce cauterization (Wallace 1827). Accordingly, a hot iron was described as "the most painful moxa" (Cothenet 1808, 11). Others viewed "cauterization" as the primary heading that included moxa *and* red-hot irons (Lecointe 1812). For Tavernier (1829), the choice lay between moxa or lighted charcoal, on the one hand, and a hot iron, hot oil, or hot water, on the other. The issue involved choosing a cautery of the right shape, and determining whether merely to pass it over the parts to be stimulated or to apply it directly.

"Moxa," wrote Larrey (1819, 459), referred to "a cylinder formed out of a cottony substance that one extracts from the ground leaf or the pith of a type of mugwort (*Artemesia chinensis*)." Larrey received a

Chinese moxa stick from von Klaproth. Dunglison detailed the process for preparing the leaves, "formerly kept a great secret by the Chinese, [moxa] being sold in their shops, ready prepared, only" (Larrey 1822, xxxix). Lisfranc (1835, 339) used artemesia moxas, writing, "They burn quickly . . . and hence cause less irritation than the ordinary moxa." A Mr. William English of Seething Lane sent the *Lancet* "foy-cong" or the "true moxa" used "for the purpose of burning eschars on the surface of the body" (Wakley 1827c, 285).

Sarlandière (1825), too, received moxas from von Klaproth, resembling cinnamon sticks cut into pieces (69). Attempts to produce his own failed—they either wouldn't burn, or burned too hot. He wrote, "It is in vain that I used various glutinous and resinous bodies, with or without the addition of nitrate, etc." (58–59). Simple down, pressed into cones, worked better. He recommended *Artemesia latifolia,* gathered after sundown in summer, and shade-dried. One either separated the down with a mortar and pestle, or carded the leaves to extract the fibers. He criticized his peers for not testing Chinese procedures. Would a people as ancient and observant as the Chinese not have employed another substance, had a better one been available? Should not European doctors follow their lead "in a subject that we have from them, and in which we are still so new and so far from equaling them?" (63). He directed his readers to M. Sallé, a pharmacist, who sold boxes of artemesia moxa for fifty *centimes* and who had taught Sarlandière to card down from the leaves.

For most surgeons, including Larrey, however, "moxa" meant any burnable substance producing cauterization: "From the earliest ages, the Nomades employed, for this purpose, the fat wool of their flocks, as well as certain spongy substances growing upon oaks, and springing from the hazel—the Indian, the pith of the reed, and flax, or hemp, impregnated with some combustible material—the Persian the dung of the goat—the Armenian the agaric of the oak—the Chinese and Japanese the down of the Artemesia—the Thessalian, dried moss— the Egyptian, Arracanese, and several oriental nations, cotton—the Ostiaks and Laplanders, the agaric of the birch—and the Aborigines of North America, rotten and dried wood, which they called *punk*" (Larrey 1822, xxxv–xxxvi). The description repositioned Chinese practice in a compendium of world medicines. Implicitly, as often occurred with eighteenth-century writers, this suggested that Western surgeons could choose or invent at will.

Cotton impregnated with saltpeter burned better, observed Morel. Such moxas were available "and very artistically ornamented and colored . . . at the shop of the pharmacist Bataille, on Baune Street . . . in Paris." One could also purchase Morel's own design "of nankeen cotton, or of an apricot color" (Morel 1813, 102–103). Familiar with ten Rhijne and Kaempfer, Percy (1819) favored cotton wick used by military gunners, as had Fabricius of Aquapendente. Tavernier (1829) preferred carded cotton—plant matter burned too quickly, and resulted in a less effective superficial wound. Larrey (1822, 4) recommended a cylinder of cotton wool, wrapped in linen stitched closed. He included drawings of both Chinese moxas and his own. John Moore Neligan's *Medicines* explained that in England moxas were made from the pith of sunflower stems, "or by soaking cotton-wool in a concentrated solution of nitre," pressed into cones like Chinese moxas. "More recently," he added, "Professor Osborne, of Dublin, has proposed the use of fresh-burned quicklime as a substitute" (Neligan 1844, 201).

How to apply moxa? One could, wrote Jourdan ([1816]1819), adhere it with saliva. Guersent (1826a) used cardboard with an opening the size of the moxa, to protect the surrounding skin. Larrey (1822) promoted his own invention—a *Porte-Moxa* (moxa holder). One inserted a lit cone into the holder's metal ring, which three small ebony supports prevented from touching the skin directly. The implement gained currency. (See Figure 25.)

Ten Rhijne and Kaempfer continued to influence the idea that virtually any surface of the body would serve, excepting more delicate areas. Nor, thought Larrey (1822), should one apply moxa to the skull, for fear of injuring the brain. Fleshy parts were preferable. Chinese diagrams influenced both Larrey and Sarlandière. "I have subjoined a plate containing the back and front views of a doll," wrote Larrey (1822, 3–4), "with the places proper for the application of the Moxa marked upon it." Dunglison's translation omitted the plate, originally drawn by Sarlandière, remarking that the figures were "executed in such a careless manner in the original work . . . that no correct idea could be obtained from them" (Larrey 1822, 3–4). Larrey's verbal description should suffice.

Sarlandière traced his interest in moxa to working in a military hospital. He observed patients suffering from cotton moxa burns and speculated that Chinese procedures worked better. Von Klaproth

(1825) connected him with Isaac Titsingh's *Tsoe-Bosi*, or *jingluo* figurine, and manuscripts. Through trial and error, Sarlandière developed the approach of encircling the painful site with ten to forty cones. They burned down, generating scabs that fell off ten to fifteen days later. He then made a second circle of cones inside the initial ring. Gradually, he moved toward the center, achieving cures "that I would not hope to realize using cotton moxa" (Sarlandière 1825, 79).

Although Sarlandière and Wallace followed Buschof and Temple in

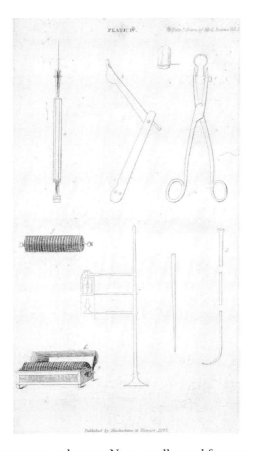

Figure 25. Acupuncture and moxa. Note needle used for acupuncture (top left), as well as moxa and *Porte-Moxa* (moxa holder) designed by Larrey (top right). William Wallace, *A Physiological Enquiry Respecting the Action of Moxa,* 1827. Courtesy of the Boston Medical Library in the Francis A. Countway Library of Medicine.

placing moxas on painful sites, both also turned to the nervous system. In neuralgias, one followed the trajectory of the affected nerves, or placed moxas at their origin. For paralysis, one positioned moxas at the origins of nerves affecting the organ deprived of movement. Wallace (1827, 68) recommended application "in paralytic affections . . . over the origin of the nerves which lead to the diseased parts, and afterwards along the same nerves in different parts of their course." This directive provided a non-Chinese rationale for treating points at a distance from the problem area—an aspect of Chinese practice that, as we have seen, regularly confounded European physicians.

Moxas were also categorized as *exutoires*—techniques producing an "issue." One raised and punctured a blister. Dressings and ointments promoted infection and pus—the sign that the body was expelling harmful influences. One could also apply a seton—a piece of horse-hair or silk thread bound onto the opened blister (Tavernier 1829, 48–50).[35] If the area was not deliberately infected, a scab formed, falling away after a week, producing pus. "It is difficult," wrote Vaidy, "to make this pus last beyond two months, and only with respect to [this aspect] is moxa inferior to a seton." One could also apply an irritant daily, to prevent the wound from healing over (Vaidy 1820a, 68; 1820b, 15). It was from this "issue," Guersent noted (1839), that all moxa's secondary advantages derived.

Few patients willingly submitted, particularly when facing a red-hot iron (Morel 1813). Consequently, few physicians outside of military hospitals—where patients were relatively at the mercy of their surgeons—used even moxa. "This is a great error," Vaidy (1820a) wrote. "I have made frequent use of it in my civil practice, and I have almost always succeeded in persuading women for whom I judged that it would be suitable" (66–67). Still, for many physicians moxa remained a treatment of last resort.

Case narratives illustrate the demographics of patients treated with moxa. Of sixty-five cases I located from a review of European and American medical journals, books, medical dictionaries, and a dissertation,[36] twenty-one involved women patients and forty-four, men. The average age was thirty-four, with more patients in their twenties and thirties. The youngest was a six-year-old boy; the eldest, a sixty-seven-year-old man. Thirty-two were working-class men: bakers, hackney coachmen, farm workers, laborers, painters, peelers, sawyers, silk workers, watchmen, or wool combers. Twelve were soldiers, some in the light infantry, one a dragoon and one a general. Four working-class women included a stocking maker and a widow who sold newspapers. Two were mothers. Only ten patients were from the upper classes—six were "gentlemen," among them a viscount; five women were discussed as "ladies." Working-class patients were treated in public infirmaries and military hospitals. Upper-class patients received treatment at home.

What conditions were described as responding? Pain, paralysis, respiratory illnesses, and sometimes problems with sight and hearing. Pain included lumbago, sciatica, rheumatism, spinal problems, and the results of accidents. Paralysis encompassed the effects of multiple causes. Respiratory conditions referred to everything from the aftermath of a cold to tuberculosis. Deafness and blindness, when not present since birth, also seemed responsive. Sarlandière (1825) used moxa for tumors, coxalgias (pain or disease in the hip), rickets, chronic rheumatism, hardenings, noninflammatory swellings of tissues, muscles, joints, glands, testicles, and viscera, and for neuralgias and nervous conditions.

The Tonic Power of Caloric

For the writers interested in explaining moxa's effectiveness, no single answer sufficed. If one located the problem in the quantity of the body's fluids, then removing fluids would solve the issue. On the other hand, if one viewed a condition as deriving from "the state of the vital properties of the solids," one would restore "the vital powers of the vessels to a natural state" (Wallace 1827, 20–21), conscious of the influence the fluids also had on those vital powers. The state of the capillaries, for example, was viewed as playing an important etiological role. Enhancing their function might help promote health-enhancing circulation.

Authors debated whether moxa's efficacy derived from the effects of fire and heat or from the discharge of pus. If the latter, then how should moxa be differentiated from other forms of cautery and blistering, especially if moxa succeeded where cautery had failed? Wallace argued that "caloric" excited the capillaries, enhancing their tonicity and increasing circulation. His *Lancet* reviewer disagreed, and doubted that moxa would win converts, even with Wallace's advocacy (Wakley 1827b). Neligan differentiated between moxibustion and other cauteries, because moxa's effects were generated more slowly.

The issue was the nature of fire. Jourdan (1819) described fire as the element "that penetrates the entire universe, which illuminates it, and which animates all of organized nature" (87). Moxa transmitted the expansive and radiating properties of fire to the body's interior. The penetrating nature of heat distinguished it from all other agents. Lecointe (1812) therefore described moxa as "carrying a stimulating heat to the organs, and insinuat[ing] itself sometimes as far as the seat of the problem, which it dislodges and which it fixes upon more superficial parts" (5). Larrey suggested that moxa communicated to the interior of the body "a very active volatile principle." The most striking point is that there was no name for this principle except through a return to the elemental term *fire* (Larrey 1822, 8). Still, the effects of the treatment—whether understood or not—led not merely to its adoption, but to its continued integration and transformation by Western practitioners.

Acupuncture

Western surgeons continued to review Chinese versions of surgery. Summarizing what was known at the time, Lepage discussed moxa, acupuncture, and the treatment of cataracts and hernias; Dr. Sue, one of his mentors, served as a primary source.

A Surgical Frame of Reference

The Chinese, wrote Lepage (1813), used massage. "This practice is not perhaps to be scorned, and, modified according to the circumstances, one could doubtless expect good effects from it" (85). Pearson (1826b) observed that the Chinese pinched and twisted the skin, bruising it, or scraping it with a coin's edge "until the same effect of excoriation ensues," complemented by moxibustion, cupping, and acupuncture. They also used liniments and *tuina*—"kneading the joints and muscular parts with the hands" (147–148). Gutzlaff (1837, 170–171) summarized a Chinese surgical text on swellings, ulcers, tumors, running sores, lung injuries, and "herpetic eruptions," but without sufficient detail for readers to analyze.

Sutleffe (1820–21) rehearsed the history of China's famous surgeons, including anecdotes about "Hwa-to" (Huatuo, ca. 110–207) and Jin Gui (6th c.). Medhurst (1838) wrote that "Hwa-to" was "said to have laid bare the arm of a wounded chieftain, and to have scraped the poison off the scapula, while the unmoved warrior continued to play at chess, and to drink wine with the other arm" (111). Huatuo was remembered, too, for his skills in diagnosis, herbal medicine, moxa, and acupuncture, and was said to have learned medicine following deadly epidemics. He became one of the divinized physicians. (His patient, General Guangong, was also deified as Lord Guan, the Supreme Warrior.) Still, for Medhurst (1838), not only was Chinese medicine "mere quackery"; Chinese surgery, in his view, did "not extend beyond puncturing, cauterizing, drawing of teeth, and plastering, without attempting any operation in which skill or care is required" (112). (All reporters conveniently omitted high mortality rates among surgical patients in Europe and the United States.)

Lay cited a Chinese work, "Great Summary of Surgery and Therapeutics in Diseases of the Eye." It explained how physicians prepared patients for surgery days in advance "to quiet the air which flows in the arteries, to disperse the venous blood in even proportions, and to equalise the weakness of the bowels." The physician sought a propitious day, because a person's *yang* and the *yin* were "identical with those in the universe." He dispensed ointments and prescriptions of "*'bright'* native cinnabar, lapis calimniaris, amber, pearl, or, perhaps, mother of pearl, and *genuine bear's liver,* in equal quantities" (Lay 1841b, 326–327).

Lockhart (1842) translated a Chinese midwifery text, the *Baochan dashengbian* (On Safe Pregnancies and Successful Births).[37] It provided advice for parturition, prescriptions for pregnancy and the postpartum period, things to avoid, and "illustrative cases." His friend Fleetwood Churchill, who eventually authored a book on midwifery (1848), commented, "We cannot say that this work inspires us with any very high idea of the state of obstetric science among our celestial *confrères*" (Churchill 1842, 566). In 1820 Dr. Walter Channing, professor of obstetrics at Harvard Medical School, had argued that no one should practice without formal medical training. Reflecting concerns for legitimizing male obstetricians, Churchill included passages where the Chinese author criticized midwives.

Western observers transposed challenges to Chinese valor of the kind described earlier into discussions of Chinese surgery. "Detesting the sight of blood," wrote Gutzlaff (1837, 156), "phlebotomy is almost unknown amongst them, and the terror inspired by bleeding renders the remedy much more dangerous than the distemper." According to Wilson, "John Chinaman is not a bold reckless character; and he therefore never goes deeper, in any of his surgical operations, than the surface" (Editor 1846h, 90). Only Williams explored the underlying logic. Bloodletting was counterindicated for fever, which was "like a pot boiling; it is requisite to reduce the fire and not diminish the liquid in the vessel, if we wish to cure the patient'" (Williams 1848, 2:184). Few observers went any deeper, given the frequent Western conviction that bloodletting rid the body of dangerous excess blood, relieving it of a pathological plethora. One sees the contrast particularly in the Western assumption that a hot plethora could cause fevers by contributing to biliousness in the blood (Kuriyama 1999). Failure to bleed was thereby directly linked to fever.

Some observers saw only deficits. "In surgical operations," wrote Wood (1830, 153), "they are entirely at a loss." Gutzlaff (1838) agreed. Wounds were sewn and dressed with ointments, supplemented by dietary recommendations. Downing reported that the Chinese disliked "the knife," never let blood, neglected fractures, left bullets in wounds, sucked out poisons, did not use cupping, and opened abscesses "often injudiciously" (Bird 1842b, 806). Even so, one writer reported that, while out for a stroll, he observed a practitioner using bamboo instead of cupping glasses: "The operator had the man bent down . . . with his hands on his knees, while he himself was applying the bamboo to his back. One application had already been made; very little blood, however, seemed to have been drawn; but I could not perceive in what way the scarification was performed, or whether indeed there was any such operation . . . The operator seemed a mere charlatan; and the only peculiarities which I noticed about him, were his broad hat, the brim full six feet in circumference, and a roll of European newspapers" (Anonymous 1835b, 44). The purpose of the roll of newspapers went unexamined, the practitioner relegated to the status of street charlatan for no apparent reason. Chinese patients with access to Western hospitals did not necessarily find them any more credible or use them. One man chose an herbal prescription instead. It worked. He was reported as saying, "Inglishman sabe outside pigeon . . . Chinaman sabe inside pigeon" (Lay 1841b, 326–27). The English know the business of externals; the Chinese, internal matters.

An Emerging Body of Sources

One exception to Western dismissal of Chinese surgery involved acupuncture. Gutzlaff (1837) wrote that it was "performed by silver needles, which are stuck into the flesh and twisted round, whilst the physician compresses the slight wound thus made" (169). In one of the few reports of direct observation, Lay (1841a) described an ambulatory doctor who clearly merged acupuncture and bleeding:

> [He] drew some needles from a paper, with an air of grave preparation, and after rubbing some . . . powder upon his own thigh, stuck one of the needles into it . . . The next step in the process was the selection of a few seeds from a paper parcel, putting them in his mouth and giving the remnant to the patient, as a pledge of his generosity. While the seeds were undergoing a process of mastication by themselves, he took a pair of wooden cylinders, and, after holding a lighted roll of paper within them, clapped them upon the breast of the old man. After they had remained a few minutes upon the spot, they were removed, and left behind them two raised *areolae,* or bumps, which the doctor, after sipping a little water, rubbed the seeds, by this time well reduced by maceration and grinding. He next pricked the bumps with the needle which had been all the while sticking in his own flesh. To extract the blood, he applied his mouth, and drew with such violence, that the old man began to heave a sigh, and the crowd to respond by a look of anxiety. (207–208)

The doctor pressed around the spot to direct the flow of blood, put a pitch plaster between the two bumps and, after rinsing out his mouth, repeated the treatment on the patient's back. Lay remarked that actual incisions would have extracted more blood, rendering "real service" (208).

Rev. George Smith (1847b) met a Dr. Chang, whose "peculiar department of Chinese surgery was acupuncture, by which he professed an ability to perform cures for rheumatism and similar diseases. At the time of our visit, he was eking out his scanty means of subsistence by instructing three pupils" (213–214). Chang's poverty may have reflected acupuncture's standing. In 1822 an imperial edict prohibited the Imperial Medical Academy from teaching or practicing acupuncture, as inappropriate for gentleman-scholars (Andrews 1999, 2). Though it regulated only the Academy, the edict reflected elite sentiment.

Acupuncture gradually became a byword among European and American surgeons. To understand the range of representations of acupuncture by physicians and other authors during this period, I reviewed all volumes from 1805 through 1848 of French, English, Irish, Scotch, German, Italian, and American medical journals in the Harvard University library system. I also reviewed medical dictionaries, encyclopedias, dissertations, textbooks, and books dedicated to the topic during this period. The sole inclusion criterion was reference to "acupuncture or" "acupuncturation." (I address "electro-puncture" separately.) I located 248 sources: eighty-six primary articles; 112 reviews of these articles (some reproducing substantial sections or the entirety of the primary article); five encyclopedia articles; eight dictionary definitions; seven books or treatises; nine sections in medical textbooks; ten sections in books other than textbooks; and eleven dissertations. I then developed data fields based on issues addressed in the sources.

In addition to citation information, these fields included: whether or not the article was a review or reprint of an earlier source (and, if it was, the original source); the physicians using acupuncture in the cases described; a definition of acupuncture; acknowledgment of Chinese origins; European sources cited; the treatment setting; patient information (name, gender, age, occupation, and social class); the chief complaint and its cause(s); other therapies tried; the particulars of the treatment (number of needles; number of treatments; kind of needles used; point location; and method, depth, and length of insertion); resulting sensations; conditions determined to be treatable or untreatable; explanation of acupuncture's "action"; modifications to the practice; outcome; physician and patient comments on the process or results; and any other miscellaneous notes.

Acupuncture was explicitly identified with the Chinese and often the Japanese, although some surgeons doubted "the Chinese marvels reported by travelers" (Bedor 1812, 150). Others argued that, given China's medical history, "we cannot but conclude, that observation and experience must therefore have brought to light many important remedies, of which, however, we are almost entirely ignorant" (Editor 1821a, 431). James Morss Churchill was persuaded by successful outcomes "witnessed by European spectators on its native soil, and at length experienced in our own hemisphere; and even, latterly, in our own country" (Churchill 1821, 5; see also Churchill 1825). In 1825, Pierre Pelletan Jr. (1825a, 75) reported hearing of recent operations in England by a Chinese doctor. James Copland (1825) speculated that Pelletan meant Churchill. The matter remains unclear, as no other sources discussed a Chinese physician at work in England.

Ten Rhijne and Kaempfer remained primary sources. Surgeon Louis Berlioz—regularly credited with introducing acupuncture into European practice—concluded that both had rightly praised it (Berlioz 1816). Both were repeatedly cited and excerpted. Other surgeons reiterated Berlioz's surprise that, although acupuncture had long been known in Europe, no one appeared to have tested it (Churchill 1821; Haime 1819). Coley went uncited. Dujardin and Vicq-d'Azyr, on the other hand, were cited disproportionately often, despite their own dependence on ten Rhijne and Kaempfer. Only Dantu (1826) showed familiarity with discussions from the travel narratives.[38] Only Sarlandière employed a translated Japanese text—*Traité de la médecine des Japonais et des Chinois* (Treatise on the Medicine of the Japanese and the Chinese)—characterizing it as "the medical code which, among these peoples, is as revered as are the aphorisms of Hippocrates in the west" (Sarlandière 1825, 174). One editor called it "a curious Japanese manuscript" (Editor 1827g, 192).

Berlioz began experimenting in 1810, not publishing until 1816. In the interim, Bédor (1812, 149) asserted that acupuncture had never been used in France. M. Nacquart (1812) disagreed, having encountered an unpublished manuscript on the subject—possibly Berlioz's. Others positioned themselves as first in a given country or city—a Mr. Scott in England (Churchill 1821), a Monsieur Mareschal (1825) in Nantes. By 1825 Pelletan could trace a history of European practitioners and publications (Pelletan 1825a, 74). The list grew, and included France, England, Ireland, Scotland, Italy, Spain, Germany, and the United States. Of the European authors, Berlioz was most frequently cited, followed by ten Rhijne and then Kaempfer. Haime, Cloquet, Churchill, Vicq-d'Azyr, Dujardin, Demours, and Bidloo were also cited, in descending order of frequency. Other practitioners received occasional mention (Churchill's colleague Scott; Sarlandière, Velpeau, Morand, Elliotson, Pelletan, Dantu, and Bédor); still others were noted in passing. Some surgeons—like Churchill's colleague "Mr. Jukes," and Bretonneau, who performed experiments on animals— did not publish but were discussed by others.

Influential works were translated, as when Bache translated Morand's dissertation: "The growing importance of the remedy, and the great attention bestowed upon it in France" would make it "an acceptable present to American physicians" (Morand 1825b, n.p.). Sources were cited in medical dictionaries (Dunglison 1833, 1:184), encyclopedias (Elliotson [1845]1848a), and textbooks like Dunglison's *New Remedies* (1839, 28) and Elliotson's *Principles and Practice of Medicine* (1839).

France led the way in research and publications, followed by England, Italy, and the United States. Despite Edinburgh's importance in the Western medical world, Scotch journals published only four articles and two reviews. It has been argued that American interest did not surface until after 1820 (Bodemer n.d.). The same, however, was true for European countries other than France. Medical attention highlighted acupuncture between 1823 and 1826; in subsequent years there were fewer and fewer articles and reviews.

Journals exchanged issues, reproducing or summarizing articles and case histories. John Hamilton, for example, learned of surgeon-anatomist Jules-Germain Cloquet—the first to conduct extensive acupuncture trials (Editor 1827g, 193)—from reading a review of Dantu's book (Hamilton 1831). American journals circulated European medical advances (Anonymous 1820) by reviewing European journals, often within only months of their publication. This review process was practiced by medical journals throughout the United States, including journals published in Massachusetts, Philadelphia, New York, Louisiana, Georgia, Ohio, and Missouri. For example, as shown below, Pelletan's article on the history, outcomes, and theories of acupuncture (Pelletan 1825a) was followed by review articles, which were followed by reviews of the review articles:

Pierre Pelletan, fils [1825a] Notice sur l'acupuncture, contenant son historique, ses effets et sa théorie. *Revue médicale française et étrangère* 1:74–103. [primary article]

Pierre Pelletan, fils [1825b] On Acupuncture. *Medico-Chirurgical Review*, n.s. 3:257–264. [review in British journal]

   M. Pelletan [1826] On Acupuncture. *Ohio Medical Repository* 1(6):23–24. [review of British source]

Editor 1825d Acupuncturation. *Boston Medical Intelligencer* 3(3):16. [review of primary article]

James Copland [1825] On Acupuncture, &c. *London Medical Repository, Monthly Journal, and Review*, n.s. 3:340–345, 432–433. [review of primary article]

Editor [1825q] Pelletan, Bally and others on Acupuncture. *Monthly Journal of Medicine* 5(January–June):314–318. [American reprint of Copland, without his discussion of a dispute between two physicians]

Editor [1826f] Professor Pelletan Fils on acupuncture. *Ohio Medical Repository* 1(8):32. [This journal first published a reprint of a British review, above, and then this even briefer summary.]

Reviews both reprinted extensive excerpts and summarized content, the brevity of the review allowing one to see what was considered significant data. The importance of such details lies in what they reveal about patterns of dissemination and cross-fertilization of medical knowledge. For example, the United States produced little original acupuncture-related research but outstripped all other countries, combined, in reviews (sixty-three all told, as compared with twenty-one from France, twenty-nine from England, and a handful from other countries). Proportionately, these numbers held true throughout the period, indicating the reach and range of knowledge related to acupuncture.

Settings and Patients

European discussions located acupuncture almost entirely in hospital or dispensary (outpatient) settings. French hospitals included St. Louis, Hôtel Dieu, Hôpital de la Pitié, Hôpital de Charité, the military hospital of Val de Grâce, and the hospital of Caen. English ones included St. Thomas and the dispensaries at St. George and St. James. In Ireland, patients were treated at Meath Hospital, and in Italy, at

Turin Hospital. We do not know how many doctors visited affluent patients at home. Elliotson, for example, described using "*acupuncture very extensively, both in private and at St. Thomas's Hospital*" (Editor 1828a, 473).

Frontspiece plates in copies of some British medical journals containing articles about acupuncture indicate that they originally belonged to Boston physician John Warren. Given the American medical elite's familiarity with European hospitals, and their exposure to such journals, physicians like Warren might have been expected to experiment with acupuncture in hospitals, too. Those who may have, did not generally publish. Bache, who treated prisoners, was the exception. Although American almshouse and voluntary hospitals sometimes served as educational settings, most American medical schools provided only lecture-based curricula, clinical experience waiting until one studied with a preceptor (Williams 1976). American surgeons, therefore, were relatively less likely to encounter acupuncture in their training, and more likely to read about it or observe it practiced abroad.

Who were the patients? Using only the primary-source articles to avoid duplications, I identified 334 original cases from Europe and the United States.[39] Male patients (226) outnumbered female (94). (Eight other adult cases do not specify gender; two cases refer to "infants" and four to "children.") Most cases included patients' ages either as a specific year or as a category—"middle aged," "young girl," "man of advanced age." Most patients ranged from their twenties to their forties.[40] An elderly woman treated by William Markley Lee was the gardener of a friend and the only African American reported. Because the case occurred in South Carolina, she was probably a slave. The absence of racial detail for other cases suggests they involved European or European American patients. Most male patients were tradesmen, servants, soldiers, or sailors. Women patients occupied analogous social roles.[41] Only rarely did physicians describe cases involving prostitutes, and these were in relation to venereal pain.

Of Needles

Most authors quoted ten Rhijne and Kaempfer on acupuncture needles—gold or silver; four inches long; slender, polished, and tempered; spiraled ivory handles; a copper tube the size of a goose quill as a gauge; an ivory hammer with thimble-like indentations and a hollow handle containing needles. Only Guersent (1826b) commented that Chinese needles were "not . . . always of gold or silver . . . most often they are of steel and come from Holland" (553). Western physicians generally used steel—Haime (1819) thought the modest physician disdained gold or silver. Dantu (1826) observed that almost everyone carried needles and, as Lee (1836a, 1836b, 1837a, 1837b) commented, any household could furnish them.

Needles ran from an inch and a half to four or five inches long. Elliotson (1844, 174n) recommended polishing and sharpening with an emery-bag. Handles were commonly added, made of Spanish wax, sealing wax, a piece of catheter, lead, cork, or sometimes ivory. Cloquet originally used ivory handles, saying that his needles were "no different from those of the Chinese except in that the metal was steel" (Dantu 1826, 211). Over time he adopted tempered steel needles (Meyranx 1825a). Sarlandière, eager to be authentic, complained that others "use common needles, of an inappropriate metal, and with which fairly serious accidents have already happened. The needles of the Japanese that I have in my possession are formed of an extremely fine, straight metal shaft, with the caliber, form, and elasticity of a fine boar's bristle. This shaft is composed of several metals, and the amalgam that results seems similar to that of the gong of the Chinese . . . [like those] in the museum in Madrid, and which I have thoroughly examined." The amalgam included gold, silver, and copper. The needles were three inches long, with a handle "nine lines [3/4 inch] long, over a half-line [1/24 inch] wide, ending in a small button."[42] Fine grooves made the handle easier to roll between one's fingers (Sarlandière 1825, 174–175).

Few sought such needles. One writer said that because gold and silver needles were thicker and duller, they afforded little advantage (Editor 1827g). Churchill (1821) announced that his needles—designed by Edward Jukes, surgeon accoucheur to the Westminster Medical Institution—were sold at Mr. Blackwell's Bedford-Court, or Mr. Laundy's at St. Thomas's Street. Mlle Delaunay's, at the office of *Annales de la médecine physiologique*, carried Sarlandière's. A case held five, with a small guide tube. Sarlandière (1825) added, "The same proportions of metal as those that make up the indigenous Japanese needle have been found by the artisan who has made up these needles after the same model" (175). Five with gold handles cost 47 francs; five with silver were 26. In a pinch, one ad-libbed. As John Renton (1830) wrote, "Not having my case of needles with me, I used half-a-dozen common ones of different sizes" (103).

Missionary discussions appeared during the 1830s and '40s. By then, most Western physicians had ceased researching acupuncture. There were, therefore, few eagerly awaiting readers when Lay presented a paper on Chinese surgery (Wakley 1840a, 1840b) or published on acupuncture (Lay 1841b). These pieces, like his *The Chinese as They Are,* reviewed in the *Lancet* (Wakley 1841), not only discussed the nine needles but included drawings (see Figure 26). Lay (1841a, 229) explained that each needle had specific uses. The explanation came too late for the height of the discussion.

Point Location

Most practitioners administered "a single acupuncturation" sometimes followed by a second. Further treatments occurred less frequently.[43] However, "a single acupuncturation" could mean (1) one needle inserted either once or multiple times, or (2) one treatment involving multiple needles. Hamilton cited Renton using "as many as ten" and Elliotson, "a considerable number" (Hamilton 1831, 446). Elliotson (1844, 173), in contrast, described preferring one needle, left for

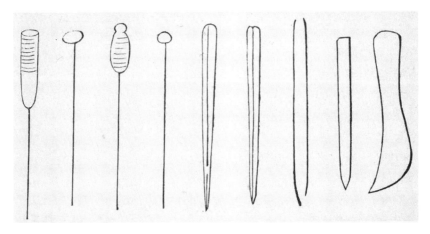

Figure 26. The nine needles. George Tradescant Lay, *The Chinese as They Are,* 1841. Widener Library of the Harvard College Library.

some time and then moved. "If the patient does not bear the needle well," he wrote, "it is at once withdrawn: but if he does, and the disease proves obstinate, it is introduced two, three, four, five, or six times" (Elliotson 1848a, 55).

Some physicians experimented on animals—Bretonneau (Editor 1820a) and Pierre Béclard (Académie 1825a) used puppies. Such experiments appeared to demonstrate the safety of inserting needles into arteries and nerves, contrary to ten Rhijne's and Kaempfer's arguments (Guersent 1826b). Antonio Carraro (1826) held a kitten under water until it went still. Plunging a needle into its heart, he resuscitated it, suggesting that acupuncture might offset asphyxiation or drowning.

Cloquet inserted needles into the chest, liver region, stomach, and intestines (Dantu 1826). Elliotson (1830a) protested sticking them into joints or below the knees. Mr. Brett (1831, 1832), a British surgeon in India, disagreed, having treated "natives" for rheumatism by inserting needles in joints (a case of globalization, where a British physician practiced Chinese acupuncture on Indian patients). Still, Dunglison (1839) avoided larger nerves and arteries, the heart, stomach, and intestines.

Many surgeons used pain-point acupuncture, needling the pain as it moved from one site to another, the shifts construed as signs of efficacy (Haime 1819; Elliotson 1830a; Longhi 1839; Emiliani 1845a). Doctors using Kaempfer cited the *senki* case, with its three rows of three points (Churchill 1821; Dantu 1826; Elliotson 1848a). Béclard (1821) believed the Chinese inserted needles randomly, avoiding nerves, tendons, and vessels. Haime (1819) wrote that they pricked the head for headaches, diseases characterized by stupor, ophthalmia, and apoplexy, and the breast, back, and abdomen for pain, dysentery, anorexia, hysterical affections, cholera morbus, and iliac passion.[44]

Readers of Dujardin had seen ten Rhijne's drawings; the drawings led Dantu (1826) to conclude that one could insert needles over the body's whole surface. Von Klaproth commended Sarlandière's interest in Chinese sources, omitting his own role in helping Sarlandière acquire the *jingluo* figure and acupuncture treatise from the papers of Isaac Titsingh, a surgeon with the Dutch East India Company who had headed the company's Deshima offices from 1779 on and from 1794 served as Dutch ambassador to Beijing. Entitled *Tchin kieou ki pi tchhao*

(Transcription of the Best Secrets for the Use of the Needle and the Caustic), the treatise had been composed in 1780 by a Chinese doctor, "Tai-tchoung-youan" (von Klaproth 1825, 374–375).[45] Sarlandière described having made three drawings of the figurine, two of which were lost, forcing him to delay publishing his book.[46] "M. Rehmann, physician to the emperor of Russia, had told me in 1817 or 1818 about having seen my lost drawings at the home of one of the doctors of the king of Prussia; I don't know how they ended up with him, and I waited for the occasion to be able to recover them, since the recent vogue of acupuncture had caused me to research it" (Sarlandière 1825, iv). Eventually he redid the drawings, without which the treatise "would lose all its value" (iv). (See Figure 27.) Numbering all 337 points, he added a corresponding romanized list of Chinese names and an index locating clusters of points. Points 1 through 20, for example, were on the side of the face. The treatise described 110 conditions, each detailing groups of points to needle in relation to specific conditions. Each point was given by both name and number, allowing one to locate it on Sarlandière's meridian diagram. For example: "*Nitisju* is an unexpected [and] very dangerous indisposition, often followed by death, without prompt [medical] help: if one perceived that a numbness in the shoulder set in, followed by pain in the chest and swelling in the face, one would prick *Kensy*[265] (4 lines [1/3 inch] deep), *Kioktje*[132] (7 lines [slightly over 1/2 inch]), and *Sjaktak*[131] (3 lines [1/4 inch]) doing, in addition to the pricking, a strong bloodletting" (106).

Finally one could study point combinations, identify their locations on the body, and link them to actual conditions, as defined from within Chinese medicine—together with at least a basic description of symptoms to assist the clinician in linking Chinese and Western diagnoses. Yet the unprecedented level of detail failed to persuade. Physician Guérin de Mamers (1825) wrote, "The manuscript . . . is composed of 110 aphorisms, where are found displayed, unhappily in a very obscure manner, the state of medicine among one part of the peoples of Asia" (283). De Claubry (1825) commented: "Here is a sample: 'in jaundice, one pricks *tjuquan* and *riomon;* in pain in the kidneys, one pricks *etju* and *bozo,* following which, one burns moxa on *fatsriu-no-kets.*' All these Japanese names designate different parts of the body, corresponding anatomically to certain organs, or rather, the places upon which experience has taught that revulsive methods

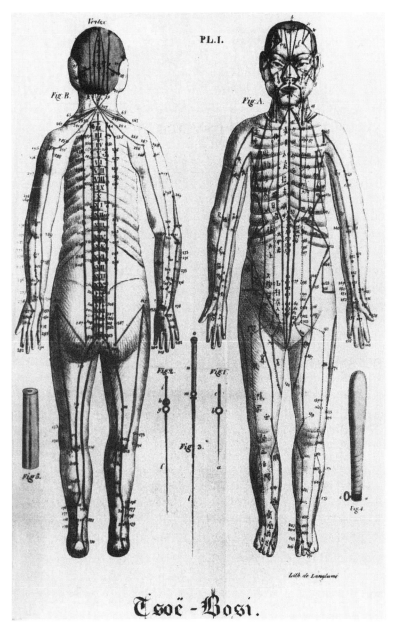

Figure 27. Tsoë-Bosi. Jean Baptiste Sarlandière, *Mémoires sur l'électro-puncture*, 1825. (Old Negative no. 72–225.) Courtesy of the National Library of Medicine, History of Medicine Division.

must be brought [to bear]" (124).[47] He dismissed the book, ignoring Sarlandière's painstakingly assembled lists, tables, drawings, and prescriptions.

Years later, Lay (1841b) connected the *jingluo* to acupuncture. "Each important spot along the course of the internal vessels," he wrote, "has its particular designation; and hence the native physiology and anatomy serve as guides to the surgical operator as they do among us" (238–239). If moxa or a needle could not be applied directly to the affected site, where should it be placed? Lay acknowledged that the Chinese physician studied such questions, but "so refined and recondite are his reasonings, and so great is the natural hebetude [dullness or lethargy] and tardiness of my own mind, that I seldom feel much inclination to follow him" (328). Here Lay touched directly on the practice of inserting needles at a distance from a painful site. The heyday of acupuncture research had passed, however; the connection was not pursued.

The Operation

Portrayals of acupuncture mallets led Berlioz (1816) to explain that he instead rolled needles between his fingers, introducing them gradually, pausing to inquire about the patient's comfort. His approach influenced Churchill (1821), who feared a mallet might break the needle or cause greater pain. Similar concerns led Cloquet to stretch the skin to prevent it from twisting around the needle (Morand 1825b). Sarlandière (1825) used a glass guide tube, again alluding to contemporary Chinese practice: "One next taps the head of the needle with the tip of the index finger (the modern Chinese have abandoned the hammer that they used to use), just until the handle is engaged in the guide, which one then withdraws, to continue tapping it until the point of the instrument penetrates to the depth desired" (175). Wallace (1827) positioned moxa at the top of a needle, which conducted the heat—also a practice in China. The combination functioned as a "local tonic," acting "on the immediate seat of the disease" (81). A Prof. Recamier modified a needle holder developed by Cloquet, mounting needles of different lengths on a "port-stone." Held by a screw, the needle fit into a groove, allowing the operator to adjust its length (Morand 1825b).

A. Demours attached a syringe to a cupping glass and pumped out the air, creating a vacuum. A shaft descended through the glass. Its base contained either a single-bladed lancet or four blades, which one plunged down to let blood (Demours 1819a, 1819b). Few other physicians identified acupuncture with bloodletting. Indeed, Berlioz (1816) believed that if blood was released, the effectiveness was nullified. Haime (1819, 29n) suggested striking acupuncture from the list of evacuants. Churchill (1821, 8–9) agreed, "not only by the consequences of the operation, but by the manner in which it is performed, and the nature of the diseases to which it is applied." One American construed acupuncture as a Chinese *alternative* to bloodletting (Editor 1823h).

Depths of insertion varied. Ten Rhijne had described needles as lightly inserted in afflicted sites. One could insert them more deeply in adults than in children and elders, and in plump persons more than in thin (Morand 1825; Dantu 1826). Based on Kaempfer, some surgeons advocated inserting to a depth of "a few lines." John Tweedale (1823, 313) passed a thread around the needle, "at rather less than a quarter of an inch from the point" to control the depth. More surgeons preferred three-quarters of an inch to a full inch or an inch and a half, or in some cases two or three inches. Few penetrated the stomach (Berlioz 1816; Haime 1819). Only Sarlandière (1825) defined the Chinese measure *sun:* "the length of the second phalange of the middle finger on the left hand (on men, and of the right hand for women) of the person upon whom the operation is to be practiced" (102n).

Elliotson (1839) argued that outcomes depended less on the depth of insertion than on its duration. Pelletan (1825a) read Kaempfer as recommending a duration of one or two breaths, and ten Rhijne, thirty. Accordingly, some surgeons left needles in for less than a minute, or from three to four minutes. Others chose between fifteen minutes to an hour, up to three hours, and even between seven to ten hours. Cloquet was credited with the innovation of leaving needles in for hours and sometimes days (Dantu 1826). Elliotson reported nine days (Hamilton 1831, 510). In such cases, one editor recommended insertion up to the wax head and covering with "an adhesive plaster" to prevent the clothing from pulling it out (Editor 1827g, 194). "One immediately understands," added de Claubry (1825, 103), "how this procedure differs from the old method, and must have different effects."

Additional modifications appeared. Military surgeon George Bushe (1832) once used "a red hot needle" to puncture arteries, for aneurisms. (Staff surgeons prevented him from repeating the procedure on another patient.) Surgeon William Home (1839, 1840) used an "acupuncture" needle to probe for a bullet surrounded by a "tumor." M. Wiesel described a fracture that resisted healing. He introduced two needles into the "false joint," leaving them for six days, then removing them due to pain and swelling. He reinserted them fifteen days later. After six weeks, the fracture had healed, which he attributed to the needles (Anonymous 1844a; Editor 1844h, 1845c, 1845d, 1847j). Medical journals published these accounts under the rubric of acupuncture, suggesting the minimalist approach at work in classifications.

The Chinese Apply It to Everything

Berlioz (1816) observed that the Chinese sometimes used acupuncture prophylactically. According to Sarlandière (1825), they applied it to "rheumatismal" pain, gout, and violent colics, as well as vomiting, and diarrhea, convulsions, paralysis, hysteria, syncope (fainting), and all "nervous" afflictions. Elliotson initially used it for such cases (1827; see Editor 1828c). Twenty years later, he had developed a more varied list: "In tetanus, convulsions of all kinds, apoplexy, gout, rheumatism, swelled testicle and gonorrhoea, and in fevers both intermittent and continued, it is also celebrated among them; enjoying credit, like all remedies of undoubted efficacy in certain diseases, for power which it does not possess over others" (Elliotson 1848a, 55).

It has been argued that Western practice largely involved pain-point application, bearing little resemblance to Chinese applications (Haller 1973; Veith 1975). The particulars reveal a more complex scenario. "Pain" was a broad category, covering specifics that might now be categorized differently. It included chronic, uterine, ophthalmic, and cancer-related pain, and pain caused by hip-joint disease, diseases of the muscular structures, bruises, or sprains. Various authors cited Chinese applications for abdominal and intestinal conditions—especially colics, including cholera morbus, iliac passion, diarrhea, dysentery, flatulence, flux, gastroenteritis, inflammatory irritations, vomiting, and anorexia (understood as a want of appetite). Following suit, Western practitioners reported using acupuncture for old abdominal pains, cramps, chronic inflammation of the digestive organs and intestines, gastralgia, and phlegmasia (a chronic intestinal problem). Each of these conditions was classified as a variety of pain.

The Chinese were characterized as applying acupuncture to "affections" and "morbid action."[48] Western correlates included chronic diseases and organic disorders. One could virtually map the body with acupuncture. The Chinese, for example, were thought to use it for headaches, including cephalalgia; coryza—runny nose from a cold, and the heaviness that sometimes accompanied it; and head and abdominal congestions. Western applications included not only headaches in general, but also specific varieties—hemicrania, pericrania, and migraines, as well as pleurisy.[49] Cases detailed treatments for pain in the neck, chest, pericardium, uterus, kidneys, back, and lower back. Shoulders, arms, hands, every part of the hip, leg, and foot, and even the sites of amputations were included. Two cases of paralysis resulted in cure.

Occasionally, women sought help for pain related to venereal disease. Morand (1825) described one woman who, "aware of her disease, and driven to despair . . . determined to destroy herself, and, seizing a razor, inflicted a dangerous wound on herself in the neck" (75). She had syphilitic genital lesions; the physician inserted a needle there. The pain was relieved for six days, but returned; then she was treated with "baths of the vapour of cinnabar" (76).

"Rheumatism" and "neuralgia" represented two broad pain-related conditions, linked with Chinese use of acupuncture for "nervous affections." Beginning with Berlioz and Haime, doctors applied acupuncture to cases related to nerves. One medical dictionary explained: "Rheumatism is distinguished by *acute* and *chronic*. The acute is preceded by shivering, heat, thirst, and frequent pulse; after which the pain commences, and soon fixes on the joints. The chronic rheumatism is distinguished by pain in the joints, without pyrexia, and is divided into three species; *lumbago,* affecting the loins; *sciatica,* affecting the hip; and *arthrodynia,* or pains in the joints" (Hooper 1825, 1038). Many pain-related conditions clustered under the rubric of rheumatism or, sometimes, lumbago and sciatica. Of the 334 cases I located, for example, sixty-one were variations on rheumatism, and ten, on lumbago. According to Gutzlaff (1837), however, although lumbago was common among the Chinese, especially among the poor, Chinese doctors treated it "by putting adhesive plaster, composed of a variety of ingredients, upon the spine" (161).

Classificatory ambiguities appear in relation to sciatica, which is defined sometimes as a form of rheumatism, and sometimes as a form of neuralgia. Of the fifty-four neuralgia cases I found, twenty-eight involved sciatica, also called *"névralgie sciatique,"* or "sciatic neuralgia" (Morand 1825; Dantu 1826). Another common neuralgia was *tic douloureux,* sometimes simply known as "the tic," a form of facial neuralgia causing excruciating pain (twelve neuralgia cases involved *tic*). Western doctors found acupuncture effective for rheumatism. Lee wrote, "I frequently employ it, much to the surprize of my patients, from the trifling pain which it causes, and the promptness of the relief; and equally to the astonishment of the attendants, who rarely have faith in the remedy, until proved by positive demonstration" (Lee 1836a, 132; see also Namias 1840).

Elliotson (1830b) differentiated between rheumatisms eased by heat and those worsened by it. Acupuncture, he said, benefited only cases "attended by coldness or relieved by heat" (337) and was best used in "rheumatism of parts." Hamilton (1831, 447) countered that Drs. Renton and Graves had not found this distinction germane. M. Lallemand, of Montpelier, used acupuncture to good effect with neuralgia, but found it ineffective for rheumatic pain (Editor 1843a).

But use did not stop here. The Chinese reportedly used acupuncture for ophthalmia (an eye inflammation), lippitude (soreness or blearedness of the eyes), and cataracts. Western doctors, in turn, applied it to cases of "eye illnesses," ophthalmia, amaurosis (a partial or total loss of sight), diplopy (double or triple vision), and some neuralgia-related cases of blindness. The Chinese were said to use it for fevers; Western physicians tried it for intermittent fevers, phrenitis, and erysipelas (a febrile disease that caused skin lesions).[50]

Where the Chinese were thought to use acupuncture for cephalitis (a brain inflammation) and pneumonia (a pulmonary inflammation), Western practitioners tried it for inflammations including phlegmasia, phlebitis, carditis (of the heart), periostitis (of the periosteum), and pleurisy. The Chinese were said to treat muscular "contractures," spasms, convulsions, and epilepsy. Western surgeons extended acupuncture to chronic hiccoughs, muscle contractions, spasms, palsy, and chorea.[51]

If the Chinese were said to use acupuncture for paralysis, tetanus, and tetanus-related conditions such as emprosthotonos (where the body is drawn forward by excessive action of the anterior muscles of the trunk) and opisthotonos (spasm of the muscles of the neck, back, and legs, in which the body is bent backward), Western doctors applied it to paralysis, paraplegia and hemiplegia, and tetanus. The Chinese were described as using it for dizziness, syncope, coma and comatose affections, somnolence, and soporose conditions (characterized by morbid sleep or stupor); I found one Western case using it for comata, a soporose affection. The Chinese were thought to treat tympany, a morbid swelling classified as a tumor.[52] Western users applied it to other swellings (also categorized as "tumors"), including erectile tumors, aneurisms, and ganglions.[53] If the Chinese treated testicular swellings, Western doctors addressed cases of inguinal hernias, inflamed testicles, neuralgic conditions in the spermatic cord, and varices (varicose veins; Hooper 1825). Even affective problems were addressed. The Chinese were said to treat cases of hysteria and melancholy; in two cases, Morand (1825b) treated hysteria and grief-induced pain.

Some Western doctors went beyond their understanding of Chinese applications, experimenting in cases of toothache, sore throats and swollen glands, asthma, dyspnea (laborious breathing), "suffocations," convulsive cough, and whooping cough. Cloquet (1826) twice attempted to reverse mercury poisoning, without success. Dunglison and Elliotson, presumably in the interest of thoroughness, cited the horror story of a Parisian midwife who, in the eighteenth century, was reported to have murdered infants by inserting a needle into the infant's brain as the child emerged from the womb, with the intent "of peopling heaven more and more" (Dunglison 1833, 17; Elliotson 1848a, 56). Léopold Deslandes (1842) and François Lallemand ([1847]1848) applied it against "spermatorrhea" (involuntary semen emission, often while sleeping)—including the insertion of needles into the scrotum, in part as a deterrent.

Some Western physicians also used needles to treat different kinds of fluid retention, or dropsy, including edema, anasarca, ascites (in the abdomen), and hydrocele (an edema in the testicle or scrotum). One or more punctures allowed the gradual release of fluid. Such cases blurred the lines with the older practice known as tapping, which also involved inserting a needle to release fluid. Elliotson argued a thin connection with Chinese practice, writing: "The most obvious purpose of this operation, is to allow the escape through the skin of the fluid of oedema or anasarca; or of the blood, when superficially accumulated; but,—from an idea that disorders arise from a kind of subtle and acrid vapour pent up,—it has been had recourse to by the Chinese, for the purpose of giving vent to this vapour, from time immemorial" (Elliotson 1839, 1080).

The Chinese were also thought to use acupuncture for conditions related to drunkenness, apoplexy, and verminose affections and related pain, and for wind-related illnesses. As we saw in Chapter 1, winds represented a way of talking about external influences that could injure systems already in a state of imbalance, as well as evil winds that harmed one's system. This heading included illnesses dependent on the presence of malignant vapors (harmful *qi,* which Western physicians might have construed as miasmas), as well as intestinal conditions caused by winds. Dunglison (1833) expressed the closest Western analogy: "Winds exert considerable influence on the animal economy; acting by their temperature, which necessarily modifies that of the circumambient air, as well as by their moisture or dryness; and by the emanations of different kinds, which they transport to greater or less distances" (2:435). Wind, that is, could cause illness.

The evidence suggests that acupuncture was broadly characterized as being used for pain. However, "pain" had a more comprehensive meaning at the time, and it is clear that the application of acupuncture approximated early nineteenth-century Western understandings of Chinese usage more extensively than has previously been thought. With experience, Western doctors arrived at their own understanding, too, that acupuncture "only suit[ed] particular cases, and you have to make a very careful diagnosis, or you will be disappointed in it" (Elliotson 1832a, 692). Nevertheless, in important respects Western practitioners worked closely from what they recognized as Chinese practice, even when they introduced modifications.

Case Experiences

Some patients found treatments painful or ineffective (Morand 1825b). Lee (1836a) described a man who "suffered so much from the extraction [of the needle], that no persuasion could induce him to submit to any variation of the experiment" (131). Patients who experienced partial results sometimes waited before returning (Banks 1831). Churchill (1821) described one man who could not believe the relief would last. "I heard nothing of him for two days, when his daughter called on me, and informed me that her father was quite well, and had resumed his employment as a wine-merchant's cellar-man" (373).

Some patients learned about acupuncture from others. One such man sent for T. W. Wansbrough "to come to him immediately, and bring my 'needles' with me'" (Wansbrough 1826, 846). Patients who recovered suddenly, expressed astonishment (Meyranx 1825a). Thion (1826) described a patient who "said to me with amazement, 'I'm no longer suffering'" (9). Wansbrough (1828) reported an emotional scene. When the patient's wife heard he was free of pain, "her eyes were filled with tears of grateful joy, and her hands were clasped in wonder and astonishment; the old man himself, when he returned home, 'cried for joy,' exclaiming, 'He has cured me!'" (367). Other patients found it difficult to believe their doctor had not "employed a magical procedure" (Berlioz 1816, 308), witchcraft (Morand 1825), "magical effects" (Wansbrough 1826, 847), or enchantment (Bergamaschi 1827; Editor 1841a).

Few cases described upper-class patients. One involved the Earl of Egremont, "a martyr to rheumatism." Hearing of acupuncture's successes, he summoned a surgeon, who inserted two needles for twenty minutes. For the first time in weeks, the Earl slept well. As one of the surgeon's friends told the tale, "Filled with joy, he gave the fortunate practitioner a check for a large sum, sent him home with post horses, and that day bestowed on one of his favourite racers the name of 'Acupuncture.' The event made my friend's fortune" (Kingdon 1833, 817–818).

Surgeons occasionally described receiving treatment. Renton (1830), who suffered from rheumatism, wrote, "The introduction into the muscle of four needles for three minutes, at once completely removed the affection" (105). Similarly, Lee (1836a) found that after fifteen minutes, he was free of rheumatic pain and could move his arm with ease. Months passed before the symptoms returned.

Of the 334 cases I reviewed, 304 specified an outcome. Thirty ended in failure; 12 provided partial, temporary cures; 41 were partial but lasting; and 220 were both complete *and* lasting. Accidents occasionally occurred. Needles sometimes broke (Wakley 1830) or were inadvertently inserted all the way (Berlioz 1816), one episode proving fatal (Editor 1827g). Even when acupuncture yielded effects, there could be side effects. In nineteen cases, for example, patients experienced syncope; Cloquet estimated that one in thirty of his patients fainted (Morand 1825). Lee (1836a) commented, "This uncommon symptom would have caused me some alarm, had I not previously met with such a case in a French journal" (31). One of Peyron's patients experienced violent contractions, and ten minutes of delirium "such as the magnetizers are pleased to depict" (Peyron 1826, 279). Even so, De Claubry (1825) decided, "If experience confirms only a quarter of the hopes that the first trials have conceived, it will be necessary to acknowledge that we possess one of the most energetic therapeutic methods" (103). Side effects meant little when weighed against cure.

Acupuncture's Action

Nobody succeeded in resolving how or why acupuncture worked. Some investigators focused on phenomena generated by treatments—a reddened areola accompanied by slight swelling (Thion 1826), or a burning feeling (Goupil 1825; Bache 1826; Elliotson 1832b). Bertolini compared it with a flow of warm water (Editor 1826d), others with a flow of cold water (Most 1829). Still others noted "a numb and prickly sensation," generally preceding successful outcomes (Renton 1830, 106). Hamilton (1831) experienced "great itching . . . and a numb aching sensation" (446; see Brett, 1832). It appears not to have occurred to anyone that Chinese practitioners might have identified these descriptions as indications that a needle had "caught" the *qi (de qi)*.

Instead, surgeons drew on their own pet theories. Electricity entered the discourse. Churchill (1823a, 177; 1823b) observed something like "the passage of the electric aura." Récamier felt a shock when he touched needles inserted in a patient's back (Morand 1825b). Some patients experienced "shooting pains in the region of the needle" (Dantu 1826, 236). One of Bache's patients felt a pain shoot "with the velocity of lightening." He screamed, and his body shook as though receiving a powerful shock (Cassedy 1974, 898). Lee's patient reported "an acute tingling sensation" (Lee 1836a, 130). Such phenomena appeared to accompany efficacy (Pelletan, 1825a); explaining it remained the challenge.

There was always Kaempfer on air or wind, with needles providing a vent (Churchill 1821). Wansbrough disagreed. Needles blocked air, and cures often occurred before they were removed, making the escape of air unlikely. He believed the action must "depend on some of those mysterious operations of nature that will ever be beyond the reach of human ken" (Wansbrough 1826, 848).

Vicq-d'Azyr had classified acupuncture as an irritant, like blistering or moxa (Moreau 1805). Yet its effects seemed disproportionate to the slight irritation it caused. Sarlandière (1825) wondered whether needles modified tissue vitality, denaturing the pain and deactivating the irritant. Wallace (1827) classified acupuncture as a stimulant, because of its mechanical influence. Hamilton (1831) thought *how* needles were inserted made the difference.

Berlioz (1816) turned to theories of sympathy, where all parts of the body lent each other mutual assistance and alterations to one part affected the entirety. He speculated that acupuncture stimulated certain nerves, restoring some principle of which the pain had deprived them. If nerve-related pain resulted from the accumulation of fluid running through the nerves, then acupuncture promoted "the free circulation of this fluid . . . thereby clearing these organs of the surplus that heightened or distorted their sensibility" (Haime 1819, 42).

Cloquet and others wondered whether inflammation resulted from an accumulation of nervous fluid. Did needles withdraw excess fluid and, therefore, the pain? Might one transfuse such excess from one person into another in whom it was deficient? (F. 1825). Were nervous and electric fluids one and the same? Meyranx concluded they were (1825b). Pelletan (1825c) reverted to "imponderable" fluids (caloric, light, and electricity)—infinitely small particles without discernible weight that penetrated the body freely. To test the theory of nervous or electric fluid, Cloquet adopted steel needles, adding a ring at one end and attaching a conducting wire. He submerged the other end in muriatic acid to intensify the effects. Sometimes, he placed it in the patient's mouth, creating a galvanic circuit. Morand (1825) wondered whether needles functioned like a lightning rod. Pelletan experimented with a galvanometer, claiming to show that small quantities of electrical fluid were released with the needle (Editor 1825j).[54]

Such theories proved problematic. If accumulated electrical fluid caused pain, no benefit could derive from a needle whose head was covered with wax—an assertion contradicted by case experience. Furthermore, because soft tissues conducted electricity, they were probably not the site of its accumulation. Electric current appeared to oxidize the needle (Editor 1827g).[55] Yet Boston doctor Henry Carpenter penciled in his copy of Morand that electricity seemed "rather doubtful, or perhaps very much so, for the fact that needles of gold, silver, and plated have been used with as much success as the steel."[56]

In 1812 Bédor suggested that the Chinese had so often witnessed acupuncture that their confidence contributed to its efficacy. He doubted it would have similar effects in the West, where people had no "partiality for painful means of healing" (Bédor 1812, 150). Surgeon Edward Jukes worried, "lest the ember of animal magnetism might be rekindled in the discussion, and the operation from being associated with an exploded theory, sink into undeserved and premature oblivion, from preconceived prejudice" (Churchill 1821, 71–72). Indeed, during the height of acupuncture's popularity, one editor wrote, "At present it is the fashion among the knowing ones of this Metropolis to rank acupuncture and moxibustion with metallic traction and animal magnetism" (Editor 1825f, 562–563). Another editor was troubled by the absence of "any rational way of accounting for its effects." A philosophical mind could not help but "sentence acupuncture to banishment from regular practice, as being nothing else than a variety of animal magnetism" (Editor 1827g, 191–192). Many cases in which acupuncture proved most effective were the sort susceptible to "strong impressions of the mind" (Editor 1827g, 337).

One critic wrote that in some cases acupuncture's *modus operandi* should "be considered as similar to that of incantations, cauls, &c. for it is notorious that many a malady has yielded to the potent spell of some old beldame, which had long resisted the professional skill of the regular descendents of Hippocrates." Bread pills sometimes produced salivation when the patient was told they contained calomel (Editor 1829b, 167). Even so, another later editor reminded physicians that the body obeyed "the high behests of the intellectual powers. Men are often cured, and frequently killed, through the imagination" (Editor 1844g, 253). Here we see precursors of mind/body medicine.

Three arguments undermined this argument. First, Cloquet's success rate was roughly 83 percent—more than "so feeble an influence" would be expected to yield. Second, the permanence of many cures seemed inconsistent with "the effects of confidence in an imaginary remedy." Third, whether treatments failed or patients lost confidence, temporary relief might still result (Editor 1827g, 338). Elliotson—a defender of Mesmerism—argued that one could not reduce acupuncture's action to imagination, "for the same good is done, whether the patient has any fear of the operation or not; nor on faith, for the relief is equal, whether the patient believes in its efficacy or laughs at it, and merely suffers you to try it, because he sees you are anxious to afford him relief" (Elliotson 1830a, 272). He conjectured that efficacy might depend on electricity.

One British doctor reminded his audience that many therapies left physicians in the dark (Eberle 1822). Wakley proffered an alternative, echoing the Chinese model. A friend experienced success treating chronic neuralgias. When asked how it worked, he answered: "'that it all happened by letting out the wind.' This explanation gave perfect satisfaction, and perhaps we may adopt it with as much propriety as any other which has yet been offered" (Wakley 1825, 183). Ultimately, it proved difficult to explain acupuncture's action without appealing to something resembling an imponderable fluid. Yet again, no physician exploring these issues ever resorted to explaining them in terms of *qi*.

Vitalism, Electricity, and Electro-puncture

Whether electrical, nervous, and even magnetic fluids were identical was only part of the discussion. Most of the parties involved had rejected Mesmerism, despite its continued public popularity. Mesmeric metaphors made medical researchers nervous, particularly when "magnetizers" and biologist adherents of *Naturphilosophie* monopolized discussions of electricity. Ironically, some China observers reiterated Amiot's claim that Mesmerism of a sort was alive and well in China. Gutzlaff (1838, 2:213), for example, wrote, "Animal magnetism was known amongst them from time immemorial." *Pidding's Olio*, like Amiot, linked the practice with barbers. The paper quoted a M. Borget, who had noticed many clients falling asleep while being shaved, a phenomenon that puzzled him. One morning he observed a man sit on a stool, and began to sketch him: "The barber, instead of commencing his operations, placed himself before his customer, and, first of all, took hold of his hands, then passed his own several times over the shoulders, and before the face of the sitter, who shortly fell into a state of quiet drowsiness, if he did not actually go to sleep. He then moved his customer's head about in every direction he pleased, to facilitate the operation of shaving" (Anonymous 1844d, 91). Upon completing his work, the barber roused the customer. (See Figure 28.) Borget regularly observed the practice after that. Yet such stories did not enter Western discussions either of Mesmerism or of subtle fluids.

In 1820 Danish physicist and chemist Hans Christian Oersted published a pamphlet translated as "Experiments on the Effect of a Current of Electricity on the Magnetic Needle." Increasingly, electrophysics became the language of vital forces. Work by Michael Faraday (1791–1867) on electromagnetism also allowed researchers to examine vitalism without appearing to have drifted into Mesmerism. By midcentury, a broad belief had emerged that the world of phenomena manifested a "single force" that could appear in electrical, thermal, dynamical, and other forms (Kuhn 1977, 68). The medical version was

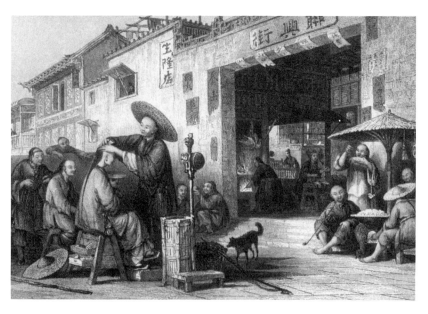

Figure 28. A Chinese barber. Thomas Allom and G. N. Wright, *China: Scenery, Architecture, Social Habits, Etc.,* 1843. Widener Library of the Harvard College Library.

often couched as "vital power" and sometimes was assigned sacred dimensions, as when Michael La Beaume (1820) wrote, "The electric principle is the apparent means by which the Deity acts throughout the universe" (92).

Developments in how the human system's dynamic dimensions were conceptualized had crucial implications for how European and American surgeons formulated and conducted experiments with acupuncture. If we review lists of conditions for which electricity was seen as effective—as one 1806 treatise illustrates—they intersect strikingly with conditions to which acupuncture was applied. For example, one treatise on medical electricity indexed the following cases: abscess, ague and fever, pains in the breast, bronchocele or tumor in the forepart of the neck, bruises, burns, cancer, catarrh, coldness of the feet and hands, colic, consumption, costiveness, cramp, convulsions, earache, epilepsy, fever, headache, hypochondria, hysterics, incubus or nightmare, inflammation, locked jaw, jaundice, nerves affected, numbness, pain in the ankle, arm and shoulders, back, and temple; palpitation of the heart, palsy, phlegmatic, piles, pleurisy, quinsy, rheumatism, pain in the side, sleepwalking, sore, scrofula, sprains, swellings, pain or cramps in the stomach, stiffness, Saint Anthony's fire (a local febrile disease), Saint Vitus's dance, tumor, vertigo, ulcer, and wounds (Hall 1806).[57] Parallels abound.

By 1812, despite concern that advocates of electricity had "gradually extended its supposed efficacy to almost every disease incident to the human system" (Cleaveland 1812, 26), galvanism continued to be tested into the 1820s, overlapping with acupuncture experimentation and continuing for decades thereafter.[58] It is possible, for example, that electrical experiments in cases of suspended animation or drowning inspired Carraro's experiments with kittens.[59] M. Pallas (1847), chief physician to the French armies in Algeria, suggested that excessive atmospheric electricity might cause disease, particularly of the nervous system. La Beaume (1826) was only stating a widely held view when he wrote, "*All* substances in nature, whether solids or fluids, animate or inanimate, have *inherent* in them a certain portion of the electric principle . . . the just proportion of this elementary matter exactly preserving the balance—so that its mutual attraction and repulsion, should *maintain* the equilibrium of their being—*preserve* their characteristic differences, and *prevent* disorganization and decay" (81).

Small wonder that physicians compared the sensation from acupuncture needles with "electric aura" (Churchill 1823a, 177), "shock" (Morand 1825, 32), "galvanic phenomena" (Ferussac Bulletin Général 1825), and "a sort of electric shooting pain" (Dantu 1826, 235), or that they linked acupuncture's efficacy with "the transmission of the galvanic fluid" (Lee 1836a, 132). Balance and equilibrium occurred not as *yin* and *yang,* but as electricity.

Berlioz—whose dissertation (1800) had explored the effects of electrical fluid—proposed enhancing acupuncture with electricity (Berlioz 1816). Sarlandière (1825) reported being the first to do so, calling it "electro-puncture" (it was also called "galvano-puncture"). Physicians Guillaume Duchenne, M. Pétrequin, and M. Leroy d'Etoiles and physiologist F. Magendie conducted related experiments, often using modified needles like Cloquet's. Italian doctors followed suit (Da Camino 1834, 1847; Strambio, Quaglino, Tizzoni, and Restelli, 1847). As Pelletan (1825a, 104) observed, gold or silver made the best conductors. Sarlandière connected them to an electrical machine with gold wire.

Electro-puncture was applied to rheumatism and lumbago, neuralgia, aneurisms, paralysis, amaurosis, deafness, intermittent fevers, pleurisy, asthma, colics, headaches, stomachaches, and uterine pain. Others used it with varices, the obliteration of arteries, and hydrocele.[60] Yet apart from Sarlandière (1825), much of this work occurred during the 1840s, almost two decades after the height of acupuncture experimentation. A whole branch of Westernized acupuncture persisted, therefore, in the form of electro-puncture.

Remembering and Forgetting

Acupuncture underwent cycles of flourishing, fading, and renewal. In 1805 Moreau, commenting on Vicq-d'Azyr, observed that those versed in physiology would have to determine whether Europeans' failure to employ acupuncture would prove regrettable. Béclard (1821) described acupuncture as known to the West for over a century, but recommended leaving it to its inventors. A cool response to Berlioz's preliminary findings from Paris's Société de Médecine in 1811 prompted him to wait before publishing his research.

Churchill (1821) initially published only a few cases, arguing that the open-minded would be receptive but the skeptical would "not be persuaded, though one rose from the dead" (72–73). Various journals responded favorably to his restraint (Editor 1821b; Copland 1822; Editor 1822a). One Boston journal explained its initial resistance to acupuncture: "We reckoned, erroneously, it would seem a kin to the famous *tractors* . . . But we have probably been mistaken—Acupuncturation is likely to become, employed with discretion and directed with skill, a valuable resource in many cases where our present means fail" (Editor 1822b, 441). Shortly thereafter, Churchill (1823a) reported hearing about "successful cases from respectable members of the Profession," leading him to promise "a body of evidence . . . which shall dissipate the most obstinate scepticism" (372). He produced this five years later (Churchill 1828).

N. Chapman of Philadelphia had encountered the case of the Earl of "Egmont" (Egremont), and was aware of the possible social repercussions of its being endorsed by nobility. "And therefore we should not be surprised if it becomes fashionable in rheumatism, which so often resists every means of cure" (Chapman 1824, 459–460). The *London Medical Repository* confirmed the perception: "We need not advert to the employment of acupuncture in this country; the extent to which it has been tried must be well known to the readers of this journal" (Copland 1825, 341). By 1825 most Parisian hospitals practiced acupuncture. The journals "fill their columns with observations and reflections on this new method of curing diseases. Even men of the world are not content to remain ignorant of this triumph of Medicine in our days: in short, every where acupuncturation is spoken of; in the drawing room as well as at the Institute" (Morand 1825, 1–2). Popular writers like Balzac employed the term metaphorically in his "Physiology du Mariage" (Lu and Needham 1980). Abel-Rémusat summarized the state of the field in 1825, writing that acupuncture had become the subject of general attention, although enthusiasm had already diminished and might be replaced by indifference. Still, he reviewed Berlioz, Haime, Churchill's colleague Scott, Churchill himself, Morand, Pouillet, Magendie, and Velpeau. In particular, he focused on his own involvement with Sarlandière and electro-puncture. Yet, as he anticipated, within a year one editor suggested that acupuncture had faded from view and "one appears almost ridiculous currently when one sustains that one can obtain happy effects from acupuncture" (Editor 1826d, 485).

By 1827, however, Wallace described acupuncture as gaining attention on the Continent, and a Scotch editor published a lengthy review (Editor 1827g). In 1828 Wakley wrote of this "remedy which, in despite of the sneers of certain learned sages, has come into general use" (Wansbrough 1828, 366). Yet a Mr. Lawrence again asserted in 1830, "We do not hear much now of diseases being treated by acupuncturation" (962). John Banks (1831) noted having witnessed it in Paris, and used it for rheumatism. He submitted an article to the *Lancet* (Banks 1830), adding with apology that he believed acupuncture was now little used in England. Lee (1836a) argued that the modality deserved far more American attention than he thought it had received. A French editor, reviewing Lee's work, noted that it recalled well-known ideas now forgotten or neglected (Editor 1837i). Although one editor referred to acupuncture's "comparatively recent revival in Europe" (Cormack 1842, 46), Costelli (1846) wrote that it was often forgotten and merited remembering, while Lallemand (1848) suggested that it had fallen into disrepute due to over-application to every form of pain. What should we make of this apparent ebb and flow?

The Routinizing of Practice

In 1829 the *Boston Medical and Surgical Journal* commented that the acupuncture rage had not crossed the Atlantic (Editor 1829a). Yet the evidence suggests otherwise. As noted earlier, there was the widespread reprinting and reviewing of European journal articles on acupuncture. American editors dropped only topics that "no longer represented novelties" (Editor 1841g, 1). If publication volume diminished over the years, it may have had less to do with diminished interest and more with acupuncture's no longer representing innovation. Nor was access restricted to larger cities. Even less central American medical libraries carried publications that discussed acupuncture. For instance, the library of the Medical School of Maine at Bowdoin College not only owned European medical journals that published articles on acupuncture; it also acquired the works of Vicq-d'Azyr and Churchill (Bowdoin College 1825). Almost a decade later, it had Bache's translation of Morand's dissertation on the topic (Bowdoin College 1834).

Nor did published cases reflect the full extent of acupuncture practice. Bretonneau, for example, had used acupuncture several times, and Dupuytren commended it to medical students (Haime 1819).

Nine students were involved in cases described by Dantu (1826). A Mr. Salmon and a Mr. Dendy discussed using acupuncture for rheumatism (Kingdon 1833). None of them published. Cloquet's cases numbered no less than three hundred (Pelletan 1825a), while Morand (1825) witnessed acupuncture practiced at St. Louis on more than twenty patients daily. Elliotson referred to, but did not publish, all of forty-two rheumatism cases—a figure cited in multiple reviews. As late as 1839, Da Camino noted having treated 105 patients, primarily for neuralgia (179–180). Only a fraction of these cases saw publication.

Some American physicians also appear to have used acupuncture without publishing. Bache referred to his friend Dr. Harris, who "operated for me in several of the first cases in which I resorted to the remedy" (Cassedy 1974, 905; see also Greenwood 1976). Three unpublished medical theses on acupuncture—one by Thomas A. Elliott (1826) in South Carolina, and two from the University of Pennsylvania, by John Jefferson Hall (1826) and John M. Galt (1831), both of whom were from Virginia—reinforce the argument.

Elliott's thesis thoroughly reviewed current knowledge regarding the Chinese and Japanese origins of acupuncture, needles and needling technique, modifications introduced by various practitioners, cases and treatable conditions, and theories regarding action. Elliott (1826), describing himself as "a tyro [beginner] in the science" (20), detailed some of his own successes treating acute and chronic rheumatism, ophthalmia, and cephalalgia. He referred to a Prof. Dickson, whom he had observed treating ophthalmia, and a Prof. Ramsay, "to whom I am much indebted for a number of the cases on which I have experimented," and who had noticed certain galvanic phenomena "when holding the needle in his fingers" (14). None of these doctors published, which suggests the difficulty of determining the extent of American use.

Just as medical journals published less on acupuncture as it became less novel, medical encyclopedias and textbooks—although they still included focused articles—also began folding acupuncture into other topics in less overt ways. For example, Chapman (1834) included acupuncture among fourteen therapies for *tic douloureux*. Elliotson's *Principles and Practices* contained a section on acupuncture, which one reviewer selected as the single extended excerpt (Cormack 1842); his encyclopedia article on neuralgia (Elliotson 1848a, 1848b) embedded acupuncture and moxa among related therapies. Dunglison's annotated bibliography for medical students (1837) included his own *General Therapeutics* and *Medical Lexicon* and Tavernier's *Elements of Operative Surgery*—all containing discussions of acupuncture. The Boston-based booksellers W. D. Ticknor and Fields (1844, 1847) advertised Dunglison, Elliotson, Larrey, Velpeau, and Tavernier. The continuing availability of such books indicates that medical readers had ongoing access to information on acupuncture (and also on moxa).

Finally, medical supply catalogs yield telling evidence. S. Maw of London sold surgical instruments. A copy of his catalog, owned by Joseph Wightman of Boston, offered an "acupuncturation needle" in an ivory case for one shilling (Maw 1839). George Washington Carpenter's 1835 catalog included acupuncture and moxa, under treatments for chronic rheumatism. His free medical advertiser cited Dunglison's *New Remedies* (1839) as a source. "All the remedies in his valuable work we propose keeping on hand to supply the orders of Physicians"— among them, "acupuncturating needles," described in relation to rheumatism, anasarca, and other diseases (Carpenter 1844, n.p.).[61]

Suppliers would not have advertised a commodity they did not believe would sell—and this, even after acupuncture appeared to have faded from view. Therefore, the ongoing, albeit more sporadic, publication of journal articles on the topic might demonstrate the incorporation of acupuncture into standard works, and the sale of acupuncture needles indicate a routinizing of the practice. Years later, physician William Osler would recommend acupuncture for lumbago (Veith 1975). Is it not possible that he did so from within this tradition of routinized use?

Religious Healing

In addition to comparing Chinese and Western forms of "surgery," foreign observers continued to witness the Chinese fascination with life-extending activities and to comment on what they construed as religious forms of healing. Some pointed to *changsheng*, or longevity, practices. Lepage (1813), for example, summarized the related section in Du Halde. Captain Pidding reprinted "The Art of Preserving Health and Beauty and Securing Long Life, Free from Infirmity and Disease, in All Climates" in full (Celebrated Chinese Physician 1844).[62] This work characterized such practices as involving "the regulation of the heart and its affections" (10:77), dietary practices (11:83), and regulating one's actions by day (13:99), and rest at night (14:106–107). Pidding editorialized, "We may no doubt be surprised to find the Chinese (who are so little versed in the science of anatomy reasoning as if they understood it" (14:107). Experience, coupled with pulse reading and medicines, nevertheless restored patients to health, and as for the celebrated Chinese physician, Pidding added, "some little allowance being made for the differences of climate, there is no doubt but that his rules may be of as much benefit in England as they were in China" (14:107). Personally, though, he judged the approach so "dry and rigid a piece of morality" that he would have preferred attempting "to introduce the use of Chinese characters into Europe" (Cibot 1844, 4).

Pidding also serialized an article by "the celebrated Doctor Chang" from the Tang dynasty, advocating vegetarianism (Chang 1844–1845). "According to him," Pidding commented, "medicine has said, facts have proved, and a long experience has forever decided, that the daily or even frequent use of meat is not only very unprofitable, unwholesome, but even very dangerous and hurtful in the southern provinces" (Chang 1844–1845, 35:276). Plagues were blamed on the Tartars, "great eaters of flesh" (36:285). He republished the account, Pidding explained, to illustrate that Chinese notions were still popular, despite being centuries old. Other reporters in the West called *changsheng* practices sensible (Coldstream 1848).

Attitudes toward Daoist longevity thought and practice, however, remained mixed. Where Confucius had been represented as the voice of Reason in the eighteenth century, Laozi now occasionally did the honors. "Dao" was translated as though synonymous with Reason. Chinese texts, describing how multiplicity had come into being, characterized the Dao as having produced "one," one having given rise to two, and two having produced three. Sinologist M. G. Pauthier (Williams 1848, 2:244–245) triumphantly lauded this metaphor as a Chinese form of the Trinity, claiming that it showed intuitions of Christianity.

Despite occasional medical articles by Western physicians on "liquors of life" purported to promote longevity (Editor 1817), no observer registered sympathy for analogous Chinese practices. Gutzlaff (1838) wrote of the "many who eagerly drink the ambrosia, and are soon numbered with the dead" (213), arguing that alchemy had made its practitioners the only group in China familiar with chemistry. "Expert in finding out herbs for the cure of various diseases," he wrote, "they often pass for very great physicians" (213). Observers like journalist Wood (1830) ridiculed the ingredients. Having purchased two wild cats for their skins, as zoological specimens, he agreed to return the bodies to the seller, only to observe them later stewing in wine. The preparation was intended to prolong the life of the vendor's aging father.

The observers did not understand that the pursuit of such formulas was a statement not only about life on earth, and the wish to enter into a different relationship to it, but also about the relationship with death and with the dead. If becoming an ancestor depended upon the largesse of one's descendants, the future assumed some uncertainty. Becoming an immortal nullified the more fragile dimensions of human bonds. One gave only the impression of dying. To make the point, it was said that the body was magically replaced with a sword or a cane, in which case the living could never be fully certain whether or not the adept had actually succumbed to death.

Grave and Ghosts

Rituals accompanied the journey into death: silver coins were placed on the mouth of one close to death to allow the person to die more quickly. Following death, a hole was sometimes made in the roof of the head to allow spirits to exit more readily. Priests opened the way into the realm of the dead.

> The soul, when once out of hell, has to pass over a bridge, built across a river of blood, filled with serpents, and other venomous creatures. This passage is dangerous, because . . . there are devils lying in wait to throw it into the accursed stream. But at length, the soul passes over, and the priests give it a letter of recommendation to one of the ministers of Budha, who will procure it a reception into the western heavens. According to the doctrine of the priests, every man has three souls; the first comes to live in the body; the second goes to hades; and the third resides in the tablet, which has been prepared for it. (S.R. 1840, 619)

Bodies might be handsomely dressed and "coffined"—the body put on quicklime, the boards sealed against odors—and kept in the house or in the ancestral hall, or in a common hall for the poor, until the family could afford a site selected by a *fengshui* practitioner (see Figure 29). (One of the worst British offenses during the Opium Wars occurred when troops opened coffins in such buildings and mutilated corpses; Williams 1848, 2:271.) One of Fortune's Chinese acquaintances characterized *fengshui* diviners as rogues who called on families after the body had been buried for a time, urging them to relocate it. If the relatives objected, the practitioner replied, "Very well, I don't care, but

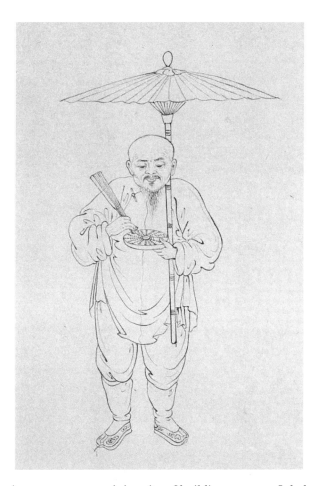

Figure 29. A geomancer examining site of building or grave. Ink drawing by Tinqua, ca. 1830s. Chinese artists produced sets of such drawings, depicting different professions, which foreign visitors purchased, and which were also sold abroad (see Huang and Sargent 1999). Photograph courtesy of the Peabody Essex Museum.

your children and relations will also be regardless of your remains when you die, and you will be miserable in your graves" (Fortune 1979, 322). Williams (1848, 2:265) described a practitioner who fell ill after recommending a grave site. Suspecting the family of poison, he had large rocks put near the grave, ruining the site's balance.

Smith (1847b, 409) described veneration of the dead as "one of the most formidable barriers" to missionizing. (See Figure 30.) Williams (1848) wrote vindictively, "It forms one of the subtlest phases of idolatry, essentially evil with the guise of goodness, ever established among men" (2:259–260). Monasteries supported themselves by selling incense,

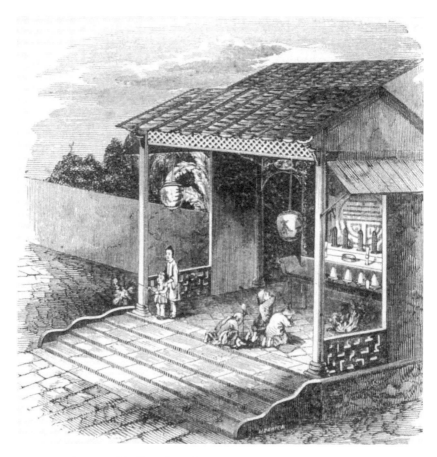

Figure 30. Ancestral hall, and mode of worshipping the tablets. Samuel Wells Williams, *The Middle Kingdom,* vol. 2, 1848. Widener Library of the Harvard College Library.

gilt paper, candles, and fees for funeral services, as well as hostel services. Smith (1847b) complained that his next-door neighbors hired such priests to attend to the departed, describing related cases involving illness. "The inmates commence beating drums and gongs, and set out a feast, in the superstitious belief that some deceased member of the family is starving in the world below, and that, in revenge of their neglect, his spirit has come to feed on the body of the sick person. Hence they seek, by the bribe of a feast, and the intimidation of sounds, to expel the unwelcome author of their calamity" (183).

The dangers of angry ghosts remained alive and well, as illustrated in a letter to the editor of the *Indo-Chinese Gleaner* from "Amicus" (1818) detailing the recent death of the wife of a wealthy man. Ten years earlier she had had two slave girls beaten to death after the older one was impregnated by the woman's husband. She then had the girls hung up by the neck so it would appear that they had committed suicide. Bribes followed, and the case was dismissed. Possessed by the girls' spirits, who declared her guilt, the mistress went mad. Her fits became so severe that her husband confined her, tended by an old serving woman. Prevented from publicizing their wrongs, the angry ghosts possessed the servant. The mistress died; her husband offered to support the servant, provided she entered a convent. She consented, but only after the ghosts had extracted a promise that the husband would venerate her as a goddess, as would his two daughters, who had assisted in the murder. Their conditions having been met, the ghosts were finally satisfied and departed. Amicus concluded that what Europeans would attribute to the power of conscience, the Chinese would diagnose as "demoniacal possession" (145). Even so, ghosts with grievances had a long presence in European and American folklore. The *American Magazine of Wonders,* for example, printed stories of "proofs of spirits and apparitions" (Fraser 1809a, 1809b), and the *Boston Medical Intelligencer* published a discussion of "ghostology" (Anonymous 1824b).

In 1844, 373 British troops died in Hong Kong of various diseases. Such large-scale death also occurred in Amoy, leading locals to fear the unquiet spirits of the British dead. Villagers claimed to have witnessed barbarian ghosts "running up and down the hills at night, and 'talking English most fearfully'" (Smith 1847b, 336–337). Daoist priests were brought to expel the dangerous influences with processions, gilt paper—spirit money—and incense, this time up against literal foreign demons *(fangui).*

Charms and Talismans

"P.P.T." (1820b), possibly a Protestant missionary, translated from a manual for converts to "the Romish religion" describing 380 common violations of Christian moral law, along with protective measures. Such practices were, in a word, "Sin." The translator explained that many Chinese children's caps had the two characters for "eight immortals" embroidered on them, to ensure longevity. Almanacs also contained "a charm for every year in the cycle . . . which are annually pasted as preventatives against pestilence; as well as twelve charms for the cure of various diseases" (360). The practice dated back to a "Chang keo," who pasted charms on walls to fend off contagion.

Gutzlaff (1837) alluded to "thirty-six to ninety-nine maladies arising from the influence of evil spirits" (158–159), many of the complaints resembling consumption, and requiring amulets. Morrison donated three kinds of amulet to the Royal Asiatic Society—those worn on one's person or sometimes hung up; small sacred books known as "girdle-scriptures," usually containing Buddhist sutras; and written spells *(fuzhou)*. The first included "money swords"—copper cash strung on a piece of iron shaped like a sword, and hung over a bed so the ruler under whose authority the coins were minted would keep away ghosts and spirits. They were used in houses where there had been suicides or violent deaths, as well as in response to illness. One could also request three or four cash from one hundred friends, stringing and hanging them around a child's neck to "lock" him to life and bind the hundred persons to ensure he reached old age. Women used a corresponding "neck-ring lock." A certain brass mirror healed madness brought on by the sight of a spirit or demon. There were peach and gourd charms for longevity.

Different deities required different spells, which might be pasted on a wall or over a door, or burned, the ash drunk in a liquid. A "triangular spell" was written down, folded into a triangular shape, and pinned to a child's clothes to ward off harmful spirits and sickness. Pictures of deified individuals hung in people's houses to protect children and other family members (Morrison 1835). Still, added Williams (1848), "Although these people are almost as superstitious as the Hindus or North American Indians, they do not depend in case of sickness upon incantations and charms for relief, but resort to the prescriptions of the physician" (2:179–180)—a claim that was only partly true.

And yet rituals, amulets, and charms against harmful influences were not the exclusive province of religious authorities. Physician Sun Dejun (fl. 1826), who defined and described afflictions by demons and other "pathogenic agents," provided medicinal responses. One could, for example, take "a pill . . . of tiger skull bones, cinnabar, realgar, rhizomes of the demon-vessel plant *(kuei-chiu)*, feathers of the demon-arrow plant, black hellbore, orpiment, and elm fruit" (Unschuld 1985, 222–223). Herbs could modify the *qi* of bodies and demons.

Divinations

Medicine entered the divinatory constellation as well. A writer for the *Chinese Repository* wrote of walking through the permitted section of Canton: "Passing through the street to-day, about two o'clock P.M., I counted *twelve* of these fortune-tellers, ten medical establishments, and five money-changers. Two of the first were priests, one a Budhist, and the other of the Taou sect. They were all poor, filthy, and beggerly in their appearance; and each had gathered around him a circle of idlers of the same description" (Anonymous 1835b, 45). A person was as likely to visit a diviner to discover the whereabouts of stolen property as to determine "which of a dozen doctors shall be selected to cure his child" (Williams 1848, 2:277). Even the body—particularly one's face—could be divined. Ruschenberger (1838) described a Chinese friend who was a self-styled physiognomist. Ruschenberger responded by explaining phrenology and examining his friend's head. The friend had him repeat the performance with several merchants. For the duration of Ruschenberger's stay in Canton, he received daily requests for phrenological consultations.

"P.P.T." observed divination using birds. Eight were kept in a cage subdivided into three sections. Some sixty folded cards were spread on the table. A petitioner seeking an answer related to sickness drew a bamboo slip from a cylinder. The diviner opened one of the three sections, releasing a bird, which then picked up one of the cards, receiving a grain of cooked rice in exchange. The diviner opened the card, pulling out two slips of paper—one informing the inquirer that he would recover; the other, a print of a doctor feeling his patient's pulse and pointing out his disease. To demonstrate the prediction's reliability, he wrapped two cash in the folded card, returned it with the others, reshuffled them, and released another bird, which proceeded to select that very card. Shortly thereafter, the petitioner observed precisely the same dynamic with another inquirer, causing observers to challenge the fortuneteller. The latter, to demonstrate "the omniscience of his bird," put one cash in the card, allowed the questioner to shuffle the pack, and covered the front of the cage before laying out the cards again. However, "on removing the board, the bird came out, and to the astonishment of all, the same card was chosen again" (P.P.T. 1820a, 319–320). The diviner left, having established his avian assistants' infallibility.

Western observers sometimes compared Chinese practices with analogues marginalized in the West. Downing cited Culpeper to illustrate that Western physicians had once believed in planetary influences over health. Sometimes Protestant prejudice exploited parallel Chinese sentiments. For example, the throne outlawed healers who claimed to call spirits, produce charms, or transform water with spells. Missionaries condemned "the power of priestcraft," as when a man whose wife was dying sought help at a Daoist temple. A red-turbaned priest, holding burning paper, performed ritual dances around a table of offerings. "At one time he prayed in softly-uttered tones; soon again he employed scolding accents to the deity whom he invoked. At one moment he would endeavor to coax away the angry spirit; at another he would terrify it away by whipping the air. After half an hour's frantic noise, and persevering somersets on the ground, he rose and placed a hairpin on the head of the anxious husband, after binding the hair into the peculiar tuft of the Taou sect" (Smith 1847b, 313–314). More spirit money was burned, the man bowed to the altar, paid his fees, and went home comforted.

The planchette *(jixian),* a board or table covered with sand or incense ash, was used for spirit writing, medical applications being common. Diviners might take a divining stick to the home of the patient, pass it over his or her body, and then return to the planchette to generate advice, which often involved a charm or prescription. Missionaries equated it with Spiritualism, which has often been identified as beginning in 1848 with the Fox sisters in upstate New York. It actually occupied a much older place in Western occultism, alongside apparitions, knockings, and related phenomena (Versluis 2000).

Gods associated with healing drew attention as well. Morrison's Chinese-language glossary included Kwan-yin (Guanyin), "a merciful goddess, much spoken of, and frequently represented." He also included "T'hëen hwa Shin-moo, the Sacred Mother who superintends children ill of the small pox," and "Hwü-füh Foo-jin, the patronness of barren women" (Morrison 1817, 111). These images of "a woman with a male child in her arms" inevitably led to comparisons with the Virgin Mary that had troubled even the earlier Catholic missionaries (Smith 1847b, 180). Abeel (1836) caustically described an unnamed god associated with healing who occupied a place on the wall opposite entrances. "He is painted in the act of conjuring an invisible being, with his face toward the heavens, and a small wand in his outstretched hand, while a hideous figure answering to their idea of a dragon . . . answers the summons, and appears in the clouds" (170).

For years, the Jesuits had insisted on Confucius's identity as a philosopher, arguing that he had not been divinized. During this period that representation was problematized, as when one reviewer of Dunn's exhibition wrote: "From one of the native books it appears there are upwards of 1500 temples, dedicated to Confucius, and more than 60,000 bullocks, pigs, sheep, and deer, are annually offered to the manes of the sage. Not only every province, but every minor district, of which there are more than seventy in some of the provinces, has a temple dedicated to the philosopher, where sacrifices are offered by the officers of government, scholars, and others" (Wines 1840, 586). Protestant missionaries increasingly disparaged Confucius as one who "did not like to retain God in his thoughts, because he was fain to be thought a God himself" (Lay 1841a, 150)—a distortion of the posthumous process of deification. Yet the Chinese had never attempted to conceal the fact that Confucius was venerated, his ancestral mantle spread over China as a whole.

Observers commented on city gods processed through the streets to expel afflictions. An epidemic of cholera morbus struck Canton in 1821. "Cha-ta-jin," head of the Salt Department, selected three days in the lunar cycle during which to go to the temples of "Teen-How" *(Tianhou)*, Queen of Heaven, and "Ching-wang" *(Jingwang)*, god of the city, to set up altars and pray. The daily paper reported that, in Macao, people processed the figure of the god through the city while banging gongs and setting off firecrackers to "expel noxious influences" (Editor 1821c, 231).

Fortune (1979) described a god and attendants dressed like the "highest mandarins," and "ill-looking executioners with long, conical, black hats on their heads, and whips in their hands for the punishment of the refractory." Although he found the sight interesting, Fortune added, "no Christian could look upon [it] without feeling the deepest commiseration" (191–193). Such accounts filtered into the popular media. The *American Magazine of Useful and Entertaining Knowledge* printed stories about Chinese temples (Dwight 1846a, 1846c). It frustrated the missionaries that even Chinese scholars resorted to these practices. Their own religious solutions to illness, suffering, and death seemed obvious to them, and they never understood why such solutions were not equally self-evident to the Chinese. That boxes of medicine were occasionally stolen from Western dispensaries and that patients came for treatment did not translate into the widespread acceptance of Western religious and medical worldview, thwarting missionary hopes.

Williams (1848, 2:235), like many missionaries, criticized the Chinese for lacking "a well understood and acknowledged standard of doctrine." If Western writers could not arrive at clear explanations of Chinese beliefs, he thought, it was either because the Chinese themselves were indefinite about their own ideas or because they had so many of them—not that Westerners failed to grasp an alternate worldview. One of the few religious qualities of the Chinese that impressed some observers was the peaceful coexistence of different religious groups. "The toleration of the Chinese is a phenomenon in the moral history of the world," wrote Lay (1841a, 100–101), "and deserves investigation." Generally, however, as Davis (1836a) observed, missionaries were "accustomed habitually to view the heathen almost exclusively on the side of their spiritual wants" (1:316).

The same held true for Western understandings of Chinese healing. Lepage's discussion, framed as "historical research," suggested an academic approach to Chinese medicine that did not mine it for possible applications (Grmek 1962). (For that matter, Lepage's work was rarely cited.) Abel-Rémusat had challenged his contemporaries for assessing Chinese medical texts and constructs when they could not read the originals. Edward Sutleffe issued similar critiques: "There has never been a medical man in Europe, who could, in conscience say, he thoroughly knew what the Chinese taught and practiced in medicine. A few garbled extracts from Wang-Shuh-Ho, by no means one of the first names in China, and the hasty reports of embassy travellers, are the data on which learned and scientific men venture to pronounce their sentence of condemnation on things which they know not, and to flatter into a pernicious self-conceit both themselves and their young Edinburgh pupils" (Sutleffe 1820–1821, 3[17]:127). Sutleffe both agreed with the low assessment of Chinese medicine and charged his peers with conceit. Critics, he argued, should visit China and conduct actual research, rather than succumb to complacency and contempt.

Few took up the challenge, although one must also acknowledge that the period saw unprecedented engagement with specific practices, like acupuncture. The resulting experiments, assimilation, integration, and synthesis both built on existing Western theory and stretched it. Still, even those involved in this cross-cultural project—like Sarlandière, himself a surgeon who worked closely with von Klaproth—were ultimately unable to override the weight of their own paradigms.

George T. Staunton (1822) had cautioned Western observers to divest themselves of prejudice either against or in favor of the Chinese. Most, however, were so steeped in the apparently self-evident truths of their own convictions that they failed even to recognize their own biases. If anything, some insisted they had gone to China with nothing but prejudices in favor of the Chinese—"romantic illusion," as Wood put it (1830)—only to find themselves disappointed by what they encountered. The acuteness of their disappointment appeared to corroborate its truth. Rooted in the conviction of Western rightness, it seeped into accounts sent West, emerging in works produced by writers who had never gone to China, whether in relation to material culture, racial representation, or the many versions of healing.

Conclusion

I have argued that healing traditions provide a window onto how understandings of humankinds, religion, medicine, and healing intersect over time—and that this intersection, in turn, is expressive of broader cultural trends. Normative views of humanness, for example, enabled one generation of Westerners to define the Chinese as white and another to define them as yellow, with attributions of monstrosity mapped at the margins. The early presence of polarized meanings—of Mongol hordes and images of disease in the social body, on the one hand, and of paragons of civilization on the other—stands out as a forerunner of anti-Chinese rhetoric in tension with stereotypes of model minorities. In tracking the genealogies of these meanings, we see where we have come from.

When I began this study, I had no idea how much information about Chinese healing traditions had entered the West between the thirteenth and nineteenth centuries. I presume the same holds true for many readers. Although the volume of information was slim when compared with our own time, the content was far more comprehensive than we credit. Not to exaggerate, however: As I noted in the introduction, few readers had access to the full range of what was disseminated, making this current work both artificially systematic and unprecedented.

Continuity and Change, Classifications and Categories

Looking at complex interactions over time involves conceptualizing both continuity and change, and how both shape and are shaped by the imagination. Both endeavors entail risks. Foregrounding continuity can result in focusing on recurrent phenomena as though they retain an unchanging power. Humoral theory and anatomical reading of the body come to mind. Both coincided with early reports on Chinese healing and remained influential. It is, of course, important to trace how the power of certain concepts leads people to work and rework them over time. At the same time, it is equally important to examine how discontinuity weaves its way throughout what is sometimes only the appearance of continuity. When do new content, experience, and surrounding events so suffuse a continuing practice that it both is and is not what it was before? Theories of humoral fluids, for example, both persisted as part of a core medical paradigm, while gradually intersecting with anatomical interpretations of the circulatory system *and* theories of imponderables such as magnet, electrical, and nervous fluids. Each, in turn, was brought to bear in Western efforts to understand the "action" of Chinese practices.

I prefer holding these ostensibly paradoxical processes together, rather than privileging one over the other. Indeed, I suggest drawing on *yin-yang* and *bian* representations of change. Accordingly, one looks for dimensions of continuity embedded in discontinuity, and *vice versa,* recognizing that both undergo a persistent process of reconfiguration. Change is the constant, in multiple forms. *Bian,* as a concept, entails asking whether a phenomenon is undergoing an internal change, or shifting from one form to another—resulting, potentially, in an outcome that appears to look nothing like its original form, as with a frog that becomes a quail, or a piece of jade that becomes a boy. I have found it useful to keep these paradigms in mind, in tracing the cross-cultural interchanges between Western and Chinese understandings of healing.

A related issue involves how Western commentators conceptualized and classified Chinese practices. If the material I have discussed in this book illustrates nothing else, it should remind us that people encounter difference through inherited classifications and categories, many of which operate on unconscious levels to structure thought, perception, and experience. World-making, Mary Douglas and David Hull (1992) suggest, involves manipulating, modifying, and sometimes jettisoning such received schema. Encounters between cultures can challenge, nuance, and even explode those categories. In other words, the classification of experience, and the concepts that underlie classificatory models, are historical phenomena. As Émile Durkheim and Marcel Mauss (1963) observed, "Not only has our present notion of classification a history, but this history itself implies a considerable prehistory" (5).

The most prominent instances in this study include typologies of humankinds and emergent theories of race; the defining of religion in tension with interreligious encounters, combined with efforts to resist and accommodate; and the changing definitions of science, medicine, and related knowledge. Each case illustrates how valence and meaning become attached to difference, modulating classificatory schemes in the process. It is what Roy Wagner (1981) refers to as the process of "symbolization": representations of other cultures are never simply descriptive, but involve locating the other culture within the symbolic frameworks—including the classes and categories—of the observing culture. This process implies potential action: one categorizes in order to formulate a response *to* and, potentially, an action *upon*. For example, by inserting the Chinese within Christian understandings of sacred time and history and, gradually, a construction of progress influenced by millenarian underpinnings, the Chinese were rewritten as objects of conversion.

An implicit dimension of classification involves determining what constitutes similarity. It begins with identifying common properties. Sinophiles and proponents of chinoiserie did it regularly when comparing Western and Chinese practices. How, though, are true common features identified and assigned significance in ways that contribute to the formation of categories? This involves more than just the number of common features. It also involves the value systems that define what is viewed as *important* commonality. To say that "important" commonalities matter begs the question of who determines "importance" and how. Nor can context or vantage point be forgotten. Nelson Goodman (1992, 21) provides an everyday example: "Consider baggage at an airport check-in station. The spectator may notice shape, size, colour, material, and even make of luggage; the pilot is more concerned with weight, and the passenger with destination and ownership. What pieces of luggage are more alike than others depends not only upon what properties they share, but upon who makes the comparison and when." In relation to classifying the Chinese, the Jesuits linked Confucian literati with the category "philosopher" to avoid identifying them as religious and to expedite papal support for the order's missionizing strategy. Voltaire, on the other hand, seized on the category of philosopher to support his criticism of religious institutions in Europe. Facile identification of similarities—a persisting problem in earlier phases of comparative studies of religion—generally overlooks these kinds of underlying differences (Patton and Ray 2000). Here I return to the role of the imagination, which inevitably is involved when one observes another culture. In the process, one's perception of one's own culture undergoes a transformation.

Mixtures and Mélanges

More recently such transformations have been conceptualized under a plethora of rubrics—criollization, *mestizaje,* hybridity, synergy, syncretism, synthesis, pluralism, and *bricolage*—all of them current vocabularies of intersection, interface, and exchange. The particulars of the periods addressed in this book reflect their own versions of such outcomes of exchange. The many examples I have reviewed lead us to ask what facilitates the movement of a healing system from one culture into another. What characterizes the kind of porousness in and between systems that enhances the potential for understanding and even crossover? Chinese healing traditions represent a particularly interesting case study precisely because Chinese practitioners themselves picked, chose, adapted, rejected, and combined at will. Structurally, their process appears the same as those of the Western observers and commentators; conceptually, however, it was not.

I suggest that at least six kinds of hybridity emerged in relation to Chinese healing practice in the West. The first appeared in the reporting of practices by foreign observers, as the result of seeing, discussing, and/or experiencing those practices. This act of reporting converged with the influence of imagined representation. This group is far and away the largest.

The second type involved the translation of texts, such as those produced by Michael Boym, Julien Hervieu, A. Pearson, and William Lockhart. Here, translation effected the blending. The use of familiar Western terms camouflaged profound conceptual and paradigm differences, as was initially the case with comparative discussions of pulse taking. The objectives of economic, political, and religious expansion further colored the process. Lord Macartney, for example, was truly interested in China but was, at the same time, informed by a model of imperial expansion, butting up against a counterimage of empire held by the Chinese. Moreover, as both Fr. Amiot and Jean Pierre Abel-Rémusat forcefully pointed out, actual translation was routinely hamstrung by the translators' lack of fluency, not only in classical, medical, and vernacular Chinese from different periods, but also in Chinese conceptual frames.

The third type drew on direct inquiries from Western observers and commentators directed to Chinese practitioners. Willem ten Rhijne and Engelbert Kaempfer created precedents for individuals like Amiot, John Livingstone, Robert Morrison, Charles Gutzlaff, Toogood Downing, and George Tradescant Lay as direct inquirers, and like Jean Astruc, Charles Jacques Saillant, Henri Bertin, and Pierre Sue who relied on correspondence, channeled through others. Such correspondence represented attempts to approximate direct interchange, subject again to the vicissitudes of translation.

A fourth type involved reviews and discussions of Chinese concepts, theories, and practices, based on readings of the first three versions of hybridity. Voltaire, François-Albin Lepage, Abel-Rémusat, and Ralph Waldo Emerson represent this approach. A fifth and closely related form of hybridity entailed adopting selected aspects of a practice. Such adaptations varied in the degree to which the adapters attempted to make sense of Chinese theory and incorporate it, as did John Floyer, or simply took up a form, gutted of Chinese content, as did Sir William Temple and many surgeons who experimented with moxibustion and acupuncture. In no known cases did anyone seek to bring a Chinese doctor to Europe or the United States. Prohibitions on emigration notwithstanding, missionaries succeeded in getting Chinese seminarians and even a Chinese patient to Europe. Had there been an interest in extending an invitation and maneuvering the visit, it could have happened, one suspects.

What also virtually never seemed to happen was a sixth type of hybridity, in which the Chinese worldview came to inform a Western individual's perspective so profoundly as to represent a quasi conversion. The two clearest examples are Amiot and Jean Baptiste Sarlandière. Neither transformation was absolute; both men rejected significant dimensions of Chinese religious and medical thought. Nevertheless, Amiot's embracing of the *qi* paradigm—his dependence on Mesmeric theory notwithstanding—signals his years of immersion in and acceptance of Chinese life and thought. Sarlandière, not having this advantage, nevertheless approximated Chinese practice as authentically and comprehensively as he could, and took its vitalist dimensions seriously, albeit through theories of electricity. As I have shown, there were other scattered instances in which resources and practices were made available such that, had the recipients been so inclined, they could have moved into a more complete adoption of Chinese approaches to healing.

I began by proposing that cultural, racial, religious, and medical formulations constitute a network of mutually informing signs, each allowing us entrée into dimensions we might otherwise miss. I conclude by suggesting that China continues to serve as an ongoing reference point, requiring us still to inquire into how China, the Chinese, and Chinese healing practices are imagined. China remains a vehicle for reflection on, and critique of, Western cultures. Increased complexity in racial discourse further complicates the issue, but does not remove it. Both Europe and the United States confront religious landscapes characterized by growing pluralism, of which multiple forms of Chinese healing have become an integral part (Barnes 1998, 2005). A fascination with the world's "mysticisms" has led to interest in Daoism and minimal attention to Confucius. The dominance of biomedicine creates a context within which all therapeutic modalities are assessed and practitioners define their identities (Barnes 2003). Perhaps most of all, the generations of the late twentieth- and early twenty-first centuries have, themselves, wrestled with ways to make sense of time and change, which are no longer so absolutely equated with paradigms of progress and modernity. This concern has led some not only to revisit the heritage of Western vitalism, but also to look beyond it to alternate formulations—in this case, through a language of energy to the paradigm of *qi*. All of which is to say that the interpretive lenses upon which I have drawn over the course of this book continue to matter when imagining China, healing, and the West.

Notes

1. First Impressions: Until 1491

1. Nestorian Christianity grew from the doctrines of Nestorius (d. ca. 451) of Syria, who argued that there were two separate persons in Christ, one human, one divine. The Roman Church rejected Nestorius's position as heretical (Cross and Livingstone 1974).
2. A printed edition appeared in 1468.
3. Polo sent a revision in 1307 to Thibaud of Cepoy, agent of Charles of Valois of Venice.
4. Chaucer named five Greeks: Aesculapius (Asclepius), central figure of an ancient Greek healing cult; Hypocras, or Hippocrates (fourth or fifth century BCE); Rufus of Ephesus, a first-century physician and medical author; Dioscorides, author of a treatise on *materia medica* (ca. 77); and Galen. The other physicians were from the Islamic medical world: Haly (Haly, or Ali Abbas, 930–994), a Persian medical encyclopedist; Serapion (Ibn Sarabiyun), a ninth-century Syriac physician; Rhazes (al-Razi, 865?–925?); and Avicenna, a medical encyclopedist and systematizer. Averroes was another Arab Islamic writer. Damascien probably was Ibn-el-Nafis (Alī ibn Abī al-Hazm, ca. 1210–1288), a famous physiologist from Damascus. Constantyn was Constantinus Africanus, a medical translator. Bernard of Gordon (ca. 1258–ca. 1320), a noted medical author, taught medicine at Montpellier. John of Gaddesden (ca. 1280–1361?), court physician to British king Edward II, compiled the *Rosa anglica* during the mid-fourteenth century, drawing on writers like Galen, Dioscorides, Avicenna, Averroes, and Gilbertus Anglicus. Gilbertyn was Gilbertus Anglicus (Gilbertus del Egle, dates unknown), an English medical writer.
5. In 1272, *fulin* (Franks) were said to have founded a charity hospital in Beijing, although little information about them remains (Wu 1931).
6. *Jingluo: Jing* referred to the warp of a loom; *lo* referred to fibers or cords, and meant "to connect."

7. During the Song dynasty, the *Shanghanlun* was divided into three separate books: *Shanghanlun, Jingui yuhanjing* (Canon of the Golden Casket and Jade Cases), and *Jingui yaolue fanglun* (Essentials and Discussions of Prescriptions in the Gold Casket). For discussion of Shanghan conceptions of disease, see Epler 1988 and Ågren 1986.

8. Through connections with Iran, Avicenna's *Qanun fi al-tibbi* (Muslim Medicinal Recipes) entered China. Written primarily in Persian, the work cited Galen as an authority and source of recipes (Buell and Anderson 2000).

9. Tombs in China's Hubei and Hunan provinces have yielded manuscripts from the Warring States (400–220 BCE), Qin (221–206 BCE), and early Han (206 BCE–220 CE) dynasties. In 1973 a large collection was discovered in tomb 3, dating from 168 BCE, in Mawangdui in the northeastern part of the city of Changsha, Hunan (Harper 1998).

10. Even this theory does not appear consistently throughout the *Neijing* (see Harper 1998, 90).

11. Only over time did greater ambivalence toward bloodletting emerge, due to concerns over losing primordial *qi;* see Epler 1980 and Kuriyama 1995.

12. Polo observed astrologers and diviners, some of whom treated Qubilai for gout.

2. A New Wave of Europeans: 1492–1659

1. The Chinese had analogous perceptions of Europeans. "To paint an ugly man, they paint him with a short coat, a beard, and big eyes and nose" (Pantoja 1606, 17).

2. Europeans also encountered Africans in China. Most Portuguese households in Macao had African slaves. Some slaves escaped, establishing a community in Canton (Dikötter 1992). Mundy (1919, 192) described such a man, "Antonio, A Capher Eathiopian Abissin, or Curled head." "Blacke Antonio" spoke his own language, Portuguese, Chinese, and English, and taught Mundy to pronounce two hundred "China Characters."

3. Spanish physician Nicolás Monardes (1565) wrote about plants from the Americas.

4. For discussion of Ricci's critique of vegetarianism, see Reinders 2004.

5. Wind blockage is a disorder with symptoms similar to those of migratory arthralgia.

6. The Duke of Zhou was an ancient culture hero.

7. Pu Songling's *Liaozhai zhiyi* (Strange Stories from a Chinese Studio) was completed in 1679 (P'u 1925).

8. Bodhisattvas are individuals so dedicated to the virtue of compassion that they delay their own enlightenment in order to further the awakening of all sentient beings.

9. The female bodhisattva Guanyin is the Chinese version of a male Indian counterpart, Avalokiteshvara. She was also said to have been the third daughter of a northern ruler during the Zhou dynasty. "Omitoffois" referred to A-mi-to-fo, or Amitabha, Buddha of the Western Pure Land Paradise (Ch'en 1964).

3. Model State, Medical Men, and "Mechanick Principles": 1660–1736

1. Chinese medical works in the Vatican library include: the first chapter of the *Daguan bencao*, a *materia medica;* two copies of chapter 7 of the *Daguan bencao;* chapters 3 and 5 of the *Yixue rumen;* six fascicles of Wang Ren-an's *Bencao yifang hebien*, on *materia medica* and medicine; the *Bencao beiyao* (1682), a *materia medica* by Wang Ang; the *Tangtou gejue*, on medicine; Li Shizhen's *Bencao gangmu;* the *Qiongxiang bienfang*, Zhang Binyu's medical advice for peasants; chapter 7 of the *Bianzu yixue rumen waiji*, a medical work (an edition from the first half of the seventeenth century); and a 1578 copy of Wang Shuhe's *Mojue* (cataloged in Pelliot 1995).

2. Fr. Ripa introduced copperplate engraving to China at the Kangxi emperor's request, producing thirty-six vistas of the imperial summer resort garden at Chengde. These engravings, which Ripa brought to Britain in 1724, helped bring Chinese gardens into fashion.

3. Most medical texts in Manchu were translated Chinese sources and remained in manuscript form. That these works were largely unpublished indicates how quickly sinification occurred (Walravens 1996).

4. Originally chapter 42 of the *Liji* (Book of Rites), the *Daxue* characterizes the profound person as putting the affairs of state in order by first putting his family in order, which he accomplished by first putting himself in order.

5. The terms *ti* and *yong* appeared in the *Yijing* and the *Laozi*, but thinker Wang Bi (226–249) first joined them as *tiyong*.

6. Hugh Shapiro (n.d.) observes that the history of nerves in the West dates to Herophilus (early third century BCE), who called motor nerves *prohairetika*, "capable of choosing, purposive." Shapiro argues that volitional activity was a core component of Western formulations of identity, with emphases on the individual as a choice-making agent.

7. The character for *jing* in *jingluo* is also used for "classic" (as in *Yijing*, "Classic of Change"). In both cases, *jing* signifies the warp threads in cloth—metaphorically, that which weaves things together.
8. "Mechlin" referred to Malines, Belgium.
9. Controversy surrounds Cleyer's authorship, multiple scholars over the years charging him with plagiarism, others defending him (see Abel-Rémusat 1829, Chabrié 1933, Pelliot 1934, Szczesnik 1949–1955, Grmek 1962, and Golvers 2000). As I read the evidence, in 1654 Paris publisher Sebastian Cramoisy announced Boym's projected publications, including a work to be entitled *Medicus sinicus* (Chinese Medicine). Since at least 1643, Boym had collected Chinese medical sources, including Wang Shuhe's *Mojue* and other works on tongue diagnosis. In 1656 Boym left Rome for China, accompanied by Philippe Couplet. Boym eventually asked for Couplet's assistance in sending his work back to Europe. In 1658 Couplet relayed Boym's materials to Jesuits in Batavia, to have them forwarded to Europe. Instead, they came into Cleyer's hands. In 1659 Boym died in Vietnam.

While under house arrest with Couplet in Canton in 1665, Domingo Navarrete (1676, 58–59) wrote that Couplet "is most passionate about the Chinese physicians . . . he is trying to translate several books, so they may be of use in Europe." In 1669 Cleyer wrote to Couplet from Java, asking him for sources and translations related to Chinese medicine. Physician-sinologist Abel-Rémusat (1788–1832), who wrote his dissertation on Boym, believed that Cleyer joined Boym's translations with subsequent translations he received in 1669 and 1670, and that Cleyer published the whole under his own name in 1680 as *Clavis medica*.

In 1682 Cleyer's name appeared alone on the title page of *Specimen medicinae sinicae*, as the editor of materials on Chinese medicine sent from China, and some that an "erudite European" had sent from Canton between 1669 and 1670. This "European" described himself as having studied Chinese books and consulted with local Chinese doctors when possible. Couplet seems the likeliest candidate. Cleyer's own role is disputed: some scholars view *Specimen* as a compilation of materials once belonging to, translated by, and/or written by Boym; others conclude that it is a composite volume, in which Boym's work was joined to that of others (Golvers 2000, 176). Lu and Needham (1980) are persuaded by sinologist Paul Pelliot (1934) and others who exonerate Cleyer of having plagiarized Boym; I am less convinced, and therefore I cite works as Cleyer's with reservations. Either way, Boym's original role appears to have been minimized, if not concealed.

Between 1682 and 1692, while in Europe, Couplet appears to have retrieved Boym's manuscript from Cleyer. In 1686, Boym's translation of a version of the *Mojue* appeared as *Clavis medica ad Chinarum doctrinam de pulsibus* (The Medical Key to the Pulse Doctrine of the Chinese), listing Cleyer as the editor. This *Clavis* so differed from Cleyer's 1680 work as to seem entirely separate. But Cleyer's 1682 title suggests that it consisted of fragments from Boym's medical translation project, while the 1686 work represented a more finished version, drawn from Boym's other materials.

The strongest evidence that Boym authored much of *Specimen* appears in the preface to the 1686 version of *Clavis*. There, Boym described preparing Latin translations alongside Chinese medical texts with added romanization, inserting Chinese technical terms into the Latin text. The *Specimen* appears to have been produced in the same way, although Cleyer retained the romanization and omitted Chinese characters that could not be printed in Nuremberg at that time (Szczesnik 1949–1955). In 1758, excerpts from the 1686 *Clavis* were translated as *Clef de la Doctrine des Chinois sur le pulse*, appearing in *Le Conservateur* with related commentary (Anonymous 1758).

10. For additional discussion of Du Halde on Chinese pulse diagnosis, see Hsu 2000a, 2000b.

11. Previously, Santorio Santorio (1561–1636) had adapted a pendulum to measure pulse frequencies, "reversing the well-known experiment of Galileo who, with his own pulse, measured in the cathedral of Pisa the duration of the oscillation of various chandeliers" (Grmek 1962, lxxxvi).

12. Grosier (1788, 1:556) reported the emperor as having been given "a confection of kermes"—the pregnant female of the insect *Coccus ilicis*, previously thought to be a berry—by missionaries for his heart palpitations.

13. Similarities may be due to (1) acupuncture's origins in bloodletting, (2) possible exchange through Greco-Chinese trade routes, and/or (3) the possibility that bloodletting produced real relief (Kuriyama 1999).

14. "Gravel" referred to visible urinary crystals, the condition they characterized, and pain or difficulty passing urine with or without such a deposit.

15. For a history of epidemics in China, see Leung 1993.

4. Sinophiles, Sinophobes, and the Cult of Chinoiserie: 1737–1804

1. He published two additional volumes between 1814 and 1816.
2. For other contributors, see Huard and Wong 1966.
3. Li had studied at Matteo Ripa's Chinese college in Naples.

4. Nevertheless, both Macartney and Staunton lamented not having spent more time with Fr. Amiot while in Beijing, due to his failing health, and recognized his role in the *Mémoires.*

5. For an analysis of British interpretations of bowing, see Reinders 2004.

6. Fuxi (Ox-Tamer) is one of the Three Sovereigns, the other two being Shennong (Divine Husbandman) and Huangdi (Yellow Emperor).

7. For a list of Chinese seminarians, see Duhergne 1964, 395–396.

8. The spelling "Hwang-a-tung" is used by a Sackville descendant. I have also encountered "Whang-At-Ting." Sir Joshua Reynolds painted him as "Wang Y-Tong."

9. Such topics included the history of Chinese medicine; theory and practice; examples of *materia medica;* longevity practices; smallpox; astrology, superstition, and idolatry; the Imperial College of Medicine; *gongfu;* and the order and method of Chinese medicine compilations (Missionaries of Beijing 1784, 10:314–315).

10. A lay brother wrote, years earlier, that Portuguese men in Macao frequently married Chinese women, or the daughters of these couples (Boxer 1974). It is not clear whether Vandermonde's wife was of Chinese descent. Charles Augustin Vandermonde (1727–1762) founded the *Journal de médecine, chirurgie et pharmacie.*

11. It is not clear whether Cibot meant Michael Ettmüller (1644–1683) or his son, Michael Ernst Ettmüller (1673–1732). Both were members of Leipzig's medical faculty.

12. Cold-damage disorders, gynecology and obstetrics, pediatrics, smallpox, other pox diseases and related methods of inoculation, external medicine, ophthalmology, acupuncture and moxibustion, and orthopedics (Hanson 2003, 138). Topics covered by books in the French Bibliothèque Nationale, Catalogue 31:375 and 58:381, closely parallel this list.

13. The "Paripatetic school": Literally, *peripatetic* means "itinerant." Here it refers to members of the school of Aristotle interested in materialism and empiricism. An Aristotelian revival, from the first century BCE through roughly 200 CE, influenced Galen.

14. In contrast, Barrow's 1847 autobiography described his sole remarkable memory of Chusan as involving having his pulse read. "A venerable Chinese physician made his appearance," he wrote, "felt my pulse very carefully, and told our missionary that he would cure me: a person went with him on shore, brought back a packet containing, among other things, a large proportion of rhubarb, and after about twenty-four hours of acute suffering I was myself again" (62).

15. For in-depth discussion of the Macartney party's observations regarding Chinese doctors and acupuncture, see Bivins 2000.

16. In 1737 Parennin also sent a letter about venereal disease in China to the St. Petersburg Academy of Sciences, where it reached court physician Antonio Ribeiro Sanchez (1699–1793) (Huard and Wong 1968).

17. Later published in the *Mémoires de la Société impériale des naturalistes de Moscou* (1812–1813).

18. "A Grain is a pretty large Grain of Barley. A Scruple, or 20 Grains. A Dram contains 3 Scruples. An Ounce contains 8 Drams. A physicall Pound is 12 Ounces. Half a pound, or 6 ounces. A Quarter, or three Ounces, Quart. A Handfull as much as your hand holds. A Pugil, what you hold with the tops of your fingers" (College of Physicians of Amsterdam 1659, 179).

19. Parennin, when sent a questionnaire about Chinese drugs by Russian academicians, referred them to Jartoux's letter (Dumoulin-Genest 1995).

20. According to Lu and Needham 1980, French doctor Pierre Pelletan witnessed Hwang's explanation, although they refer to a point figurine. If so, it must have been Pelletan Sr., as Pelletan Jr. wrote about acupuncture fifty years later.

21. *Tabula seu index rerum ad compescendam vulnerum tyrannidem idonearum,* French national library, Catalogue 59:381.

22. Sue cited the French Bibliothèque Nationale, Catalogue 31:375 and 58:381.

23. I have found no records indicating that these authors either experienced or experimented with the meridian charts or, apart from Coley, with acupuncture.

24. A fistula is an abnormal duct, from an abscess, cavity, or hollow organ, to the body surface; a *fistula lachrymalis* is a fistula near the eye.

25. Peripneumony was inflammation of the lungs; intermittents were intermittent fevers; felons were infections at the fingertips; bronchocele was a hernia in the throat; chlorosis, an anemia sometimes resulting in a greenish skin tone; ganglions were cystic lesions; gravel was the granular material of urinary calculi; quinsy was an acute inflammation of the tonsils; shingles were a skin eruption; Saint Anthony's Fire was Erysipelas; Saint Vitus's dance was chorea; mortification was the death or decay of part of living tissue; and wens were cysts filled with fatty matter.

26. "Mr. Desvoyes" was the pseudonym of Abbé Louis-Auguste Bertin (1717–1788), brother of the minister and secret protector of disenfranchised Jesuits.

27. Bertin also informed Amiot about electricity, even sending him an electricity machine.

28. Patterns resulting from the casting of coins or yarrow stocks were recorded as patterns of six lines, unbroken (yang) or broken (yin). For example:

```
      ___  ___
      ___  ___
      _____
      ___  ___
      _____
```

Each hexagram corresponded to a description of a type of change in process, enabling one to align oneself with the nature of the time and come closer to enacting the Dao.

29. Delatour attributed the discussion of *gongfu* to Cibot; other sources attribute it to Amiot, who discussed it in additional contexts.

30. In contrast, Cibot wrote, "What attracts me among the Chinese, is that they do not seize upon change. Instead of looking for complicated, rare, and expensive remedies; they apply themselves to simplifying remedies and to finding them in what grows everywhere; and in that, unless I am mistaken, they enter better into the intentions of Providence" (Delatour 1803, 264–265).

5. Memory, History, and Imagination: 1805–1848

1. References to Staunton in this chapter refer to George Thomas Staunton, unless otherwise indicated.

2. The term *coolie* originally referred to laborers in India and eventually was also identified with the Chinese term *kuli*, "harsh/bitter labor." It might derive from the Hindi *quli*, "hired servant," or *Kuli*, a tribe in Gujerat.

3. Barrow became second secretary of the Navy for forty years, also authoring *The Mutiny and Piratical Seizure of H.M.S. Bounty* (1831).

4. An *olio* is a miscellany collection of articles.

5. Abel-Rémusat signed his name "Abel Rémusat," but used "Abel-Rémusat" in publications.

6. Franklin Bache studied medicine at the University of Pennsylvania after serving as a surgeon in the War of 1812. A chemistry professor, he also taught at the Franklin Institute and the Philadelphia College of Pharmacy and Science.

7. Foreigners were characterized by some Chinese as drinking menstrual blood, "which they regarded as a precious gift conferred by God"—and which explained their stench (Dikötter 1992, 47).

8. The history of such visits was retained. Lepage (1813) and Abel-Rémusat (1829) discussed Chinese visits to France.

9. The catalog drew on Barrow, Sir George Leonard Staunton, and John Francis Davis.

10. John Livingstone, surgeon to the British Factory, also described "A-ke" in the *Indo-Chinese Gleaner* (1821b).

11. The eleven cities were Boston, Salem, Monson, and Plymouth in Massachusetts; Portsmouth, New Hampshire; Newport and Providence in Rhode Island; Cornwall, Connecticut; New York City; Philadelphia, Pennsylvania; and Baltimore, Maryland.

12. Abel-Rémusat (1833) elaborated on this argument.

13. Toogood Downing published this article in the *Lancet* (1842) under his own name, without crediting Gutzlaff. Therefore, all references to Gutzlaff's comments imply parallel citations for Downing, whose plagiarism reached physicians.

14. A twentieth-century catalog of Chinese books in the Bibliothèque Nationale (Courant 1912) indicates that the collection included five Chinese encyclopedias with volumes on medicine, as well as 296 multivolume texts on medicine published prior to 1848. In addition to multiple editions of the *Huangdi neijing,* the collection also housed works on cold-damage disorders, women's illnesses, obstetrics and gynecology, pediatrics, smallpox and other skin eruptions, *materia medica,* ophthalmology, pulse theory and diagnostic principles, dentistry, general works, and other topics. (It is beyond the scope of this book to list the titles.) The catalog does not, however, include accession dates. Von Klaproth, although not involved in medicine, owned ten Rhijne 1683; Sarlandière 1825; Abel-Rémusat 1813; Cleyer 1682; and a recipe book for different illnesses translated into Chinese from Spanish, based on journal notes taken during a voyage to Yedo in 1774 (the author is not given) (Maciet 1839, 27).

15. Reprinted in *Captain Pidding's Chinese Olio and Tea Talk,* reaching traders (Sutleffe 1844), without naming Sutleffe. Pidding also reprinted a 1782 selection from Cibot, again unattributed, as "Medical Science in China" (Cibot 1844, 4).

16. The original appeared in *L'Experience* (I could not locate this source).

17. Medhurst's wording sometimes appears to lift directly from Sutleffe 1820–1821.

18. Evidently Lockhart, and perhaps Lay, read Chinese. Newly arrived missionaries were expected to learn to speak it; some also studied the written language to facilitate translation projects and tract writing.

19. Other journals reviewed the work, excerpting passages (Editor 1846e, 1846g, 1846h, 1846i, 1848d).

20. On smallpox vaccination, see Sprengel 1815, vol. 1; Page 1815; Pearson

1826a, 1826b; de Malpière 1825, vol. 2; Gutzlaff 1837; and Downing 1838, vol. 2.

21. Livingstone (1819b) described Kerr's ineffectual labors.

22. Other journals reprinted the piece (Carson 1847b; Editor 1847i, 1848c), illustrating international circulation of medical knowledge.

23. A probang was a thin flexible rod with a sponge at the end, used to remove objects from the esophagus or larynx.

24. Abel-Rémusat believed Cleyer had plagiarized Boym's work (see Chapter 3).

25. Deobstruent was purgative; diaphoretic, causing perspiration; emmenagogic, aiding menstruation; anthelmatic (anthelmintic), expelling worms; and corroborant, strengthening.

26. Hufeland's article may originally have been published in the *Journal der Praktichen Heilkunde* (April 1824). See also Editor 1824a, 1825l; Hufeland 1824b, 1825; Elliotson 1836.

27. Barton (1817–1818) traced knowledge of North American ginseng to Michel Sarrasin, Lafiteau, Bartram, and Kalm.

28. *Carpenter's Annual Medical Advertiser* included Shaker medicines.

29. See Parker 1836, 1839; Bell 1843, 1844; and Editor 1839b, 1839c, 1841e, 1844a, 1848e.

30. The following narrative draws on Morrison 1839, vol. 2 (which was reprinted from Livingstone 1819a, 1821a; and Morrison 1819b).

31. "Native Chinese Books" were contributed, as were works by Staunton, Barrow, Abel-Rémusat, Kircher, Semedo, Kaempfer, and others (Editor 1819b, 1819c).

32. Pearson provided a detailed translated prescription, illustrating that, had Western observers taken Chinese pharmacology seriously, they could have communicated it in accessible ways.

33. Dates are unknown for most of these individuals.

34. See Blanc 1799–1800; Cothenet 1808; Lecointe 1812; Jourdan 1819; and Larrey 1822.

35. "Seton" also referred to drawing a needle and thread through skin at the nape of the neck, on the chest, or in the scrotum, leaving the thread to cause an infection.

36. All in the Harvard University library system. The inclusion criteria were the words *moxa* or *moxibustion* in the title or body of the source.

37. It was translated from Manchu into Russian, German, and Polish.

38. Dantu cited Boym, Martini, Cleyer, Grosier, Du Halde, Sue, Macartney, and his own physician contemporaries. See also Dantu 1825.

39. This number does not include allusions to hundreds of other unpublished cases. I was also unable to secure a copy of a second collection of

cases published by James Morss Churchill (1828). The title indicates that the cases included treatments for rheumatism, lumbago, sciatica, "anomalous muscular diseases," and "dropsy of the cellular tissue," suggesting that Churchill continued his earlier circumscription of acupuncture to cases involving a particular category of pain-related afflictions.

40. Of male patients with specified ages, 1 was eleven, 3 were in their teens, 29 in their twenties, 31 in their thirties, 28 in their forties, 11 in their fifties, 13 in their sixties, and 4 in their seventies. Ninety-seven men had no specified age. There were 1 "boy," 5 "young men," 2 "old men," and 1 of "advanced age." Of the female patients with specified ages, there were 9 in their teens, 18 in their twenties, 14 in their thirties, 14 in their forties, 6 in their fifties, and 2 in their sixties. Descriptors for 14 other women included "young girl," "young woman," "middle-aged," and "old woman." Seventeen women had no age specified.

41. Occupations specified for men included: Artisan, Bookkeeper, Bricklayer, Business broker, Butcher, Carpenter (2), Carver and gilder, Chef, Clerk, Clockmaker, Coachman/cab-driver (2), Cobbler/bootmaker (3), Concierge/doorman, Countryman (4), Customs house officer, Door-keeper, Dyer, Errand boy (2), Farmer (3), Fisherman, Gardener (5), Gentleman, Guard, Gunsmith workman, Hatter, Herborist, Hosier, Jeweler, Kitchen assistant, Laborer (9), Lathe worker (2), Locksmith (3), Marine, Mason (3), Mattress-maker, Mechanic, Medical student (2), Mirror maker, Nurse (3), Office-boy, Prisoner (20), Quarrier/quarryman, Saddler/harness maker, Sawyer, School master, Seaman, Servant (3), Shoemaker, formerly a painter on porcelain, Soldier (16—including line soldiers, dragoons, officers, and veterans), Stableboy, Stone cutter, Student, Tailor (2), Tanner, Timber merchant employee, Tinsmith, Water carrier, Wigmaker, Wine merchant's cellar man, Wood sawyer. Only one peer—the Earl of Egremont—was included. Two patients were physicians and one was a surgeon.

Women's social roles, if described, appeared in relation to either income-generating work or marital and/or maternal status (a detail never included for male patients): Cook, Dressmaker, Embroiderer (4), Hatter, Laundress/washerwoman (3), Upholsterer, Weaver, Servant, Married (4), Married mother, Widow. Only one woman was described as a "lady."

42. A line was 1/12th of an inch.

43. A review of cases specifying the number of treatments, and of needles used in each treatment, yields the following results (the number or sequence of numbers of needles is followed by the number of cases in pa-

rentheses). The case data do not detail how often a single needle was inserted in a single treatment. Therefore, a single treatment using a single needle could refer to multiple punctures. In other cases, the numbers are vague.

One treatment (126 cases): 1 needle (51 cases); 2 (37); 3 (14); 4 (10); 5 (4); 5–6 (2); 6 (3); 8 (1); 10 (1); 12 (1); 20 (2).

Two treatments (32 cases): 1, 2 (2); 1, 4 (1); 1, unspecified (1); 2, 4 (1); 2, 1 (5); 2, 6 a year later (1); 2, 2 (8); 3, 1 (1); 3, 3 (3); 3, 4 (1); 4, 4 (4); 4, 5 (1); 4, unspecified (1); 5, 6 (1); 12, 12–14 (1).

Three treatments (2 cases): 3, 6, 9 (1); 8, 8, 8 (1).

Four treatments (2 cases): 4, 3, 2, 2 (2).

Five treatments (1 case): 1, 6, not clear, 2, not clear (1).

Multiple treatments, not clear how many, two needles each time (5 cases).

44. "Cholera morbus" was said to be "characterized by anxiety, gripings, spasms in the legs and arms, and by vomiting and purging" (Dunglison 1833, 1:186). "Iliac passion" was described as a colic that "arises to a violent height, and is attended with obstinate costiveness [constipation], and an evacuation of faeces by the mouth" (Hooper 1825, 346).

45. Von Klaproth (1825) reported that a Paris bookseller later acquired the original. He also cited a Chinese treatise in the Bibliothèque du Roi (Catalogue de Fouremont, no. 522).

46. Sarlandière began experimenting with acupuncture roughly concurrent with Berlioz, but Berlioz published first and received credit for it.

47. "Revulsive methods" involved "the act of turning the principle of a disease from the organ in which it seems to have taken its seat." Such methods included blistering and bleeding (Dunglison 1860, 799).

48. "Affection": "We say febrile affection, cutaneous affection . . . using the word affection synonymously with disease" (Hooper 1825, 37).

49. "Cephalalgia": "Every kind of headache" (Dunglison 1833, 1:172).

50. Phrenitis: "Characterized by strong fever, violent head-ache, redness of the face and eyes, impatience of light and noise, watchfulness, and furious delirium" (Hooper 1825, 934).

51. Chorea is Saint Vitus's Dance, which involves convulsive motions of the limbs as if the person were dancing.

52. "Risings or prominences, of greater or less size, developed by a morbific cause in some part of the body . . . Tumors differ greatly from each other; according to their seat, the organs interested, their nature" (Dunglison 1833, 2:388).

53. Erectile tumor: "a tumor, produced by the development of a soft, vascular tissue . . . susceptible of dilatation and depression" (Dunglison 1833, 2:388–389). Velpeau experimented by penetrating arteries. A ganglion

was "an encysted tumour, formed in the sheath of a tendon, and containing a fluid like the white of an egg" (Hooper 1825, 542).

54. This piece was frequently reprinted (Editor 1825m–p; Ferussac 1825).

55. Some needles had blackened and corroded when extracted (Meyranx, 1825b; Wallace 1827).

56. Carpenter's copy of Morand is in the Boston Medical Library of the Francis A. Countway Library. Carpenter might have had in mind a *Lancet* article that advanced the same argument, reprinted in the *Boston Medical Intelligencer* (Editor 1825s).

57. For similar lists, see Mongiardini 1807 and Brown 1817.

58. See Editor 1834a, 1836b, 1837d; Grantham 1837; Bird 1841a, 1841b; James 1841; Raciborski 1846a, 1846b; de Puisaye 1846.

59. See Ricketson 1806; Cocke 1809; Ure 1819; Morus 1998.

60. Electro-puncture: Sarlandière 1825; Raciborski 1846a, 1846b. Neuralgia: Pelletan 1825a; Editor 1841d; Dunglison 1842; Gruggen 1843; Hermel 1844. Aneurisms: Phillips 1845; Pétrequin 1845a (this piece was repeatedly reprinted and summarized in Ireland, England, and the United States); Anonymous 1846a; Hamilton 1846; Ciniselli 1846; Restelli 1847a, 1847b; Cappelletti 1848. Paralysis: Stokes 1834; Hamilton 1835a, 1835b, 1835c; Da Camino 1835; Editor 1839f; Dunglison 1846a. Amaurosis: Hamilton 1835a, 1835b; Rosas 1836; Person 1844. Asphyxia: Dunglison 1846a. Deafness: Jobert 1843a, 1843b, 1844. Intermittent fevers, pleurisy, asthma, colics, headaches, stomachaches, and uterine pain: Sarlandière 1825. Varices: Milani 1846; Gamberini 1847; Bertani and Milani 1847a; McCarthy 1847; Bertani and Milani 1847b. Obliteration of arteries: Namias 1846, 1847. Hydrocele: Stewart 1843, 1844, 1846; Ogier 1846.

61. Although Carpenter started the catalog in 1833, I located only the 1844 edition and cannot be sure whether he sold acupuncture needles prior to *New Remedies* (1839) or, if not, how soon thereafter he added them.

62. Lepage reviewed in detail Amiot's discussion of *gongfu;* see Lepage 1813, 85–89.

Abbreviations

AA	*Acta asiatica*
AGM	*Archives générales de médecine*
AHSI	*Archivum historicum societatis Iesu*
AJ	*Asiatic Journal*
AJFM	*American Journal of Foreign Medicine*
AJMR	*Asiatic Journal and Monthly Register for British and Foreign India, China, and Australasia*
AJMS	*American Journal of Medical Science*
AJP	*American Journal of Pharmacy*
AMag	*American Magazine*
AMed	*Anthropology of Medicine*
AMI	*American Medical Intelligencer*
AMM	*American Monthly Magazine*
AMP	*Annales de la médecine physiologique*
AMPR	*American Medical and Philosophical Register*
AMRec	*American Medical Recorder*
AMRev	*American Medical Review*
AMRJ	*American Medical Review and Journal*
AMUEK	*American Magazine of Useful and Entertaining Knowledge*
AMW	*American Magazine of Wonders*
AN	*American Naturalist*
ASEM	*Atheneum: Spirit of the English Magazine*
ASRS	*Annales de la Société royale des sciences, belles-lettres et arts d'Orléans*
BGHJAS	*Boston Guide to Health and Journal of Arts and Sciences*
BGTMC	*Bulletin général de thérapeutique médicale et chirurgicale*
BHM	*Bulletin of the History of Medicine*
BM	*Biologie médicale*
BMI	*Boston Medical Intelligencer*
BMJ	*British Medical Journal*
BMPR	*Baltimore Medical and Physical Recorder*
BMR	*Botanico-Medical Recorder*

BMS	Bulletin of Medical Science
BNYAM	Bulletin of the New York Academy of Medicine
BosMSJ	Boston Medical and Surgical Journal
BPSA	Bulletin de pharmacie et des sciences accessoires
BrMSJ	British Medical and Surgical Journal
BSM	Bulletin des sciences médicales
BWM	Boston Weekly Magazine
CA	Colored American
CPCOTT	Captain Pidding's Chinese Olio and Tea Talk
CR	Chinese Repository
CReg	Canton Register
CS	Chinese Science
DAPM	Dwight's American Penny Magazine
DAPMFN	Dwight's American Penny Magazine, and Family Newspaper
DJMCS	Dublin Journal of Medical and Chemical Sciences
DJMS	Dublin Journal of Medical Science
DMP	Dublin Medical Press
DQJMS	Dublin Quarterly Journal of Medical Science
EC	Early China
EJMS	Edinburgh Journal of the Medical Sciences
EMSJ	Edinburgh Medical and Surgical Journal
ENPJ	Edinburgh New Philosophical Journal
ERAR	Eclectic Repertory and Analytical Review, Medical and Philosophical
FEQ	Far Eastern Quarterly
FMR	Foreign Medical Review
GM	Gentleman's Magazine
GMP	Gazette médicale de Paris
GSPPT	Giornale per servire ai progressi della patologia e della terapeutica
HLCR	Hongkong Late Canton Register
HS	History of Science
ICG	Indo-Chinese Gleaner
IIMSJ	Illinois and Indiana Medical and Surgical Journal
IMSJ	Illinois Medical and Surgical Journal
IPQ	International Philosophical Quarterly
JAARTS	Journal of the American Academy of Religion Thematic Studies
JAH	Journal of American History
JA	Journal asiatique
JAMA	Journal of Asian Martial Arts
JAS	Journal of Asian Studies
JASB	Journal of the Asiatic Society of Bengal

JCDSM	*Journal complémentaire du dictionnaire des sciences médicales*
JCM	*Journal of Chinese Medicine*
JGMCP	*Journal général de médecine, de chirurgie et de pharmacie*
JGMCPFE	*Journal générale de médecine, de chirurgie et de pharmacie, françaises et étrangères*
JHI	*Journal of the History of Ideas*
JHM	*Journal of the History of Medicine*
JHMAS	*Journal of the History of Medicine and Allied Sciences*
JMCP	*Journal de médecine, de chirurgie et de pharmacologie*
JNCBRAS	*Journal of the North-China Branch of the Royal Asiatic Society*
JPCP	*Journal of the Philadelphia College of Pharmacy*
JPEP	*Journal de physiologie expérimentale et pathologique*
JRASGBI	*Journal of the Royal Asiatic Society of Great Britain and Ireland*
JRS	*Journal of Ritual Studies*
JSCMA	*Journal of the South Carolina Medical Association*
JSMSADL	*Journal de la section de médecine de la société académique du département de la Loire-inférieur*
JSPP	*Journal de la Société des pharmaciens de Paris*
JUSM	*Journal universel des sciences médicales*
LECAAA	*Lettres édifiantes et curieuses concernant l'Asie, l'Afrique et l'Amérique*, vol. 3, ed. M. L. Aimé-Martin. Paris: Société du Panthéon Littéraire.
LEMJMS	*London and Edinburgh Monthly Journal of Medical Science*
LFGHCM	*Lancette française: Gazette des hôpitaux civils et militaires*
LL	*London Lancet*
LMG	*London Medical Gazette*
LMPJ	*London Medical and Physical Journal*
LMR	*London Medical Repository*
LMRMJR	*London Medical Repository, Monthly Journal and Review*
LMRR	*London Medical Repository and Review*
LMSPR	*London Medical, Surgical, and Pharmaceutical Repository*
MABR	*Monthly Anthology and Boston Review*
MAR	*Medical and Agricultural Register*
MCHSAMUC	*Mémoires concernant l'histoire, les sciences, les arts, les moeurs, les usages, &c. des chinois*. Paris: Nyon l'aîné, Libraire.
MCJR	*Medico-Chirurgical Journal and Review*
MCR	*Medico-Chirurgical Review*
MCRJMS	*Medico-Chirurgical Review, and Journal of Medical Science*
MCRJPM	*The Medico-Chirurgical Review, and Journal of Practical Medicine*
MCT	*Medico-Chirurgical Transactions*

ME	Medical Examiner
MERMS	Medical Examiner and Record of Medical Science
MJFM	Monthly Journal of Foreign Medicine
MJM	Monthly Journal of Medicine
MJMS	Monthly Journal of Medical Science
MJMSci	Monthly Journal of the Medical Sciences
MM	Medical Magazine
MMSJ	Missouri Medical and Surgical Journal
MNL	Medical News and Library
MNP	Medical News-Paper; or The Doctor and The Physician
MOI	Medical Observations and Inquiries
MPC	Medical and Philosophical Commentaries by a Society in Edinburgh
MPJ	Medical and Physical Journal
MQR	Medical Quarterly Review
MRec	Medical Recorder
MRep	Medical Repository
MRJ	Medical Review and Journal
MROEI	Medical Repository of Original Essays and Intelligence
MROPIMS	Medical Recorder of Original Papers and Intelligence in Medicine and Surgery
MS	Medical Sciences
MSer	Monumenta serica
MT	Medical Times
MTrans	Medical Transactions (College of Physicians, London)
NAMSJ	North American Medical and Surgical Journal
NAR	North American Review
NEJMS	New England Journal of Medicine and Surgery and the Collateral Branches of Science
NEQM	New England Quarterly Magazine
NJA	Nouveau journal asiatique
NOMJ	New-Orleans Medical Journal
NRRSL	Notes and Records of the Royal Society of London
NYD	New York Dissector
NYJM	New York Journal of Medicine
NYJMCS	New York Journal of Medicine, and the Collateral Sciences
NYJMS	New-York Journal of Medicine and Surgery
NYL	New York Lancet
NYMCB	New-York Medico-Chirurgical Bulletin
NYMPJ	New York Medical and Physical Journal
NYMSR	New-York Medical and Surgical Reporter

NYSJM	*New York State Journal of Medicine*
OMR	*Ohio Medical Repository*
PAPS	*Proceedings of the American Philosophical Society*
PEW	*Philosophy East and West*
PJMPS	*Philadelphia Journal of the Medical and Physical Sciences*
PJT	*Pharmaceutical Journal and Transactions*
PMJMS	*Philadelphia Monthly Journal of Medicine and Surgery*
PMPJ	*Philadelphia Medical and Physical Journal*
PT	*Philosophical Transactions*
PTRSL	*Philosophical Transactions of the Royal Society of London*
REAP	*Revue de l'École d'anthropologie de Paris*
RIHSC	*Rhode Island Historical Society Collections*
RMCP	*Revue médicale-chirurgicale de Paris*
RMFEJC	*Revue médicale française et étrangère et Journal de Clinique de l'Hôtel-Dieu et de la Charité de Paris*
RPSMP	*Recueil périodique de la Société de médecine de Paris*
RS	*Revue de synthèse*
RSSCW	*Research Studies of the State College of Washington*
SHP	*Semaine des hôpitaux de Paris*
SJMP	*Southern Journal of Medicine and Pharmacy*
SM	*Scientific Monthly*
SMSJ	*Southern Medical and Surgical Journal*
SSM	*Social Science and Medicine*
TAMA	*Transactions of the American Medical Association*
TCMCS	*Transactions of the China-Medico-Chirurgical-Society*
TJMAS	*Transylvania Journal of Medicine and the Associate Sciences*
TM	*Transactions médicales*
TMPSC	*Transactions of the Medical and Physical Society of Calcutta*
TR	*Thomsonian Recorder*
TRASGBI	*Transactions of the Royal Asiatic Society of Great Britain and Ireland*
WJAMMA	*Western Journal of Agriculture, Manufactures, Mechanic Arts, Internal Improvements, Commerce, and General Literature*
WJMS	*Western Journal of Medicine and Surgery*
WL	*Western Lancet*
WMCQHM	*William and Mary College Quarterly Historical Magazine*
WMG	*Western Medical Gazette*
WP	*Winterthur Portfolio*

Bibliography

For some early sources I have cited editions published several years after a work's original publication date, as the texts were the same and only these other versions were available to me. With non-English-language sources, if I had access to English translations published close to the time of the original work, I quoted from them, to stay closer to English of the same period. All other translations into English from Latin, Portuguese, Spanish, French, Italian, or German are mine.

A-Z. 1824. Chinese visits to Europe. *AJMR* 17 (Jan.–June):242–243.

Abeel, David. 1836. *Journal of a residence in China, and the neighboring countries*, 2nd ed. New York: J. Abeel Williamson.

Abel, Clarke. 1818a. *Narrative of a journey in the interior of China*. London: Longman, Hurst, Rees, Orme, and Brown.

———. 1818b. Dr. Abel's narrative. *ASEM* 4(4):152–156.

Abel-Rémusat, Jean Pierre. 1813. *Dissertatio de glossosemeiotice, sive de signis morborum quae è linguâ sumuntur praesertim apud sinenses*. Paris: Didot.

———. 1825. *Mélanges asiatiques*, vol. 1. Paris: Librairie Orientale de Dondey-Dupré.

———. 1829. *Nouveaux mélanges asiatiques*, 2 vols. Paris: Schubart et Heideloff.

———. 1833. Observations sur l'état des sciences naturelles chez les peuples de l'Asie orientale. *Mémoires de l'Institut Royal de France, Académie des Inscriptions et Belles-Lettres* 10:116–167. Paris: Imprimerie Royale.

———. 1843. *Mélanges posthumes d'histoire et de littérature orientales*. Paris: Imprimerie Royale.

Abercromby, David. 1685. *De variatione, ac varietate pulsus*. London: Samuel Smith.

Académie Royale de Médecine. 1824. Acupuncture. *AGM* 6 (Sept.):619.

———. 1825a. Acupuncture. *AGM* 7:140.

———. 1825b. Accidents de l'acupuncture. *AGM* 7:143.

———. 1825c. Variétés: Acupuncture. *RMFEJC* 2:148–149.

———. 1825d. Note sur l'acupuncture. *AGM* 7:149–151.

———. 1825e. Section de médecine.—Séance du 25 janvier.—Acupuncture. *AGM* 7:305–306.

———. 1825f. Acupuncture [M. J. Cloquet]. *AGM* 7:308–309.

———. 1825g. Acupuncture [M. Ségalas]. *AGM* 7:309.

———. 1825h. Acupuncture. *AGM* 7:464–465, 469.

———. 1827. Sciatique guérie par l'acupuncture. *AGM* 15:450.

Acosta, Cristóvão. [1582]1964. *Tratado das drogas e medicinas das Indias Orientais, no qual se verifica muito do que escriveu Doutor Garcia de Orta*. Lisbon: Junta de Investigações do Ultramar.

Ågren, Hans. 1986. Chinese traditional medicine: Temporal order and synchronous events. In *Time, science, and society in China and the West*, ed. J. T. Fraser, N. Lawrence, and F. C. Haber, 211–218. Amherst: University of Massachusetts Press.

Ai, Gongzhe. 1819. Chinese poetry. *ICG* 2(8):63–68.

Alemand, Louis Augustin, Michael Boym, and Julien Hervieu. 1671. *Les secrets de la médecine des Chinois, consistant en la parfaite connoissance du pouls. Envoyez de la Chine par un françois, homme de grand merite*. Grenoble: Philippes Charuys.

Alexander, William. 1792–1794. Journal of Lord Macartney's embassy to China. British Library. Manuscript. Additional 35174.

Aliquis. 1830–1831. Arguments against apprenticeships. *Lancet* 2:42–45.

Allnatt, R. H. 1843–1844a. The "best remedies" for neuralgia. *LL* 2:67–68.

———. 1843–1844b. Remedies for neuralgia. *LL* 2:545.

Allom, Thomas, and G. N. Wright. 1843. *China, in a series of views*, vols. 1–2. London: Peter Jackson.

Altick, Richard D. 1978. *The shows of London: A panoramic history of exhibitions, 1600–1862*. Cambridge, MA: Harvard University Press.

Ames, Roger T. 1984. The meaning of the body in classical Chinese thought. *IPQ* 24(1):39–54.

Amicus. 1818. Demons. *ICG* 1(5):144–145.

Amin, Samir. 1989. *Eurocentrism*, trans. Russell Moore. New York: Monthly Review Press.

Aminicus. 1804. Mr. Clayton, on Ching's Worm Lozenges. *MPJ* 12(June–Dec.):173–174.

Amiot, P. 1779. Notice du cong-fou des bonzes Tao-sée. *MCHSAMUC* 4:441–451.

———. 1791a. Extrait d'une lettre de M. Amiot, missionnaire, écrite de Pékin le 16 Octobre 1787, sur la secte des *Tao-sée*. *MCHSAMUC* 15:208–259.

———. 1791b. Extrait d'une lettre de M. Amiot, écrite de Pékin le 26 Juin 1789. 2: Sur la médecine chez les Chinois. *MCHSAMUC* 15:v–xv.

Anderson, Aeneas. 1795. *A narrative of the British embassy to China, in the years 1792, 1793, and 1794*. New York: Rogers and Berry.

Anderson, Alexander. 1843. Minutes of a meeting of the committee, March 27, 1843. *CReg* 16(19):84–85.

Andrews, Bridie J. 1999. Acupuncture and the reinvention of Chinese medicine. *American Pain Society Bulletin* 9(3). www.ampainsoc.org/pub/bulletin/may99/history.htm (downloaded 3/19/02).

———. n.d. The politics of *Qi:* Changing Chinese conceptions of how the body works. Manuscript. Department of the History of Science, Harvard University.

———. Forthcoming. *The modernizing of Chinese medicine.* Cambridge: Cambridge University Press.

Andrieux, M. 1825. Rhumatisme goutteux guéri par l'acupuncture. *RMFEJC* 3:450–451.

Anonymous. 1740. *An irregular dissertation occasioned by the reading of Father Du Halde's description of China.* London: J. Roberts.

———. 1753. Account of the weather. *GM* 23(May 31):209.

———. 1758. Clef de la doctrine des Chinois sur le pouls. In *Le conservateur; ou, Collection de morceaux rares, & d'ouvrages anciens, élagués, traduits & refaits en tout ou en partie,* July, 134–154.

———. 1773. *The present state of the British interest in India.* London: J. Almon.

———. 1778. Notice de quelques plantes, arbrisseaux, &c., de la Chine. *MCHSAMUC* 3:437–490.

———. 1779a. Notice du che-hiang. *MCHSAMUC* 4:493–500.

———. 1779b. Notice du livre LXXXVI du recueil Kou-kin-y-tong. *MCHSAMUC* 5:237–242.

———. 1779c. Notice du pe-tsai. *MCHSAMUC* 4:503–510.

———. 1779d. Quelques compositions & recettes pratiquées chez les Chinois, ou consignées dans leurs livres, & que l'auteur a crues utiles ou inconnues en Europe. *MCHSAMUC* 4:484–492.

———. 1779e. Notice du mo-kou-sin et du lin-tchi. *MCHSAMUC* 4:500–503.

———. 1780a. Armoise. *MCHSAMUC* 5:514–518.

———. 1780b. Raisins secs de ha-mi. *MCHSAMUC* 5:481–486.

———. 1780c. Remèdes. *MCHSAMUC* 5:492–494.

———. 1782. Notice du sang de cerf, employé comme remède. *MCHSAMUC* 8:271–273.

———. 1786. Mémoire sur l'usage de la viande en Chine. *MCHSAMUC* 11:78–182.

———. 1803. Advertisement: Dr. Ching-Ching-Ti-Ching. *BWM* 1(Sept. 10):185–186.

———. 1804. Chinese anecdote. *BWM* 2(43):171.

———. 1816. Antique monument in China. *BWM* 1(7):26.

———. 1820. To the subscribers. *AMRec* 3.

———. 1823. Review of Rémusat's *Éléments de la grammaire chinois. NAR* 17:12.

———. 1824a. Death of the Chinese lady. *Times,* July 13, p. 3.

———. 1824b. Ghosts—Hobgoblins. *BMI* 2(23):94.

———. 1831a. Extraordinary case of a Chinese at Guy's Hospital. *Times,* Apr. 5, p. 3.

———. 1831b. Operation upon Hoo Loo, the Chinese for a tumour, in Guy's Hospital. *Times,* Apr. 11, p. 2.

———. 1833. The adventures of Le-Yuen. *Chinese Courier* 2(42):3.

———. 1835a. *Catalogue of phrenological specimens belonging to the Boston Phrenological Society.* Boston: John Ford.

———. 1835b. Walks about Canton. *CR* 4(1):42–46.

———. 1835c. Walks about Canton. *CR* 4(5):244–245.

———. 1836. *The Indian vegetable family instructer.* N.p.

———. 1839. Moxas of wafers. *AJMS* 25:465.

———. 1842. Smoking shop. *NYL* 1(16):256.

———. 1844a. Ununited fracture successfully treated by acupuncture. *NOMJ* 1(1):461–462.

———. 1844b. European medical practice in China. *CPCOTT* (22):172–173.

———. 1844c. Medical aid to the Chinese. *CPCOTT* (10):79.

———. 1844d. Animal magnetism in China. *CPCOTT* (12):91.

———. 1846a. Galvanic puncture in aneurism. *MT* 15(367):19.

———. 1846b. How the Chinese prepare tea. *DAPM* 2(16):247.

Anson, Lord George. 1748. *A voyage round the world in the years MDCCXL, I, II, III, IV.* London: John and Paul Knapton.

Appleby, John H. 1983. Ginseng and the Royal Society. *NRRSL* 37(2):121–145.

Appleton, William W. 1951. *A cycle of Cathay: The Chinese vogue in England during the seventeenth and eighteenth centuries.* New York: Columbia University Press.

Arago, M. 1844. New magnetic fluid. *NYD* 1(4):198–199.

Argens, Jean-Baptiste de Boyer, Marquis d'. 1741. *Chinese letters,* trans. Marquis d'Argens. London: D. Browne and R. Hett.

Astruc, Jean. 1777. *Traité des maladies vénériennes,* 4th ed., vol. 2, trans. M. Louis. Paris: P. G. Cavelier.

Aumont, M. 1825. Accidents arising from acupuncturation. *LMPJ* 53(Jan.–June):260.

Authors of the Ancient Part. 1759. *The modern part of an universal history,* vol. 9. London: S. Richardson, T. Osborne, C. Hitch.

Azouvi, François. 2000. Physique and moral. In Wright and Potter 2000, 267–279.

B., R. 1836. Cure of hydrocele by acupuncture (Letter to the editor). *Lancet* 2(June 25):432–433.

Bache, Franklin. 1826. Cases illustrative of the remedial effects of acupuncturation. *NAMSJ* 1:311–321.

Bailly [Bally], Dr., and Dr. Meyranx. 1825. Du galvanisme médical. *AGM* 9:66–80.

Banks, John Tatum. 1830. Acupuncturation. *Lancet* 2 (Apr. 30):129.

———. 1831. Observations on acupuncturation. *EMSJ* 35:323–328.

Barchusen, Johann Conrad. 1710. *Historia medicinae.* Amsterdam: Joannem Wolters.

Barlow, E., and Robley Dunglison. 1848. Rheumatism. In *Cyclopaedia of practical medicine,* ed. John Forbes, Alexander Tweedie, and John Conolly, rev. Robley Dunglison, 4:23–42. Philadelphia: Lea and Blanchard.

Barrow, John. 1804. *Travels in China.* London: T. Cadell and W. Davies.

———. 1807. *Some account of the public life, and a selection from the unpublished writings, of the Earl of Macartney,* vols. 1–2. London: T. Cadell and W. Davies.

———. 1847. *An auto-biographical memoir of Sir John Barrow, Bart.* London: John Murray.

Bartoli, Daniello. 1975. *La Cina.* Milan: Bompiani.

Barton, Benjamin Smith. 1806. Account of Henry Moss, a white Negro. *PMPJ* 2:3–18.

Barton, William P. C. 1817–1818. *Vegetable materia medica of the United States,* vols. 1–2. Philadelphia: M. Carey and Son.

Bartram, John, and William Bartram. 1957. *John and William Bartram's America,* ed. Helen Gere Gruickshank. New York: Devin-Adair.

Baudier, Michel. 1682. *The history of the court of the king of China.* London: Christopher Hussey.

Bayard, H. 1841. On infanticide in France. *LEMJMS* (April): 407.

Bayle, Antoine Laurent Jesse. 1828. *Bibliotheque de thérapeutique,* vol. 1. Paris: Gabon.

———. 1837. *Bibliotheque de thérapeutique,* vol. 4. Paris: Gabon.

Beck, T. Romeyn. 1848. Opium smoking. *AJMS,* n.s. 15:302.

Becket, John Brice. 1773. *An essay on electricity.* Bristol: J. B. Becket.

Béclard, Pierre Auguste. 1821. Acupuncture. In *Dictionnaire de médecine,* 2nd ed., 1:335–336. Paris: Bechet.

Bédor, M. 1812. Acupuncture. In *Dictionnaire des sciences médicales,* A–AMP, 149–150. Paris: C. L. F. Panckoucke.

Belcher, William. 1798. *Intellectual electricity, novum organum of vision, and grand mystic secret.* London: Lee and Hurst.

Belden, Louise Conway. 1965. Humphry Marshall's trade in plants of the new world for gardens and forests of the old world. *WP* 2:106–126.

Bell, Jacob. 1844. Importation of Chinese quicksilver. *PJT* 3:539.

———. 1848. Kew Gardens and Museum of Vegetable Products. *PJT* 7:150–152.

Bell, John. [1763]1965. *A journey from St. Petersburg to Pekin, 1719–22*, ed. J. L. Stevenson. Edinburgh: Edinburgh University Press.

———. 1843. On the medical mission to China. *BMS* 1:273.

———. 1844. Medical Missionary Society. *BMS* 2:174–176.

Benedict, Carol. 1996. *Bubonic plague in nineteenth-century China*. Stanford: Stanford University Press.

Bergamaschi, Dr. 1827. Acupuncturation in tic douloureux. *LMPJ*, n.s. 2:91–92.

Berkeley, Edmund. 1993. Benjamin Franklin and a "dear ould friend." *PAPS* 137(3):399–405

Berlioz, Louis. 1800. *Dissertation sur les effets du fluide électrique introduit dans l'économie animale*. N.p.: G. Izar et A. Richard.

———. 1816. *Mémoires sur les maladies chroniques, les évacuations sanguines et l'acupuncture*. Paris: Croullebois.

Bertani, M., and M. Milani. 1847a. Application de l'électro-puncture au traitement des varices. *GMP*, 3rd ser., 2:206–207.

———. 1847b. Treatment of varices by electro-puncture. *MT* 17(423):57.

Bigelow, Jacob. 1817. *American medical botany*. Boston: Cummings and Hilliard.

Bigg, William. 1847. Respecting the cultivation of English rhubarb, near Banbury. *PJT* 6:74–76.

Birbeck, Dr. 1835. Varieties of rhubarb. *MQR* 4:264–265.

Bird, Golding. 1841a. On electricity as a remedial agent. *LEMJMS* (June): 437–439.

———. 1841b. Report on the value of electricity, as a remedial agent in the treatment of diseases. *MCRJPM*, n.s. 35:239–247.

———. 1842a. New bandages.—Opium-smoking.—Action of poisons. *Lancet* 1(Feb. 19):726–727.

———. 1842b. The Chinese theory and practice of medicine. *Lancet* 1(Mar. 5):805–806.

———. 1842c. Colic from lead.—Blue mark of the gums from lead.—Chinese medicine. *Lancet* 1(Mar. 5):805

Bivins, Roberta E. 2000. *Acupuncture, expertise and cross-cultural medicine*. New York: Palgrave.

Black, William. 1782. *An historical sketch of medicine and surgery from their origin to the present time*. London: J. Johnson.

Blanc, Jean Baptiste. 1799–1800. *Aperçu sur les avantages des caustiques caloriques, et particulièrement du moxa*. Montpellier.

Blumenbach, Johann Friedrich. [1795]1865. *The anthropological treatises of Johann Friedrich Blumenbach*, ed. Thomas Bendyshe. London: Longman, Green.

du Boccage, Madame. 1786. Extrait d'une lettre de Madame du Boccage, écrite à Paris le 5 juin 1785. *MCHSAMUC* 11:xi–xxii.

Bodemer, Charles W. n.d. Traditional Chinese medicine in nineteenth century America. Manuscript.

Boerhaave, Hermann. 1719. *A method of studying physick.* London: C. Rivington, B. Creake, and J. Sackfield.

Bond, W. H., and Hugh Amory, eds. 1996. *Printed catalogues of the Harvard College Library: 1723–1790.* Boston: Colonial Society of Massachusetts.

Bondt, Jakob de. 1658. *Historiae naturalis & medicae Indiae.* In *De Indiae utriusque re naturali et medica libri quatrodecim,* ed. Willem Piso. Amsterdam: Ludovic & Daniel Elevirios.

Bonner, Arthur. 1997. *Alas! What brought thee hither: The Chinese in New York, 1800–1950.* Madison, NJ: Fairleigh Dickinson University Press.

Bonnet, M. 1837. Radical cure of varicose veins and of herniae by acupuncturation. *MCRJPM,* n.s. 27:551–552.

de Bordeu, Théophile. [1756]1764. *Inquiries concerning the varieties of the pulse.* London: T. Lewis.

Boulard, M. 1825. Deux observations d'acupuncture. *AMP* 7:193–195.

Bowdoin College Medical School. 1825. *Catalogue of the library of the Medical School of Maine, at Bowdoin College, February 1825.* Brunswick, ME: J. Griffin.

———. 1834. *Catalogue of the library of the Medical School of Maine, at Bowdoin College, February 1834.* Brunswick, ME: J. Griffin.

Bowers, John Z., and Robert W. Carrubba. 1970. The doctoral thesis of Engelbert Kaempfer on tropical diseases, oriental medicine, and exotic natural phenomena. *JHM* 25:270–310.

Boxer, Charles R., ed. 1953. *South China in the sixteenth century: Being the narratives of Galeote Pereira, Fr. Gaspar da Cruz, Fr. Martin de Rada (1550–1575).* London: Hakluyt Society.

———. 1963. *Two pioneers of tropical medicine: Garcia d'Orta and Nicolas Monardes.* London: Wellcome Medical Historical Library.

———. 1974. *A note on the interaction of Portuguese and Chinese medicine at Macao and Peking.* Macao: Imprensa Nacional.

Boyle, J. A. 1969–1970. The last barbarian invaders. *Memoirs and Proceedings of the Manchester Literary and Philosophical Society,* 4th ser., 112:5–19.

Boym, Michael. 1656. *Flora sinensis, fructus floresque humillime porrigens.* Vienna: n.p.

———. 1686. Clavis medica ad Chinarum doctrinam de pulsibus . . . In *Miscellanea curiosa sive Ephemeridum medico-physicarum Germanicarum Academiae Naturae Curiosorum, decuriae II. Annus quartus, anni 1685.* Nuremberg: Sumptibus Wolfgangi Moritii Endteri.

———. [1652]1694. Briefve relation de la Chine. In *Relations de divers voyages curieux,* ed. and trans. Melchisédec Thévenot. Paris: Thomas Moette.

———. [1656]1730. Flora sinensis; ou, Traité des fleurs, des fruits, des plantes, et des animaux particuliers à la Chine. In *Relations de divers voyages curieux, qui n'ont point esté publiées . . .* , vol. 1, no. 2, ed. and trans. Melchisédec Thévenot, 15–30. Paris: T. Moette.

Brande, William Thomas. 1817. Observations on an astringent vegetable substance from China. *PTRSL* 1:39–44.

Breton, M. 1811. *La Chine en miniature,* vols. 1–3. Paris: Nepveu.

Bretschneider, E. 1881. *Early European researches into the flora of China.* Shanghai: American Presbyterian Mission Press.

———. [1898]1981. *History of European botanical discoveries in China,* vol. 1. Leipzig: Zentral-Antiquariat der Deutschen Demokratischen Republik.

Brett, Mr. 1831. Mr. Brett's note on acupuncturation, for cure of chronic rheumatism in natives, dated Mar. 22d, 1831. *TMPSC* 5:443.

———. 1832. Acupuncturation: Insertion of the needle in a joint. *Lancet,* Aug. 25, p. 672.

Broglia, Dr. 1834. New remedy in neuralgia. *WMG* 2(7):310–311.

Brookes, Richard. 1751. *The general practice of physic,* vols. 1–2. London: J. Newbery.

———. 1754. *An introduction to physic and surgery.* London: J. Newbery.

Brooks, Dr. 1833. *The physician's assistant.* N.p.: Benjamin French.

Brown, Thomas. 1817. *The ethereal physician; or, Medical electricity revived.* Albany, NY: G. J. Loomis.

Browne, Joseph. 1703. *The modern practice of physick vindicated.* London: Nicholas Cox.

Bruce, E., and A. Taeko Brooks. 1993. Warring states texts. www.umass.edu/wsp/wst/l-r/mc/index.html (downloaded 3/27/2005).

Brugnatelli, Prof. 1812. D'une concrétion trouvée dans les racines de rhubarbe. *BPSA* 4:543–544.

Buchan, William. 1769. *Domestic medicine; or, The family physician.* Edinburgh: Balfour, Auld, and Smellie.

Buc'hoz, Pierre-Joseph. 1781. *Herbier; ou, Collection des plantes médicinales de la Chine.* Paris: Chez l'auteur.

Buell, Paul D., and Eugene N. Anderson. 2000. *A soup for the Qan.* London: Kegan Paul International.

Buffon, Georges Louis Leclerc, comte de. [1749–1788]1971. *De l'homme; histoire naturelle.* Paris: Vialetay.

Burman, Mr. 1848. Case of ununited fracture treated by galvanism. *AJMS,* n.s. 5:546–547.

Burnett, Gilbert Thomas. 1835a. *Outlines of botany.* London.

———. 1835b. Ginseng. *MQR* 3:228.

Burton, Robert. [1621]1977. *The anatomy of melancholy.* New York: Vintage.

Buschof, Hermann. [1674]1993. *Erste Abhandlung über die moxibustion in Europa.* Heidelberg: Karl F. Haug Verlag.

Bushe, George. 1832. Aneurism treated by puncture with a white hot needle. *NYMCB* 2(5):209–210.

Butler, Jon. 1990. *Awash in a sea of faith: Christianizing the American people.*
Cambridge, MA: Harvard University Press.

Byrd, William, Jr. 1929. *William Byrd's histories of the dividing line betwixt Virginia and North Carolina.* Raleigh: North Carolina Historical Commission.

Cabot, James Elliot. 1887. *A memoir of Ralph Waldo Emerson,* vol. 1. Boston:
Houghton Mifflin.

Cairn, John. 1843. Tariff of duties on the foreign trade with China. *HLCR*
16(29):1.

Calau, Fr. 1843a. On rhubarb. *PJT* 2:658–660.

———. 1843b. On rhubarb. *MT* 8(188):96–97.

———. 1843c. On rad. Ginseng. *PJT* 2:661–662.

Calhoun, Samuel. 1825a. Dr. Meyranse, on acupuncturation. *MROPIMS* 8:837.

———. 1825b. Ophthalmia cured by acupuncturation. *MRec* 8:626.

Cambell, M. 1839. Ascite guérie à l'aide de l'acupuncture. *GMP,* 2nd ser.,
7:105.

Camino, Francesco Saverio da. 1834. *Sulla ago-puntura, con alcuni cenni sulla
puntura elettrica.* Venezia: Antonelli.

———. 1835. Case of a woman who, by the means of galvano-puncture,
recovered her speech after having lost it for twenty-three years. *MQR*
4:752–753.

———. 1838. Sopra un giudizio del dottor Zerlotto; Lettera al dott. Giacinto
Namias del dott. Francesco Da Camin. *GSPPT* 8:499–507.

———. 1839. Lettera seconda al dott. Giacinto Namias del dott. Francesco
Da Camino. *GSPPT* 10:177–197.

———. 1847. *Sull'operazione dell'ago-puntura.* Venezia: Co'tipi di Gio.
Cecchini.

Cappelletti, M. 1848. Anévrisme variqueux au pli du coude; deux applications de galvano-puncture; inflammation et gangrène du sac; guérison.
GMP, 3rd ser., 3:592–593.

Carpenter, Frederick Ives. 1930. *Emerson and Asia.* Cambridge, MA: Harvard
University Press.

Carpenter, George W., and Co. 1835. *Carpenter's family medicine chest.* Philadelphia: George W. Carpenter's Chemical Warehouse.

———. 1844. *Carpenter's annual medical advertiser for 1844.* Philadelphia: T. K.
and P. G. Collins.

Carraro, Antonio. 1826. Acupuncture in suspended animation. *OMR*
1(8):30.

———. 1842. Acupuncture of the heart in apparent death. *NYL* 1(12):189–
190.

Carrubba, Robert W., and John Z. Bowers. 1974. The Western world's first detailed treatise on acupuncture: Willem ten Rhijne's *De acupunctura*. *JHM* 29:371–398.

Carson, Joseph. 1847. Pharmacy in China. *AJP*, n.s. 13:320.

Carter, Harry William. 1823. A general report of the medical diseases treated in the Kent and Canterbury Hospital, from January 1st to July 1st, 1823. *LMR* 20(120):445–457.

———. 1824. Report of cases treated in the Kent Hospital—On acupuncture. *MJM* 3(Jan.–June):87–88.

Cassedy, James H. 1974. Early uses of acupuncture in the United States, with an addendum (1826) by Franklin Bache, M.D. *BNYAM* 50(8):892–906.

———. 1977. Why self-help? Americans alone with their diseases, 1800–1850. In *Medicine without doctors: Home health care in American history*, ed. Guenter B. Risse, Ronald L. Numbers, and Judith Walzer Leavitt, 31–48. New York: Science History Publications.

Cavallo, Tiberius. 1781. *An essay on the theory and practice of medical electricity*, 2nd ed. London: P. Elmsly.

Celebrated Chinese Physician. 1844. The art of preserving health and beauty and securing long life, free from infirmity and disease, in all climates. *CPCOTT* (10):77; (11):82–83; (12):90–91; (13):99; (14):106–107.

Cervelleri, F. 1839. *De galvanismi acus-puncturae magneticae coniuncti nonnullis in nervorum morbis praestantia*. Napoli: Societ. Typograf.

Chabrié, Robert. 1933. *Michael Boym: Jésuite polonais et la fin des Ming en Chine (1646–1662)*. Paris: Pierre Bossuet.

Chamberlain, Lucia Sarah. 1901. Plants used by the Indians of eastern North America. *AN* (January):1–10.

Chambers, Sir William. [1757]1969. *Designs of Chinese buildings*. Westmead, Farnborough, England: Gregg International.

———. 1772. *Dissertation on oriental gardening*. London: Printed by W. Griffin.

Chan, Wing-tsit, ed. and trans. 1963. *Sourcebook in Chinese philosophy*. Princeton: Princeton University Press.

Chang, Doctor. 1844–1845. Abstract of the treatise of Doctor Chang on diet and regimen. *CPCOTT* (35):275; (36):284–285; (37):291–292; (38):301–302; (39):309–310.

Chang, Hui-chien. 1960. *Li Shih-chen, great pharmacologist of ancient China*. Peking: Foreign Languages Press.

Chang, Te-Ch'ang. 1972. The economic role of the imperial household in the Ch'ing dynasty. *JAS* 31(2):243–273.

Chantourelle, M. 1831. Traitement de diverses maladies par la galvano-puncture. *TM* 6:301–309.

Chapin, Howard M. 1934. The Chinese junk Ke Ying at Providence. *RIHSC* 27(Jan.):5–12.

Chapman, N. 1824. Acupuncture. *PJMPS* 8(6):459–660.

———. 1834. Remarks on tic douloureux; with cases. *AJMS* 14:289–320.

de Chavannes de la Giraudière, H. 1845. *Les Chinois pendant une période de 4458 années.* Tours: A. Mame et Cie.

Chen, Jack. 1980. *The Chinese of America.* San Francisco: Harper and Row.

Ch'en, Kenneth. 1942. Hai-Lu: Forerunner of Chinese travel accounts of Western countries. *MSer* 7:28–236.

———. 1964. *Buddhism in China: A historical survey.* Princeton: Princeton University Press.

Cheng-Tzu-Quogen-Hoang-Ti. 1783. Préface ou introduction aux instructions sublimes et familières. *MCHSAMUC* 9:65–281.

Chevallier, M. 1835. Syrup of rhubarb stalks. *MQR* 4:258–259.

Chilcote, P. 1840. Moxa, in chronic rheumatism. *Lancet,* June 20, p. 448.

China Institute in America. 1983. *Chinese in America: Stereotyped past, changing present,* ed. Loren Fessler. New York: Vantage.

China Medico Chirurgical Society. 1846. *TCMCS,* vol. 1.

———. 1847. Medicine in China. *NYJM* 8:123–124.

Chinese Traveler. 1745. Of philosophical systems: In a letter from a Chinese traveler in Paris to his friend at Pekin. *AMag* 2(Nov.):495–499.

Chinn, Thomas W., ed. 1969. *A history of the Chinese in California: A syllabus.* San Francisco: Chinese Historical Society of America.

Chomel, M. 1815. Case of a man whose skin naturally white became black. *MPJ* 33(191):73–74.

Choy, Philip P., Lorraine Dong, and Marlon K. Hom. 1994. *Coming man: 19th century American perceptions of the Chinese.* Seattle: University of Washington Press.

Christison, R. 1832a. On the effects of opium-eating on health and longevity. *Lancet,* Jan. 21, pp. 614–617.

———. 1832b. On the influence of opium-eating on health and longevity. *AJMS* 10:252–254.

Christy, Arthur. 1932. *The Orient in American transcendentalism: A study of Emerson, Thoreau, and Alcott.* New York: Columbia University Press.

Chu, Doris C. J. 1987. *Chinese in Massachusetts: Their experiences and contributions.* Boston: Chinese Culture Institute.

Chu, Hsi [Zhu, Xi], and Lü Tsu-ch'ien, comps. 1967. *Reflections on things at hand: The neo-Confucian anthology,* trans. and ed. Wing-tsit Chan. New York: Columbia University Press.

Churchill, Fleetwood. 1842. Midwifery in China. *MCRJPM,* n.s. 36:565–567.

———. 1848. *On the theory and practice of midwifery,* 3rd American ed. Philadelphia: Lea and Blanchard.

Churchill, James Morss. 1821. *A treatise on acupuncturation: A description of a surgical operation originally peculiar to the Japanese and Chinese, and by them denominated Zin-King, now introduced into European practice, with directions for its performance and cases illustrating its success.* London: Simpkin and Marshall.

————. 1823a. On acupuncturation. *LMR* 19:372–374.

————. 1823b. On acupuncturation. *AMRec* 6(3):531–535.

————. 1825. *Traité de l'acupuncture; ou, Zin-King des Chinois et des Japonais,* trans. M. R. Charbonnier. Paris: Crevot.

————. 1828. *Cases illustrative of the immediate effects of acupuncturation, in rheumatism, lumbago, sciatic, anomalous muscular diseases, and in dropsy of the cellular tissue: Selected from various sources, and intended as an appendix to the author's treatise on the subject.* London: Callow and Wilson.

Cibot, M. 1779a. De la petite vérole. *MCHSAMUC* 4:392–420.

————. 1779b. Notice du livre chinois Si-Yuen. *MCHSAMUC* 4:421–440.

————. 1779c. Notice du che-hiang. *MCHSAMUC* 4:499.

————. 1782. Essai sur la langue et les caractères des Chinois. *MCHSAMUC* 8:133–263.

————. 1786. Notice sur le cinabre, le vif-argent & le ling-cha. *MCHSAMUC* 11:304–314.

————. 1788. Essai sur la longue vie des hommes dans l'antiquité, spécialement à la Chine. *MCHSAMUC* 13:349–375.

————. 1844. Medical science in China. *CPCOTT,* May 2, p. 4.

Ciniselli, M. 1846. Case of popliteal aneurism cured by galvanism. *MJMS* (48):150–151.

Clarke, John James. 1997. *Oriental enlightenment: The encounter between Asian and Western thought.* London: Routledge.

Cleaveland, Parker. 1812. Account of the effects of electricity. *NEJMS* 2:26–29.

Cleyer, Andreas. 1682. *Specimen medicinae sinicae.* Frankfurt: Sumptibus Joannis Petri Zuybrodt.

Cloquet, Jules. 1826. Acuponcture. In *Nouveau dictionnaire de médecine, chirugie, pharmacie, physique, chimie, histoire naturelle, etc.,* 45–46. Paris: Gabon et Compagnie.

Cocke, James. 1809. Rules for the recovery of the apparently dead. *BMPR* 1:6–11.

Cohen, I. Bernard. 1980. *Album of science: From Leonardo to Lavoisier, 1450–1800.* New York: Scribner.

————. 1997. *Science and the founding fathers: Science in the political thought of Thomas Jefferson, Benjamin Franklin, John Adams and James Madison.* New York: Norton.

Coldstream, John. 1848. Note on the treatment of cholera by the Chinese. *MJMS,* n.s. 86(20):623–634.

Cole, J. 1840. Deleterious effects of tea and coffee. *BMR* 8:100–103.

Coley, W. 1802. A case of tympanites, in an infant . . . To which is subjoined, an account of the operation of the acupuncture. *MPJ* 7(37):223–238.

Collas, M. 1786. Extraits d'une lettre de Feu M. Collas, missionnaire, sur le *Hoang-fan*, le *Nao-cha* ou sel ammoniac, & le *Hoang-pe-mou*. *MCHSAMUC* 11:329–333.

Colledge, Thomas R., Peter Parker, and Elijah C. Bridgman. 1838. Medical Missionary Society: Regulations and resolutions, adopted at a public meeting held at Canton on the 21st of Feb., 1838. *CR* 7(1):32–44.

College of Physicians of Amsterdam. 1659. *Pharmacopoeia Belgica; or, The Dutch dispensatory*. London: Edward Farnham and Robert Horn.

Commager, Henry Steele. 1960. *The era of reform: 1830–1860*. Princeton, NJ: Van Nostrand.

Committee of Inspection. 1844. Report on rhubarb. *AJP*, n.s. 9:16–17.

Condie, D. Francis. 1839. Description of a singular case of nervous disease cured by acupuncturation. *AJMS* 23(46):439–440.

Confucius. 1979. *The analects*, trans. D. C. Lau. New York: Penguin.

Conquest, J. T. 1838. Results of tapping the head in nineteen cases of hydro-cephalus. *AMI* 2(3):40–43.

Conrad, Lawrence I. 1995. The Arab-Islamic medical tradition. In Conrad et al., eds., 1995, 93–138.

Conrad, Lawrence I., Michael Neve, Vivian Nutton, Roy Porter, and Andrew Wear, eds. 1995. *The Western medical tradition: 800 B.C. to 1800 A.D.* New York: Cambridge University Press.

Constant Reader. 1837. Treatment of hydrocele by puncture. *LMG*, Mar. 4, pp. 866–867.

Cook, Harold. 1997. From the scientific revolution to the germ theory. In *Western medicine: An illustrated history*, ed. Irvine Loudon, 80–101. New York: Oxford University Press.

Cooper, Bransby Blake. 1829. Anatomical description of the foot of a Chi-nese female. *BosMSJ* 2(21):330–331.

———. 1830. Anatomical description of a Chinese female foot. *MCR*, n.s. 12:494–496.

Cooper, J. A. 1830. Neuralgia treated by moxae. *Lancet* 1(Jan. 1):461.

Cooper, J. W. 1833. *The experienced botanist or Indian physician*. Edensburg, PA: Canan and Scott.

Cooper, William C., and Nathan Sivin. 1973. Man as a medicine: Pharmaco-logical and ritual aspects of traditional therapy using drugs derived from the human body. In *Chinese science*, ed. Shigeru Nakayama and Nathan Sivin, 203–272. Cambridge, MA: MIT Press.

Copland, James. 1822. Review of *A treatise on acupuncturation* . . . , by James Morss Churchill. *LMRMJR* 17(99):236–237.

———. 1825. On acupuncture, &c. *LMRMJR*, n.s. 3:340–345, 432–433.

Cordier, Henri. 1909. Les Chinois de Turgot. In *Florilegium ou recueil de travaux d'érudition dédiés à Monsieur le Marquis Melchior de Vogüé*, 152–158. Paris: Imprimerie Nationale.

Cormack, John Rose. 1841a. Review of *The elements of materia medica, comprehending the natural history, preparation, properties, composition, effects, and uses of medicines . . .* , by Jonathan Pereira. *LEMJMS* (Jan.): 33–39.

———. 1841b. Tenth report of the Ophthalmic Hospital, Canton, for the year 1839. *LEMJMS* (Aug.): 610–612.

———. 1842. Review of *New remedies,* by Robley Dunglison. *LEMJMS* (Jan.): 42–52.

———. 1843. Medical missions. *LEMJMS* 3:267.

Cornaro, Luigi. 1768. *Discourses on a sober and temperate life.* London: Benjamin White.

Costelli, M. 1846. Histoire d'une tumeur du cou, guérie par l'acupuncture. *GMP* 3rd ser., 1 (June 20):491.

Cothenet, Claude Jean Baptiste. 1808. *Dissertation médico-chirurgicale sur le moxa ou cautère actuel.* Paris.

Courant, Maurice. 1903. *Catalogue des livres chinois, coréen, japonais, etc.,* vols. 4 and 8. Paris: Ernest Leroux.

Cox, Daniel. 1771. *Nouvelles observations sur le pouls intermittent qui indique l'usage des purgatifs.* Amsterdam.

Coxe, John Redman. 1806. *The American dispensatory.* Philadelphia: A. Bartram.

Crolahan, H. 1845. Inflamed bursae treated by puncture. *LL* 2:527.

Cross, Frank L., and E. A. Livingstone, eds. 1974. *The Oxford dictionary of the Christian church.* New York: Oxford University Press.

Cruz, Gaspar da. 1570. *Tractado em qu se cõtem muito por extenso as cousas da China.* Barcelona: Portucalense Editora.

Cullen, Christopher. 1993. Patients and healers in late imperial China: Evidence from the *Jinpingmei. HS* 31:99–150.

Cullen, William. 1773. *Lectures on the materia medica.* London: T. Lowndes.

———. 1789. *Treatise of the materia medica,* vol. 2. Edinburgh: J. Crukshank and R. Campbell; Philadelphia: R. Hodge, S. Campbell, and T. Allen.

Culpeper, Nicholas. 1651a. *Directory for midwives.* London: Peter Cole.

———. 1651b. *Culpeper's astrologicall judgment of diseases.* London: Nathaniel Brooks.

———. 1653. *Pharmacopoeia Londinensis.* London: Peter Cole.

———. 1792. *Culpeper's English family physician, or, Medical Herbal Enlarged,* ed. Joshua Hamilton. Vols. 1–2. London: W. Locke.

Cumming, Dr. 1845. Medical practice in China. *BosMSJ* 33(26):519–521.

Cummins, J. S. 1993. *A question of rites: Friar Domingo Navarrete and the Jesuits in China.* Aldershot, England: Scolar Press.

Cunningham, Andrew. 1997. *The anatomical renaissance: The resurrection of the anatomical projects of the ancients.* Brookfield, VT: Ashgate.

Currie, A. 1836–1837. Enormous enlargement of the arm. Operation. *Lancet* 2 (July 15):608.

Dampier, William. [1697]1927. *A new voyage round the world.* London: Argonaut.

Daniels, Roger. 1991. Majority images–minority realities: A perspective on anti-orientalism in the United States. In *Nativism, discrimination, and images of immigrants,* ed. George E. Pozzetta, 73–127. New York: Garland.

Dantu, T. M. 1825. *Quelques propositions sur l'acupuncture.* Paris.

———. 1826. *Traité de l'acupuncture, d'après les observations de Jules Cloquet.* Paris: Bechet.

Dardess, John W. 2003. Did the Mongols matter? Territory, power, and the intelligentsia in China from the northern Song to the early Ming. In *The Song-Yuan-Ming transition in Chinese history,* ed. Paul Jakov Smith and Richard von Glahn, 111–134, 413–489. Cambridge, MA: Harvard University Asia Center.

Daser, Dr. 1841. Reduction of a strangulated hernia, apparently effected by acupuncture. *EMSJ* 56:549.

———. 1842. Reduction of a strangulated hernia, apparently effected by acupuncture. *WJMS* 5:225.

David, Dr. 1831. Identity of the nervous and electric fluids. *AJMS* 8:478–480.

Davidson, Dr. 1839. Hydrocele treated by acupuncture. *AJMS* 24:235–236.

Davis, John Francis. 1836a. *The Chinese: A general description of the empire of China and its inhabitants,* vols. 1–2. London: Charles Knight.

———. 1836b. Chinese streets and shops. *AMUET* 3:241.

———. 1841. *Sketches of China,* vol. 2. London: Charles Knight.

Davis, N. S. 1848. Report of the Committee on Indigenous Medical Botany. *TAMA* 1:341–357.

Dawson, Christopher, ed. 1955. *The Mongol mission: Narratives and letters of the Franciscan missionaries in Mongolia and China in the thirteenth and fourteenth centuries.* New York: Sheed and Ward.

Dawson, Raymond. 1967. *The Chinese chameleon: An analysis of European conceptions of Chinese civilization.* London: Oxford University Press.

Debout, M. 1844. Acupuncture. In *Dictionnaire encyclopédique des sciences médicales,* 1:670–687. Paris: P. Asselin, Sr. de Labe, Victor Masson et Fils.

de Claubry, C. 1825. Notice sur l'acupuncture. *JGMCPFE* 91:99–124.

de Fontaney, Fr. Jean. 1843. Lettre au Père de la Chaise. *LECAAA* 3:112–13.

Delano, Amasa. [1817]1994. *Delano's voyages of commerce and discovery,* ed. Eleanor Roosevelt Seagraves. Stockbridge, MA: Berkshire House.

Delatour, Louis-François. 1803. *Essais sur l'architecture des Chinois, sur leurs jardins, leurs principes de médecine et leurs moeurs et usages.* Paris: Imprimerie de Clousier.

Delunel, Citoyen. 1798–1799 [7th year of the Republic]. Observation sur la possibilité de remplacer le thé de la Chine, du Mexique, et autres, par des plantes indigènes ou de notre climat. *JSPP* (1):328–329.

———. 1799–1800 [8th year of the Republic]. Extrait d'un mémoire lu à la Société de Médecine . . . Observations sur la possibilité de remplacer le thé de la Chine, du Mexique et autres, par des plantes indigènes. *RPSMP* 8:120–127.

Demel, Walter. 1991. China in the political thought of western and central Europe, 1570–1750. In *China and Europe: Images and influences in sixteenth to eighteenth centuries*, ed. Thomas H. C. Lee, 45–64. Hong Kong: Chinese University Press.

Demours, A. P. 1819a. Note sur l'acupuncture lue [à la Société de médecine, Paris] à la séance du 2 février 1819. *JGMCPFE*, Jan.–Feb., 161–165.

———. 1819b. Seconde notice sur l'acupuncture, ou introduction de l'aiguille, sans que la ventouse soit retirée, à travers la portion du tissu cutané, soulevé par cet instrument. *JGMCPFE* 66:377–383.

———. 1819c. Notice sur l'émission sanguine dans le vide, lue à la Société de médecine de Paris, dans la séance du 18 mai 1819. *JGMCPFE* 66:335–340.

Desbois de Rochefort, M. 1793. *Cours élémentaire de matière médicale, suivi d'un précis de l'art de formuler,* vols. 1–2. Paris: Méquignon.

Deslandes, Léopold. 1842. *Manhood: The causes of its premature decline.* Boston: Otis, Broaders.

Deverell, Robert. 1805. *Andalusia.* London: S. Gosnell.

Didier, Franklin James. 1821. A sketch of the prevalent medical doctrines and of the hospitals at Paris. *AMRec* 4(2):473–481.

Dienert, M. 1765. *Introduction à la matière médicale, en forme de thérapeutique.* Paris: Pierre Fr. Didot.

Dikötter, Frank. 1992. *The discourse of race in modern China.* London: Hurst.

Dion. 1821. Chinese doctrine of the pulse. *ICG* 3(17):129–133.

Dirlik, Arif. 2002. *Across cultural borders: Historiography in global perspective.* Lanham, MD: Rowman and Littlefield.

Diver, W. Beck. 1840. History of vaccination in China. *AMI* 4(14):209–212.

———. 1841. Introduction to William Lockhart, "Medical profession in China." *AMI* 4(20):305.

Dodsley, Robert. [1750]1817. *The economy of human life.* Philadelphia: Edward Earle.

Dolan, John P. 1973. Some early European observations on acupuncture. *JSCMA* 69(5):173–177.

Double, Mr. 1837. The inapplicability of statistics to the practice of medicine. *AJMS* 21:247–250.

Doubleday, Edward. 1848. Note on the insect forming the Chinese galls. *PJT* 7:310–312.

Douglas, Mary, and David Hull. 1992. Introduction. In *How classification works: Nelson Goodman among the social scientists,* ed. Mary Douglas and David Hull. Edinburgh: Edinburgh University Press.

Downing, C. Toogood. 1838. *The fan-qui in China in 1836–7,* vols. 2–3. London: Henry Colburn.

———. 1842. The Chinese theory and practice of medicine. *Lancet* 1 (Mar. 5):792–797.

Downs, Jacques M. 1997. *The golden ghetto: The American commercial community at Canton and the shaping of American China policy, 1784–1844.* Bethlehem, PA: Lehigh University Press.

Dreisch, Hans. 1914. *The history and theory of vitalism,* trans. C. K. Ogden. London: Macmillan.

Drucker, Alison R. 1981. The influence of Western women on the anti-footbinding movement, 1840–1911. In *Women in China: Current directions in historical scholarship,* ed. Richard W. Guisso and Stanley Johannesen, 179–199. Youngstown, NY: Philo.

Dubois, Fr. 1848. *Matière médicale indigène; ou, Histoire des plantes médicinales qui croissent spontanément en France et en Belgique.* Tournai: J. Casterman.

Dubois, M. 1803. Moxas to treat loss of speech after fever. *MPJ* 9(50):389–390.

Dubs, Homer H., and Robert S. Smith. 1942. Chinese in Mexico City in 1635. *FEQ* 1(4):387–389.

Ducachet, Henry W. 1821. Case of hydrocele, in which sabulous matter was discharged by an operation. *AMRec* 4(2):638–639.

Duffy, John. 1993. *From humors to medical science: A history of American medicine,* 2nd ed. Urbana: University of Illinois Press.

Du Halde, Jean-Baptiste. 1735. *Déscription géographique, historique, chronologique, politique, et physique de l'empire de la Chine et de la Tartarie chinoise,* vols. 1–4. Paris: P. G. Lemercier.

———. 1736. *The general history of China,* vols. 1–4, trans. Richard Brookes. London: John Watts.

Duhergne, J. 1964. Voyageurs chinois venus à Paris au temps de la marine à voiles et l'influence de la Chine sur la littérature française du XVIIIe siècle. *MSer* 23:372–399.

Dujardin, François. 1774. *Histoire de la chirurgie, depuis son origine jusqu'à nos jours,* vol. 1. Paris: De l'imprimerie royale.

Dumas, M. 1847. Nervous fluid and electricity. *WJMS,* n.s. 8:21–22.

Dumoulin-Genest, Marie Pierre. 1995. Itinéraire des plantes chinoises envoyées en France: Voie maritime voie terrestre Saint-Pétersbourg ville de confluence. In *Échanges culturels et réligieux entre la Chine et l'Occident,* ed. Edward J. Malatesta, Yves Raguin, and Adrianus C. Dudink, 129–146. Taipei: Ricci Institute.

Dunglison, Robley. 1833. *New dictionary of medical science and literature,* vols. 1–2. Boston: Charles Bowen.

———. 1837. *The medical student; or, Aids to the study of medicine.* Philadelphia: Carey, Lea, and Blanchard.

———. 1838a. Acupuncture of ganglions. *AMI* 2(14):224–225.

———. 1838b. Cure of varicose veins and hernia by acupuncturation. *AMI* 1(19):317.

———. 1838c. Electropuncture in paralysis. *AMI* 1(14):265–266.

———. 1839. *New remedies: The method of preparing and administering them.* Philadelphia: Lea and Blanchard.

———. 1842. *Practice of medicine; or, A treatise on special pathology and therapeutics,* vols. 1–2. Philadelphia: Lea and Blanchard.

———. 1846a. *General therapeutics and materia medica . . . Adapted for a medical textbook,* 3rd ed., vols. 1–2. Philadelphia: Lea and Blanchard.

———. 1846b. *Medical lexicon: A dictionary of medical science,* 6th ed. Philadelphia: Lea and Blanchard.

———. 1860. *Medical lexicon: A dictionary of medical science . . . with French and other synonyms,* 6th ed. Philadelphia: Blanchard and Lea.

———. 1963. *Autobiographical ana of Robley Dunglison, M.D.,* ed. Samuel X. Radbill. Philadelphia: American Philosophical Society.

Dunn, Nathan. 1835. Adulterations of tea. *AMUET* 2:438.

———. 1836. Luishin. *AMUET* 3:207.

———. 1839. *A descriptive catalogue of the Chinese collection in Philadelphia.* Philadelphia.

Durkheim, Émile, and Marcel Mauss. 1963. *Primitive classification.* Chicago: University of Chicago Press.

Dwight, Theodore. 1846a. Chinese worshipping idols. *DAPMFN* 2(12):184.

———. 1846b. A Chinese dinner. *DAPMFN* 2(39):619.

———. 1846c. A Chinese offering to an idol. *DAPMFN* 2(47):745.

Eberle, John. 1822. Review of *A treatise on acupuncturation. AMRec* 5:331–338.

Ebrey, Patricia Buckley. 1996. *The Cambridge illustrated history of China.* New York: Cambridge University Press.

Editor. 1744. An essay on the description of China, in two volumes folio. From the French of Père du Halde. *AMag,* Nov., 615–632.

———. 1775a. Actual cautery, its use in medicine, by the Chinese. *MPC* 3(2):216–217.

————. 1775b. Review of *Disputatio inauguralis, quaedam de hominum varietatibus et harum causis exponens*, by John Hunter. *MPC* 3:367–379.

————. 1780. Review of *The materia medica of the vegetable kingdom* . . . , by Peter Jonas Bergius. *FMR* 1(4):1–36.

————. 1788. Natural history of the tea-tree: With an inquiry into the medicinal effects of that popular plant. *AMag*, May, 406–411.

————. 1802. On Perkinsism; or, The metalic tractors of Dr. Perkins, of North America. *NEQM* 1(Apr., May, and June):15–16.

————. 1806. Sir George Staunton's translation. *MPJ* 16(89):96.

————. 1810. Description of the Elgin Garden, the property of David Hosack. *MRep*, 3rd hexade, 1:292–295.

————. 1811. Elgin Botanick Garden. *MABR* 10(May): 331–335.

————. 1812. Domestic opium. *NEJMS* 1:315.

————. 1816. China ink. *LMRMJR* 5(Jan.–June):532.

————. 1817. Another project for the prolongation of human life. *MROEI*, n.s. 3(3):310.

————. 1819a. Notice sur l'acupuncture et sur une nouvelle espèce de ventouse armée de lancettes. *JUSM* 15:107–113.

————. 1819b. Contributions to the library. *ICG* 2(7):43–44.

————. 1819c. Donations to the Anglo-Chinese College. *ICG* 2(9):168–169.

————. 1820a. Acu-puncture, considered in its curative effects. *MROEI*, n.s. 5(3):324–325.

————. 1820b. Notice on acupuncture, and medical observations on its therapeutic effects. *LMRMJR* 13(Jan.–July):52.

————. 1820c. Response to "Man a microcosm." *ICG* 3(11):374.

————. 1821a. Acupuncture. *MCR* 2:431–436.

————. 1821b. Mr. Churchill's treatise on acupuncture. *MCRJMS* 2:431–436.

————. 1821c. Cholera morbus. *ICG* 3(18):231–232.

————. 1822a. Acupuncturation. *NYMPJ* 1:242–245.

————. 1822b. Review of *A treatise on acupuncture* . . . , by James Morss Churchill. *MROEI*, n.s. 7(4):441–449.

————. 1822c. Review of *On the use of the moxa, as a therapeutical agent*. *LMR* 18(105):242–248.

————. 1823a. Anasarque guérie par l'acupuncture. *RMCP* 2:89–90.

————. 1823b. Baron Larrey's *Surgical memoirs*. *EMSJ* 19:118–129.

————. 1823c. Dr. Tweedale's case of anasarca treated by acupuncture. *MJM* 2(July–Dec.):360.

————. 1823d. Mr. Churchill on acupuncture. *MJM* 1(Jan.–June):175–177.

————. 1823e. Mr. Churchill's new cases of acupuncture. *MJM* 2(July–Dec.):179.

————. 1823f. New publications. *AJMR* 16(July–Dec.):484–485.

———. 1823g. Notice sur les deux Chinois qui habitent à Berlin. *JA* 3:122–124.

———. 1823h. Review of *Mémoires sur les maladies chroniques, les évacuations sanguines et l'acupuncture.* *AMRec* 6:308–338.

———. 1823i. Sur Paul Hoange. *JA* 2:126–127.

———. 1824a. Professor Hufeland on the artimesia vulgaris in epilepsy. *MJM* 4(July–Dec.):305–307.

———. 1824b. Review of *Surgical essays,* by Baron D. J. Larrey. *NEJMS*, 3rd ser., 13:130–139.

———. 1825a. Accidents arising from acupuncturation. *LMPJ* 53(Jan.–June):260.

———. 1825b. Accidents arising from acupuncturation. *MJM* 5(Jan.–June):369–370.

———. 1825c. Accidents arising from acupuncturation. *BMI* 3(15):62.

———. 1825d. Acupuncturation. *BMI* 3(3):16.

———. 1825e. Acupuncture. *MCR*, n.s. 3:300.

———. 1825f. Acupuncturation. *MCR*, n.s. 3:562–563.

———. 1825g. Considérations sur la pratique de l'acupuncture et de l'électropuncture, par le docteur Sarlandière. *AMP* 7:174–176.

———. 1825h. Death from acupuncturation. *AMRev* 2(1):183.

———. 1825i. Médecine étrangère: Revue des journaux de médecine italiens: Acupunture. *RMFEJC* 4:496–497.

———. 1825j. M. Pelletan on the galvanic phenomena of acupuncturation. *MJM* 6(July–Dec.):172.

———. 1825k. Notice sur l'acupuncture. *JGMCP* 91:99–124.

———. 1825l. Observations on the use of the artimesia vulgaris, in the treatment of epilepsy. *AMRJ* 2(1):137–139.

———. 1825m. On the galvanic phenomena which accompany the acupuncturation. *LMPJ* 53(Jan.–June):434.

———. 1825n. On the galvanic phenomena which accompany the acupuncturation. *MRJ* 7(1):184.

———. 1825o. On the galvanic phenomena which accompany the acupuncturation. *AMRev* 2(Sept.):184.

———. 1825p. On the galvanic phenomena which accompany the acupuncturation. *MROPIMS* 8:625–626.

———. 1825q. Pelletan, Bally and others on acupuncture. *MJM* 5(Jan.–June):314–318.

———. 1825r. Rarities from China. *BMI* 2(36):148.

———. 1825s. Reflections on the nature of the action of acupuncture. *BMI* 3(32):127–128.

———. 1825t. White Negro. *BMI* 2(34):140.

———. 1826a. Acupuncture. *MCR*, n.s. 5:621–622.

———. 1826b. Acupuncture. *OMR* 1(9):34.

———. 1826c. Bibliographie: *Traité de l'acupuncture, d'après les observations de M. Jules Cloquet, et publié sous ses yeux par M. Dantu de Vannes. AGM* 11:163–164.

———. 1826d. Médecine étrangère: Revue des journaux de médecine italiens: Recueil de quelques expériences faites sur l'acupuncture, par le docteur Bertolini. *RMFEJC* 3:485–487.

———. 1826e. Mr. Sarlandiere on acupuncture. *OMR* 1(8):32.

———. 1826f. Professor Pelletan fils on acupuncture. *OMR* 1(8):32.

———. 1826g. Revue des journaux de médecine italiens: Névralgies faciales guéris par l'acupuncture: Observations recueillies par le docteur J. Bergamaschi. *RMFEJC* 3:487–489.

———. 1827a. Acupuncturation in tic douloureux. *PJMPS*, May–Aug., 164.

———. 1827b. Acupuncture. *AJFM* 1(1):39–43.

———. 1827c. Acupuncture. *MCR*, n.s. 7:279.

———. 1827d. Appendix, no. III. Donations to the Royal Asiatic Society of Great Britain and Ireland, from its institution, Mar. 15, 1823, to Mar. 15, 1827. *TRASGBI* 1:600–635.

———. 1827e. Artimesia vulgaris in epilepsy. *LMPJ*, n.s. 2:465.

———. 1827f. Artimesia vulgaris in epilepsy. *PMJMS* 1(2):100–101.

———. 1827g. Cloquet, Sarlandière, Pelletan, Carraro, and Pouillet, on acupuncture. *EMSJ* 27:190–200, 334–349.

———. 1827h. Review of *Medical botany* . . . , by John Stephenson and James Morss Churchill. *EJMS* 3(Jan.–Apr.):462–463.

———. 1827i. Sketches and abridgements: Acupuncture. *AJFM* 1(1):39–43.

———. 1827j. Boyle and Wallace on *Moxa. EMSJ* 28:136–148.

———. 1828a. Acupuncturation. *MJFM* 1(Jan.–June):473.

———. 1828b. Electro-puncturation. *MJFM* 1(Jan.–June):382–383.

———. 1828c. Revue des journaux de médecine anglais: Cas d'hystérie avec paralysie et contracture des membres, guérie par l'acupuncture; par M. Pelletier. *RMFEJC* 4:328–331.

———. 1828d. Revue des journaux de médecine français: Observation de paralysie qui durait depuis sept ans, guérie par l'acupuncture; par M. Pelletier. *RMFEJC* 4:331–332.

———. 1828e. Spina bifida cured by puncture. *BosMSJ* 1(6):89–90.

———. 1828f. Acupuncture in rheumatism. *BosMSJ* 1(7):107.

———. 1829a. Acupuncturation. *BosMSJ* 2(32):502–503.

———. 1829b. Hotel Dieu de Caen. Acupuncturation. *MCRJPM*, n.s. 11:166–167.

———. 1830a. *Edinburgh Medical and Surgical Journal* [case by Dr. Renton]. *Lancet* 2(Aug. 21):836–837.

———. 1830b. Influence of the mind over disease. *AJMS* 9(18):500.

———. 1830c. Medical anthropophy in China. *AJMR*, n.s. 1(Jan.–Apr.):254.

———. 1831a. Asiatic intelligence.—China. *AJMR*, n.s. 4(Jan.–Apr.):139.

———. 1831b. Fatal operation on a Chinese. *AJMR*, n.s. 5(May–Aug.):42–43.

———. 1831c. On the acupuncturation of arteries in the treatment of aneurism. *AJMS* 8(16):510–512.

———. 1831d. The study of anatomy legalized by the legislature of Massachusetts. *AJMS* 18(15):264–265.

———. 1831e. Case of arthritis and sciatica treated by acupuncturation with complete success. *AJMS* 9(18):508–511.

———. 1832a. An apology for human dissection. *LMG* 9:313–317.

———. 1832b. Man-eaters. *CR* 1(3):79.

———. 1832c. An angelic remedy for opium-smoking. *CR* 1(7):295.

———. 1832d. The fashionable doctor in Canton. *CR* 1(8):343.

———. 1832e. Memoirs and remarks. *CR* 1(7):249–268.

———. 1833a. Considérations thérapeutiques sur l'acupuncture et ses principales indications. *BGTMC* 5:236–241.

———. 1833b. Opium eating. *BosMSJ* 9(4):66–67.

———. 1833c. Penal laws of China. *CR* 2(3):97–111.

———. 1833d. Disposition of the Chinese towards foreigners. *CR* 2(6):277–281.

———. 1833e. Ophthalmic Hospital at Macao. *CR* 2(6):270–276.

———. 1833f. Description of the city of Canton. *CR* 2(7):289–308.

———. 1833g. An authentic account of an embassy. *CR* 2(8):337–350.

———. 1833h. The history of that great and renowned monarchy. *CR* 1(12):473–488.

———. 1833i. Chinese botany. *CR* 2(5):225–230.

———. 1834a. Galvanism for dyspepsia. *BosMSJ* 11(21):343.

———. 1834b. New moxas. *BosMSJ* 10(19):307.

———. 1834c. Early foreign intercourse with China. *CR* 3(3):107–115.

———. 1834d. Imports and exports of Canton. *CR* 2(10):447–472.

———. 1834e. Natural history of China. *CR* 3(2):83–89.

———. 1835a. Tic douloureux. *MQR* 4:243–245.

———. 1835b. The structure of the Chinese government. *CR* 4(4):181–189.

———. 1836a. Chinese rhubarb. *AJMS* 18:495.

———. 1836b. Galvanism. *BosMSJ* 15(19):306.

———. 1836c. Treatment of hydrocele by acupuncturation. *AJMS* 20(39):238–239.

———. 1837a. Chinese eye infirmary. *BosMSJ* 16(19):292.

———. 1837b. Miscellanies, original and select. *AJ*, n.s. 22(Mar.):247–249.

———. 1837c. The late Dr. Morrison's Chinese library. *AJMR*, n.s. 22(Jan.–Apr.):64–65.

————. 1837d. Medical uses of electricity. *MCRJPM*, n.s. 26:237–238.

————. 1837e. Report on the Thomsonian system of practice. *BosMSJ* 15(25):400–402.

————. 1837f. Correspondence. *Lancet* 2(July 22):784.

————. 1837g. Velpeau's treatment of hydrocele, with injections of a solution of iodine. Trial of acupuncture and compression. *Lancet* 2(Apr. 29):194–196.

————. 1837h. Animal magnetism. *AJMS* 21:268–276.

————. 1837i. De l'acupuncture comme remède contre le rheumatisme. *GMP* 2nd ser., 5(May 15):298.

————. 1838a. Radical cure of varicose veins and herniae by acupuncturation. *AJMS* 22(43):226–227.

————. 1838b. Diseases of China. *BosMSJ* 17(6):97.

————. 1839a. Chinese physiology. *BosMSJ* 20(12):194.

————. 1839b. Medical Missionary Society in China. *BosMSJ* 19(26):415–416.

————. 1839c. Medical Missionary Society of China. *BosMSJ* 19(27):432.

————. 1839d. Medical portraits—Jonathan Pereira. *MT* 1(7):49.

————. 1839e. Mr. Armstrong's answer to Lector on acupuncturation. *LMG*, n.s. 2:82.

————. 1839f. Paralysis of the arm. Utility of electro-puncture. *MCRJPM*, n.s. 31:220.

————. 1839g. Premium essay on the opium trade. *BosMSJ* 20(1):18–19.

————. 1840a. Review of *Crania Americana* . . . , by Samuel George Morton. *WJMS* 2:35–56.

————. 1840b. Tenth report of the Ophthalmic Hospital, Canton. *CR* 8(12):628–639.

————. 1840c. E Tsung Kin Keën Yu Tsoan; or, The golden mirror of eminent medical authors, compiled by imperial authority. *CR* 9(7):486–488.

————. 1841a. Cases of neuralgia treated with acupuncturation. *MCRJPM*, n.s. 34:501–503.

————. 1841b. Chinese materia medica. *BosMSJ* 24(13):209–210.

————. 1841c. Importance of the pulse with the Chinese physicians. *MT* 3(71):215.

————. 1841d. Majendie's method of treating neuralgia. *MCRJPM*, n.s. 35:202–203.

————. 1841e. Medical Missionary Society of China. *BosMSJ* 24(11):176–178.

————. 1841f. Proceedings of societies: Royal Asiatic Society. *AJMR*, n.s. 35(May–Aug.):536–538.

————. 1841g. To readers and correspondents. *AJMS*, n.s. 1:1.

————. 1841h. Journal of occurrences. *CR* 10(6):349–352.

———. 1841i. A new history of China. *CR* 10(12):641–649.

———. 1842a. The Chinese collection. *AJMR*, n.s. 39(Sept.–Dec.):341–342.

———. 1842b. Chinese midwifery. *Lancet* 50(Jan. 1):473.

———. 1842c. Physic in China and diet in India. *MCRJPM*, n.s. 37:262–264.

———. 1842d. Portrait of Shinnung. *CR* 11(6):323–324.

———. 1843a. Acupuncture in neuralgia. *MCRJPM*, n.s. 38:532.

———. 1843b. Acupuncture in neuralgia. *WL* 2(6):289.

———. 1843c. Dr. Parker's Chinese hospital. *BosMSJ* 29(21):418–419.

———. 1843d. Electro-puncture. *WJMS* 7:467–468.

———. 1843e. Electro-puncture for hydrocele. *MT* 9(215):62.

———. 1843f. The price of Chinese books in Europe. *AJMR*, 3rd ser., 1(May–Oct.):273.

———. 1843g. Root doctors and their practice. *MNL* 1(6):76–77.

———. 1843h. A visit to the Chinese collection. *AJMR*, n.s. 40(Jan.–Apr.):104–107.

———. 1843i. Government notification. *HLCR* 16(29):2.

———. 1844a. American surgery in China. *BosMSJ* 30(13):266–267.

———. 1844b. Journal of electro-magnetic medicine. *BosMSJ* 30(18):363–364.

———. 1844c. Medical Missionary Hospital in China. *BosMSJ* 29(25):506.

———. 1844d. Physic and physicians in China. *AJMR*, Nov., 27–29.

———. 1844e. Progress of surgery in China. *BosMSJ* 30(26):504–505.

———. 1844f. Progress of surgery in China. *WJMS* 6(Nov.):420–421.

———. 1844g. Review of *Superstitions connected with the history and practice of medicine and surgery,* by Thomas Joseph Pettigrew. *NRRSL* 1(1):251–254.

———. 1844h. Ununited fracture treated by acupuncturation. *AJMS*, n.s. 8:254.

———. 1845a. American translators of Chinese. *BosMSJ* 32(25):503.

———. 1845b. Quackeries of the day. *MNL* 3(27):20.

———. 1845c. Ununited fracture successfully treated by acupuncture. *AJMS*, n.s. 9:219–220.

———. 1845d. Ununited fracture treated by acupuncturation. *MT* 11(277):327.

———. 1846a. Confessions of a doctress. *PJT* 5:380–381.

———. 1846b. Galvanic puncture in aneurism. *MNL* 4(48):113–114.

———. 1846c. Notice of a memoir entitled *Sur une nouvelle méthode pour guerir certains aneurismes sans opération sanglante, à l'aide de la galvano-puncture,* by J. E. Pétrequin. *MJMS*, n.s. 71(5):373–376.

———. 1846d. Researches on galvanic puncture. *MJMS*, n.s. 68(2):152.

———. 1846e. Review of *Medical notes on China,* by John Wilson. *DMP* 15:375–376.

————. 1846f. Austrian rhubarb. *MNL* 4(43):68.

————. 1846g. Review of *Medical notes on China,* by John Wilson. *LL* 4:251–252.

————. 1846h. Review of *Medical notes on China,* by John Wilson. *MCRJPM,* n.s. 4:73–91.

————. 1846i. Review of *Transactions of the China Medico-Chirurgical Society for the year 1845–6* and *Medical notes on China,* by John Wilson. *MJMS,* n.s. 70(4):270–276.

————. 1847a. Acupuncture in aneurism. *WJMS,* n.s. 8:23–24.

————. 1847b. A black person becoming white. *MMSJ* 4(4):80.

————. 1847c. Chinese physiology. *BosMSJ* 36(10):205.

————. 1847d. Emploi de la galvano puncture dans quelques affections rebelles du système nerveux. *RMCP* 2:326–329.

————. 1847e. Galvano-puncture in aneurism. *SJMP* 2:462–463.

————. 1847f. Galvano-puncture in the treatment of aneurism. *AJMS,* n.s. 14:243.

————. 1847g. Galvano-puncture in the treatment of aneurism. *MJMS,* n.s. 75(9):696–697.

————. 1847h. Pharmacy in China. *DMP* 18(July–Dec.):176.

————. 1847i. Pharmacy in China. *MT* 17(423):68.

————. 1847j. Ununited fracture successfully treated by acupuncturation. *AJMS,* n.s. 13:455.

————. 1847k. A Chinese view of the Asiatic cholera—Chinese therapeutics. *LMG,* n.s. 4:346–347.

————. 1848a. Chinese physiology. *IIMSJ* 2:80.

————. 1848b. Commerce of the United States with China. *WJAMMA* 1:210–211.

————. 1848c. Pharmacy in China. *PJT* 7:82.

————. 1848d. Review of *Medical notes on China . . . ,* by John Wilson, part I. *WL* 7(6):351–352.

————. 1848e. Report of the Chinese Medical Missionary Society. *CR* 17(5):244–247.

————. 1848f. Small feet of Chinese females. *BosMSJ* 39(10):207–208.

————. 1848g. Subclavian aneurism cured by galvano-puncture. *MT* 17(423):260.

Edwards, Henri Milne, and Pierre Henri Vavasseur. 1829. *A manual of materia medica and pharmacy,* trans. Joseph Togno and E. Durand. Philadelphia: Carey, Lea and Carey.

Elliot, Sir John. 1786. *Elements of the branches of natural philosophy connected with medicine.* London: J. Johnson.

Elliotson, John. 1827. Acupuncture in rheumatism. *MCT* 13:467–468.

————. 1830a. Abstract of a clinical lecture: Pneumonia; The treatment of rheumatism. *Lancet* 1(Nov. 21):335–339.

————. 1830b. Abstract of the third clinical lecture: Treatment of rheumatism; Acupuncturation; Venesection; Colchicum. *Lancet* 1(Nov. 21):271–275.

————. 1832a. Clinical lecture—Lumbago. *Lancet,* Jan. 21, pp. 689–693.

————. 1832b. Clinical lecture: Rheumatism. *Lancet,* July 14, pp. 488–491.

————. 1832c. St. Thomas's Hospital clinical lecture. *Lancet,* Jan. 21, pp. 689–693.

————. 1833a. Acupuncture. *MM* 1:309–314.

————. 1833b. St. Thomas's Hospital clinical lecture—Rheumatism. *Lancet* 1:167.

————. 1836. Artemesia absinthium in epilepsy. *AJMS* 19:224.

————. 1839. *The principles and practice of medicine.* London: Joseph Butler.

————. 1844. *The principles and practice of medicine,* ed. Nathaniel Rogers. Philadelphia: Carey and Hart.

————. [1845]1848a. Acupuncture, with added notes by Robley Dunglison. In *Cyclopaedia of practical medicine,* ed. John Forbes, Alexander Tweedie, and John Conolly, 1:54–58. Philadelphia: Henry C. Lea.

————. 1848b. Neuralgia. In *Cyclopaedia of practical medicine,* ed. John Forbes, Alexander Tweedie, and John Conolly, rev. Robley Dunglison, 3:381–385. Philadelphia: Lea and Blanchard.

Elliott, Thomas A. 1826. On acupuncturation. Thesis, Medical College, State of South Carolina University.

Ellis, Benjamin. 1830. Chinese materia medica. *JPCP* 1:150–152.

Emerson, Gouverner. 1830. Bibliographical notice: *Mémoires sur l'electropuncture. AJMS* 6(12):477–479.

Emerson, Ralph Waldo. 1903–1912. *The complete works of Ralph Waldo Emerson,* vol. 3, ed. Edward Waldo Emerson. Boston: Houghton Mifflin.

Emiliani, Dr. 1845a. Case of singultis of several years' standing cured by acupuncture. *MNL* 3(26):16.

————. 1845b. Case of singultis of several years' standing cured by acupuncture. *IMSJ* 2(1):16.

Emmons, Samuel B. 1836. *The vegetable family physician.* Boston: George P. Oakes.

d'Entrecolles, François Xavier. [1734]1843a. Lettre du P. d'Entrecolles au Père DuHalde, 4 novembre, 1734. *LECAAA* 3:692–693.

————. [1734]1843b. Lettre au Père de la Chaise. *LECAAA* 3:82–113.

Epler, D. C. 1980. Bloodletting in early Chinese medicine and its relation to the origin of acupuncture. *BHM* 54:337–367.

————. 1988. The concept of disease in an ancient Chinese medical text: The discourse on cold-damage disorders (Shang-han Lun). *JHMAS* 43(1):8–35.

de Escalante, Bernardino. [1577]1958. *Primera historia de China de Bernardino de Escalante*. Madrid: Libreria General Victoriano Suarez.

———. [1577]1992. *Discurso de la navegacion que los Portugueses hazen á los Reinos y Provincias del Oriente, y de la noticia que se tiene de las grandezas del Reino de la China*. Santander, Spain: Universidad de Cantabria.

Etiemble, Réné. 1988–1999. *L'Europe chinoise*, vols. 1–2. Paris: Gallimard.

Etoille, Leroy d'. 1842. Quelques réflexions faites au sujet d'extraits des journaux italiens—Sur le traitement de l'hydrocèle par l'électro-puncture. *GMP*, 2nd ser., 10:27–28.

Eubulus [Samuel Johnson]. 1738. Letter to the editor. *GM* 8:365.

F., D. 1825. Du mode d'action et de l'emploi de l'acupuncture; par M. Jules Cloquet. *BSM* 4:139–141.

Fabricius of Aquapendente. 1649. *Oeuvres chirurgicales*. Lyon: Pierre Ravaud.

Fairbank, John K., Edwin O. Reischauer, and Albert M. Craig. 1978. *East Asia: Tradition and transformation—New impression*. Boston: Houghton Mifflin.

Fan, Fa-ti. 2004. *British naturalists in Qing China: Science, empire, and cultural encounter*. Cambridge, MA: Harvard University Press.

Fergusson, William. 1843. Account of a case of hydrocele, treated by acupuncture, in which a needle remained in the tunica vaginalis for eleven months. *DMP* 10:227–228.

Ferussac Bulletin Général. 1825. On the galvanic phenomena accompanying acupuncturation. *PJMPS*, 2nd ser., 11:164–165.

Finch, Frederick. 1823a. Mr. Finch on acupuncture in anasarca. *MJM* 1(Jan.–June):362–363.

———. 1823b. Case of trismus, &c. approaching to tetanus, supervening to a lacerated wound, successfully treated by acupuncturation. *LMR* 20(119):403–404.

———. 1824. Acupuncturation in tetanic trismus. *MROEI*, n.s. 8:334–335.

Fisher, William R. 1837. A brief sketch of the progress and present state of pharmacy in the United States of America. *AJP*, n.s. 2:271–279.

Floyer, Sir John. 1707. *The pulse watch; or, An essay to explain the old art of feeling the pulse, and to improve it by the help of a pulse-watch*, vol. 2. London: J. Nicholson.

Foley, Neil. 1997. *The white scourge: Mexicans, blacks, and poor whites in Texas cotton culture*. Berkeley: University of California Press.

Forbes, F. E. 1848. *Five years in China*. London: Richard Bentley.

Fortune, Robert. [1847]1979. *Three years' wanderings in the northern provinces of China*. New York: Garland.

———. 1848a. Opium smuggling, opium used in China, opium smoking. *PJT* 7:290–293.

———. 1848b. Opium smuggling, opium used in China, opium smoking. *AJP*, n.s. 14:74–78.

———. 1848c. Opium smoking. *MERMS*, n.s. 4:132–133.

Foss, Theodore N. 1990. The European sojourn of Philippe Couplet and Michael Shen Fuzong, 1683–1692. In *Philippe Couplet, S.J. (1623–1693): The man who brought China to Europe*, ed. Jerome Heyndrick, 121–142. Nettetal: Steyler Verlag.

Foss, Theodore N., and Donald F. Lach. 1991. Images of Asians in European fiction, 1500–1800. In *China and Europe: Images and influences in sixteenth to eighteenth centuries*, ed. Thomas H. C. Lee, 165–188. Hong Kong: Chinese University Press.

Foster, Robert D. 1838. *The North American Indian doctor.* Canton, OH: Smith and Bevin.

Fothergill, John. 1772. Of the use of tapping early in dropsies. *MOI* 4:114–122.

Foust, Clifford M. 1992. *Rhubarb: The wondrous drug.* Princeton: Princeton University Press.

Frampton, John. 1579. *A discourse of the navigation which the Portugales doe make to the realmes and provinces of the east partes of the world.* London: Thomas Dawson.

Franklin, Benjamin. 1758. An account of the effects of electricity in paralytic cases. In a letter to John Pringle, M.D. F.R.S. from Benjamin Franklin, Esq. *PTRSL* 50:1–3.

———. 1987. *Writings.* New York: Library of America.

Fraser, D. 1809a. The murder of George Villiers the great Duke of Buckingham, foretold by his father's apparition. *AMW* 1:195–196.

———. 1809b. Proofs of spirits and apparitions in the Isle of Man, from Waldron's survey, folio, 1729. *AMW* 2:222–226.

———. 1809c. Account of a Negro woman who became white. *AMW* 2:312.

French, Roger. 1989. Harvey in Holland: Circulation and the Calvinists. In *The medical revolution of the seventeenth century*, ed. Roger French and Andrew Wear, 46–86. New York: Cambridge University Press.

Friedman, John B. 1981. *The monstrous races in medieval art and thought.* Cambridge, MA: Harvard University Press.

Friend of China. 1845. Important from China. *DAPMFN* 1(34):543.

Furnivall, J. 1837. Ascites treated by acupuncture. *Lancet,* Nov. 18, p. 313.

Furth, Charlotte. 1999. *A flourishing yin: Gender in China's medical history, 960–1665.* Berkeley: University of California Press.

G—. 1806. Quack and patent medicines. *MAR* 1(5):69–72.

———. 1807. Medical extracts, no. III. *MAR* 1(16):241–246.

Gale, T. 1802. *Electricity; or, Ethereal fire, considered.* Troy, NY: Moffitt and Lyon.

Galt, John M. 1831. Acupuncturation. Thesis, Medical Department, University of Pennsylvania.

Galvani, Luigi. 1792. *De viribus electricitatis in motu musculari.* Mutinae, Apud Societatem Typographicam.

Gamberini, M. 1839. Epilepsie guérie a l'aide de l'acupuncture. *LFGHCM*, 2nd ser., 1(82):326.

———. 1847. De quelques varices guéries par la galvano-puncture. *GMP*, 3rd ser., 2:561.

Geilfus, Bernhard Wilhelm. 1676. *Disputatio inauguralis de moxa.* Marburg: Typis Salomonis Schadewitzii.

Gentleman in the Course of His Travels. 1807. *The pocket esculapius; or, Every man his own physician.* Edinburgh: Oliver.

Gentleman Who Is Now No More. 1775. A letter dated Feb. 18, 1775. *The Bee* 11 (Sept. 12).

Gernet, Jacques. 1972. *A history of Chinese civilization,* trans. J. R. Foster. Cambridge: Cambridge University Press.

———. 1980. Christian and Chinese visions of the world in the seventeenth century. *CS* 4:1–17.

———. 1985. *China and the Christian impact: A conflict of cultures,* trans. Janet Lloyd. Cambridge: Cambridge University Press.

Gerzina, Gretchen. 1995. *Black England: Life before emancipation.* London: John Murray.

Getz, Faye Marie. 1991. *Healing and society in medieval England: A Middle English translation of the pharmaceutical writings of Gilbertus Anglicus.* Madison: University of Wisconsin Press.

Gibson, James R. 1992. *Otter skins, Boston ships, and China goods: The maritime fur trade of the northwest coast, 1785–1841.* Montreal: McGill-Queen's University Press.

Gieulés, Jean. 1803. *Sur l'emploi du moxa.* Montpellier: L'Imprimerie de G. Izar et A. Ricard.

Gilbert, William. [1600]1958. *De magnete,* trans. P. Fleury Mottelay. New York: Dover.

Gillan, Dr. 1962. Dr. Gillan's observations on the state of medicine, surgery and chemistry in China. In *Britain and the China trade, 1635–1842,* vol. 8, ed. J. L. Cranmer-Byng, 279–290. London: Routledge.

Godwin, Joscelyn. 1979. *Athanasius Kircher: A Renaissance man and the quest for lost knowledge.* London: Thames and Hudson.

Goldsmith, Oliver. [1762]1901. The citizen of the world. In *Persian and Chinese letters,* ed. Oliver H. G. Leigh, 291–427. Washington: M. Walter Dunne.

Goldstein, Jonathan. 1984. Cantonese artifacts, chinoiserie, and the formation of an early American image of the Chinese. In Lim, ed., 1984, 256–258.

Golvers, Noël. 2000. Philippe Couplet, X. J. (1623–1693) and the authorship of *Specimen medicinae sinensis* and some other Western writings on Chinese medicine. *Medizin Historisches Journal* 35:175–182.

Goodman, Nelson. 1992. Seven strictures on similarity. In *How classification works: Nelson Goodman among the social scientists*, ed. Mary Douglas and David Hull, 13–23. Edinburgh: Edinburgh University Press.

Goodrich, Samuel G. 1830. *Peter Parley's tales about Asia.* Boston: Gray and Bowen; Carter and Hendee.

Gould, Stephen Jay. 1985. *The flamingo's smile.* New York: Norton.

———. 1997. The geometer of race. In *The concept of "race" in natural and social science*, ed. E. Nathaniel Gates, 1–5. New York: Garland.

Goupil, M. 1825. Pleurodynie guérie par l'acupuncture. *RMFEJC* 3:449–450.

Graefe, Dr. 1829. Case of rheumatism cured by electro-puncturation. *AJMS* 5:501.

———. 1832. Case of chronic hydrocephalus cured by puncture. *MS* 11:211–213.

Grant, Joanna. 1998. Medical practice in the Ming dynasty—A practitioner's view: Evidence from Wang Ji's *Shishan yi'an. CS* 15:37–80.

Grantham, Mr. 1837. Tic douloureux relieved by galvanism. *MCRJPM,* n.s. 27:190–191.

Graves, Prof. 1838a. Clinical lectures on medicine—Introductory lecture. *LMG*, Oct. 13, pp. 39–46.

———. 1838b. Clinical lectures on medicine, delivered at the Meath Hospital, Dublin. *LMG*, Oct. 20, pp. 103–109.

———. 1839. On the treatment of anasarca and ascites by acupuncture. *AJMS* 23(46):464–466.

Greenwood, Ronald D. 1976. Acupuncture in the United States, 1836. *JSCMA*, May, 182–183.

Griffith, R. E. 1833. Review: *The dispensatory of the United States. AJMS* 12(23):147–161.

Grmek, Mirko. 1962. Les reflets de la sphygmologie chinoise dans la médecine occidentale. *BM* 51(Feb.):1–120.

Grosier, M. L'Abbé Jean-Baptiste. 1787. *Description générale de la Chine,* vols. 1–2. Paris.

———. 1788. *A general description of China,* vols. 1–2. London: G. G. J. and J. Robinson.

Gruggen, Mr. 1843. The employment of electro-puncture in neuralgia. *LL* 2:469.

Guerin de Mamers, M. 1825. Mémoires sur l'électro-puncture et sur l'emploi du moxa japonais en France, suivis d'un traité de l'acupuncture et du moxa; par Sarlandière. *BSM* 4:280–283.

Guersent, Louis Benoit. 1826a. Moxa. In *Dictionnaire de médecine* 14:520–523. Paris: Béchet Jeune.

———. 1826b. Piqure (thérapeutique). In *Dictionnaire de médecine* 16:552–563. Paris: Béchet Jeune.

———. 1832. Acupuncture. In *Dictionnaire de médecine* 1:528–541. Paris: Béchet Jeune.

———. 1839. Moxa. In *Dictionnaire de médecine,* vol. Mie–Ner:296–299. Paris: Béchet Jeune.

Gunn, John C. 1834. *Domestic medicine; or, Poor man's friend,* 2nd ed. Madisonville, TN: J. F. Grant.

Gutzlaff, Charles. 1832. Journal of a residence in Siam, and of a voyage along the coast of China to Mantchou Tartery. *CR* 1(5):180–196.

———. 1833. Prospectus. *Chinese Courier* 2(46):2.

———. 1834. *Journal of three voyages along the coast of China, in 1831, 1832, & 1833.* London: Fredrick Westley and A. H. Davis.

———. 1837. The medical art amongst the Chinese. *JRASGBI* 4:154–171.

———. 1838. *China opened; or, A display of the topography, history, customs, manners, arts, manufactures, commerce, literature, religion, jurisprudence, etc., of the Chinese empire,* vol. 2. London: Smith, Elder.

Guy, Basil. 1963. *The French image of China before and after Voltaire,* ed. Theodore Besterman. Geneva: Institut et Musée Voltaire.

Guzman, Gregory G. 1991. Reports of Mongol cannibalism in the thirteenth-century Latin sources: Oriental fact or Western fiction? In *Discovering new worlds: Essays on medieval exploration and imagination,* ed. Scott D. Westrem, 31–68. New York: Garland.

H., C. 1824. Details sur You-Foung-Koueï, dame chinoise, morte à Londres. *JA* 4:115–118.

Hacket, W. 1837. Cure of hydrocele by acupuncture (Letter to the editor). *Lancet,* Feb. 25, p. 787.

Haime, A. 1819. Notice sur l'acupuncture, et observations médicales sur ses effets thérapeutiques. *JUSM* 13:27–42.

Hall, John Jefferson. 1826. Acupuncturation. Thesis, Medical Department, University of Pennsylvania.

Hall, Richard Willmott. 1806. *An inaugural essay on the use of electricity in medicine.* Philadelphia: Thomas and George Palmer.

Haller, John S. 1973. Acupuncture in nineteenth century Western medicine. *NYSJM,* May 15, pp. 1213–1221.

Halliday, Stephen. 2001. Death and miasma. *BMJ* 323:1469–1471.

Hamilton, Hugh. [1833]1834. *Report of proceedings on a voyage to the northern ports of China in the ship Lord Amherst.* London: B. Fellowes.

Hamilton, John. 1831. Arthritis and sciatica. Acupuncturation employed with complete success. *LMG* (July 2): 445–447.

———. 1835a. Trial of acupuncture with galvanism made by Dr. W. Stokes, one of the physicians to the Meath Hospital. *MQR* 3:472–475.

———. 1835b. Trial of acupuncture with galvanism made by Dr. W. Stokes, one of the physicians to the Meath Hospital. *DJMCS* 6:78–86.

———. 1835c. Case of arthritis and sciatica treated by acupuncture with complete success. *AJMS* 9(18):508–511.

———. 1846. Case of carotid aneurism, in which galvanism was applied to the blood in the sac by means of acupuncture. *DQJMS* 2:539–545.

Hanson, Marta. 2003. The *Golden mirror* in the imperial court of the Qianlong emperor, 1739–1742. *Early Science and Medicine* 8(2):111–147.

Harlan, Richard. 1822. Remarks on the variety of complexion and national peculiarity of feature. *AMRec* 5(4):591–605.

Harper, Donald. 1998. *Early Chinese medical literature: The Mawangdui medical manuscripts.* London: Kegan Paul International.

Hart, Roger. 1999. On the problem of Chinese science. In *The science studies reader,* ed. Mario Biagioli, 189–201. New York: Routledge.

Hay, John. 1993. The human body as a microcosmic source of macrocosmic values in calligraphy. In *Self as body in Asian theory and practice,* ed. Thomas P. Kasules, 179–211. Albany, NY: SUNY Press.

Haygarth, John. 1800. *Of the imagination, as a cause and as a cure of disorders of the body; exemplified by fictitious tractors, and epidemical convulsions.* Bath: R. Cruttwell.

He, Zhiguo, and Vivienne Lo. 1996. The channels: A preliminary examination of a lacquered figurine from the Western Han period. *EC* 21:81–123.

Heberden, Dr. William. 1785. The method of preparing the ginseng root in China. *MTrans* 3:34–36.

Heinrich, Larissa N. 1999. Handmaids to the gospel: Lam Qua's medical portraiture. In *Tokens of exchange: The problem of translation in global circulations,* ed. Lydia H. Liu, 239–275. Durham: Duke University Press.

Heister, Lorenz. 1743. *Chirurgie, in welcher alles, was zur Wund-Artzney gehöret.* Nuremberg: Widow of J. Stein.

———. [1743]1759. *A general system of surgery,* 7th ed., vols. 1–2. London: J. Clarke, J. Whiston.

Henry, M. 1814. Comparée des rhubarbes de Chine, de Moscovie, et de France. *BPSA* 6:87–96.

Henry, Samuel. 1814. *A new and complete American medical family herbal.* New York: Samuel Henry.

Hermel, E. 1844. On neuralgia, and its treatment, especially upon the cases in which electro-puncture is likely to effect a cure. *LEMJMS* 4:508–510.

Hervé, G. 1904. Notes et matériaux. *REAP.* Paris: Félix Alcan.

Heyden, Carolus Guilelmus von der. 1826. *De acupunctura: Dissertatio in-auguralis.* Bonn: Petre Neusseri.

Heyndrick, Jerome, ed. 1990. *Philippe Couplet, S.J. (1623–1693): The man who brought China to Europe.* Nettetal: Steyler-Verlag.

Higginbotham, A. Leon. 1978. *In the matter of color: The colonial period.* New York: Oxford University Press.

Hill, James. 1842. Opium-smoking in China. *Lancet* 1 (Mar. 12):820–822.

Hill, Sir John. 1812. *The family herbal.* Bungay: C. Brightly and T. Kinnersley.

Hinrichs, T. J. 1998. New geographies of Chinese medicine. *Osiris* 13:287–325.

———. 2003. The medical transformation of governance and southern customs in Song Dynasty China (960–1279 C.E.). Thesis, Harvard University.

———. n.d. Demonic infestation, populated bodies, and the spatial dimensions of contagion. Manuscript, Department of East Asian Studies, Harvard University.

Hodgson, W., Jr. 1830. Moxa. *JPCP* 1:295–296.

Hogan, William. 1845. *A synopsis of Popery, as it was and as it is.* Boston: Saxton and Kelt.

Holcombe, Charles. 1993. The Daoist origins of the Chinese martial arts. *JAMA* 2(1):10–25.

Holmes, Oliver Wendell. 1845. Illustrations of tumors among the Chinese. *BosMSJ* 32(16):316–318.

Holmyard, E. J. 1990. *Alchemy.* New York: Dover.

Home, William. 1839. Exploration with an acupuncture needle as a means of diagnosis. *AJMS,* n.s. 1:513.

———. 1840. Report on various cases of gunshot wounds received in actions in upper Canada in 1838. *EMSJ* 54:20–31.

Honour, Hugh. 1961. *Chinoiserie; The vision of Cathay.* London: J. Murray.

Hooper, Robert. 1825. *Lexicon medicum; or, Medical dictionary,* 5th ed. London: Longman, Hurst, Rees, Orme, Brown, and Green.

Hosack, David. 1806. *A catalogue of plants contained in the botanic garden at Elgin.* New York: T. and J. Swords.

Hsu, Elisabeth. 1989. Outline of the history of acupuncture in Europe. *JCM* (29):28–32.

———. 1994. Change in Chinese medicine: *Bian* and *Hua,* an anthropologist's approach. In *Notions et perceptions du changement en Chine,* ed. Viviane Alleton and Alexeï Volkov, 41–58. Paris: Collège de France, Institut de Hautes Études Chinoises.

———. 2000a. Towards a science of touch, part I. *AMed* 7(2):251–268.

———. 2000b. Towards a science of touch, part II. *AMed* 7(3):2319–2333.

Huang, Shijian, and William Sargent. 1999. *Customs and conditions of Chinese city streets in 19th century—360 professions in China. The collection of Peabody Essex Museum, America.* Shanghai: Shanghai Classics.

Huang, Yilong. 1993. L'attitude des missionaries jésuites face à l'astrologie et à la divination chinoises. In *L'Europe en Chine,* ed. Catherine Jami and Hubert Delahaye, 87–105. Paris: Collège de France, Institut des Hautes Études Chinoises.

Huard, Pierre. 1959. La médecine chinoise dans les milieux Parisiens du XVIIe siècle. *SHP* 35:3519–3527.

———. 1978. Mesmer en Chine: Trois lettres médicales du R. P. Amiot, rédigées a Pékin. *RS* 1:61–98.

Huard, Pierre, and Ming Wong. 1959. *La médecine chinoise au cours des siècles.* Paris: Roger Dacosta.

———. 1966. Les enquêtes françaises sur la science et la technologie chinoises au xviiie siècle. *Bulletin de l'École Française d'Éxtrême-Orient* 53:137–223.

———. 1968. *Chinese medicine,* trans. Bernard Fielding. New York: McGraw-Hill.

Hucker, Charles O. 1975. *China's imperial past.* Stanford: Stanford University Press.

Hufeland, C. G. 1824a. Of the efficacy of the root of the artemisia vulgaris (mug-wort) in epilepsy. *LMRMJR,* n.s. 2:343–344.

———. 1824b. Of the efficacy of the root of the artemisia vulgaris (mug-wort) in epilepsy. *NYMPJ* 3(4):511–512.

———. 1825. Mugwort a remedy in epilepsy. *MROPIMS* 8:420–421.

Hungerford, Harold. 1987. *Sheep, goats, and Chinese encyclopedias.* Chicago: Chicago Literary Club.

Hunn, A. 1832. Essay on bilious fever and the use of calomel. *TR* 1:53–54.

Hymes, Robert. 2002. *Way and byway: Taoism, local religion, and models of divinity in Sung and modern China.* Berkeley: University of California Press.

Irwin, Graham. 1977. *Africans abroad: A documentary history of the black diaspora in Asia, Latin America, and the Caribbean during the age of slavery.* New York: Columbia University Press.

Isaacs, Harold R. 1958. *Scratches on our minds: American images of China and India.* New York: John Day.

Isani, Mukhtar A. 1970. Cotton Mather and the Orient. *NEQM* 43:46–58.

Israel, Jonathan. 1980. *Razas, clases sociales y vida política en el México colonial, 1610–1670.* México: Fondo de Cultura Económica, Sección de Obras de Historia.

Jackson, Carl T. 1981. *Oriental religions and American thought.* Westport, CT: Greenwood.

Jackson, Harold, and Grandison Harris. 1997. Race and the politics of medicine in nineteenth-century Georgia. In *Bones in the basement: Postmortem racism in nineteenth-century medical training,* ed. Robert L. Blakely and Judith M. Harrington, 182–205. Washington: Smithsonian Institution Press.

Jackson, J. B. S. 1847. *Boston Society for Medical Improvement: Descriptive catalogue of the Anatomical Museum of the Boston Society for Medical Improvement.* Boston: W. D. Ticknor.

Jackson, Samuel. 1826–1827. On vitality and the vital forces. *PJMPS* (Nov. 1826–Feb. 1827): 68.

———. 1830a. Of the pulse and its modifications. *AJMS* 6(12):104–114.

———. 1830b. On rhubarb in haemorrhoids. *AJMS* 6:315–321.

Jackson, William. n.d. *The new and complete newgate calendar; or, Malefactor's universal register,* no. 16. London: Hogg.

James, M. 1841. Complete paralysis of the fifth pair on one side, with complete abolition of sight, hearing, smelling, and taste on the same side, cured by galvanism. *LEMJMS* (Oct.): 750.

Jartoux, Pierre. 1713. The description of a Tartarian plant call'd gins-seng, with an account of its virtues . . . Taken from the tenth volume of letters of the missionary Jesuits, printed at Paris in octavo, 1713. *PT* 28:237–247.

———. [1713]1762. Father Jartoux, to the procurator general of the missions of India and China. In *Travels of the Jesuits, into various parts of the world: Particularly China and the East-Indies,* 2nd ed., trans. and ed. John Lockman. 2:424–437. London: T. Piety.

———. [1713]1843. Lettre au père procureur général des missions des Indes et de la Chine: Details sur le gin-seng, et sur la récolte de cette plante. *LECAAA* 3:183–187.

Jefferson, Thomas. [1785]1971. Letter to John Adams, Nov. 27, 1785. In *Adams-Jefferson letters: The complete correspondence between Thomas Jefferson and Abigail and John Adams,* ed. Lester J. Cappon, 100–103. New York: Simon and Schuster.

Jesuits. 1562. *Copia de algunas cartas que los padres y hermanos de la compañia de Jesus, que andan en la India, y otras partes orientales, escriuieron a los de la misma compañia de Portugal: Desde el año M.D.LVII hast el de LXI.* Barcelona: Claude Bernar.

———. 1717. *Lettres édifiantes et curieuses écrites des missions étrangères par quelques missionaries de la Compagnie de Jésus.* Vols. 1–26. Paris.

Jobert, M. 1843a. On electro-puncture in the treatment of deafness, depending on a paralysis of the acoustic nerve. *BMS* 1:266.

———. 1843b. On electro-puncture in the treatment of deafness, depending on a paralysis of the acoustic nerve. *NYJMCS* 1:413–414.

———. 1844. Electro-puncture in the treatment of deafness, depending on a paralysis of the acoustic nerve. *NYD* 1(2):110.

Johnson, James. 1807. *The oriental voyager; or, Descriptive sketches and cursory re-marks, on a voyage to India and China.* London: James Asperne.

Johnson, M. 1825. Dr. Meyranse, on acupuncturation. *MROPIMS* 8:837.

———. 1837. Opium eating in Siam. *BosMSJ* 16(12):193–194.

Jourdan, Antoine Jacques Louis. [1816]1819. Feu. In *Dictionnaire des sciences medicales,* vol. Fem–Fis, 87–159. Paris: Panckoucke.

Kaempfer, Engelbert. 1712. *Amoenitatum exoticarum politico-physico-medicarum fasciculi V.* Lemgo, Germany: Henrici Wilhelmi Meyeri.

———. [1712]1996. *Exotic pleasures: Fascicle III—Curious scientific and medical observations,* trans. Robert W. Carrubba. Carbondale: Southern Illinois University Press.

Kalm, Peter. [1770]1964. *Peter Kalm's travels in North America: The English ver-sion of 1770,* ed. Adolph B. Benson. New York: Dover.

Kaptchuk, Ted J. 1983. *The web that has no weaver.* New York: Congdon and Weed.

———. 1996. Historical context of the concept of vitalism in complemen-tary and alternative medicine. In *Fundamentals of complementary and alter-native medicine,* ed. M. S. Micozzi, 35–48. New York: Churchill Living-stone.

———. 2000. *The web that has no weaver,* 2nd ed. Chicago: Contemporary Books.

Katz, Paul R. 1995. The pacification of plagues: A Chinese rite of affliction. *JRS* 9(1):55–100.

Keate, Robert. 1837. Treatment of hydrocele. *LMG,* Feb. 18, p. 789.

Keightley, David N. 1984. Late Shang divination: The magico-religious leg-acy. *JAARTS* 50(2):11–34.

Kerber, Theodor. 1832. *De acupunctura.* N.p.: Halis Saxonum.

Kiernan, Victor. 1995. *The lords of human kind: European attitudes to other cul-tures in the imperial age.* London: Serif.

Kim, Elizabeth. 2002. Race sells: Racialized trade cards in 18th-century Brit-ain. *Journal of Material Culture* 7(2):137–165.

King, Lester S. 1991. *Transformations in American medicine from Benjamin Rush to William Osler.* Baltimore: Johns Hopkins University Press.

King, Thomas. 1838a. Puncturation in ascites. *LMG,* n.s. 1:332.

———. 1838b. Puncturation in the cure of hydrocele. *AMI* 1(4):61–64.

Kingdon, Mr. 1833. Rheumatism.—Elaterium.—Acupuncture. *Lancet,* Mar. 23, pp. 817–818.

Kircher, Athanasius. [1667]1987. *China illustrata: With sacred and secular mon-uments, various spectacles of nature and art and other memorabilia,* trans. Charles Van Tuyl. Bloomington: Indiana University Research Institute for Inner Asian Studies.

Kircher, Athanasius, and the Society of Jesus. 1667. *China monumentis, qua sacris quà profanis, nec non variis naturae & artis spectaculis, aliarumque rerum memorabilium argumentis illustrata.* Amsterdam: Joannem Jansonnium à Waesberge & Elizeum Weyerstraet.

Kitts, Charles R. 1991. *The United States odyssey in China, 1784–1990.* Lanham, MD: University Press of America.

Klor de Alva, J. Jorge. 1996. *Mestizaje* from New Spain to Aztlán: On the control and classification of collective identities. In *New world orders: Casta painting and colonial Latin America,* ed. John A. Farmer and Ilona Katzew, trans. Roberto Tejada and Miguel Falomir, 58–71. New York: Americas Society Art Gallery.

Kohn, Livia, and Harold D. Roth. 2002. Introduction. In *Daoist identity: History, lineage, and ritual,* ed. Livia Kohn and Harold D. Roth, 1–19. Honolulu: University of Hawaii Press.

Komroff, Manuel, ed. 1928. *Contemporaries of Marco Polo: Consisting of the travel records to the eastern parts of the world of William of Rubrick (1253–1255), the journey of Joan of Pian de Carpini (1245–1247), the journal of Friar Odoric (1318–1330) and the oriental travels of Rabbi Benjamin of Tudela (1160–1173).* New York: Boni and Liveright.

Kraut, Alan M. 1995. *Silent travellers: Germs, genes, and the "immigrant menace."* Baltimore: Johns Hopkins University Press.

Krziwaneck, J. 1839. *De electricitate, acupunctura, Perkinismo, et frictione.* Prague: Typis Thomae Thabor.

Kuhn, Philip. 1990. *Soulstealers: The Chinese sorcery scare of 1768.* Cambridge, MA: Harvard University Press.

Kuhn, Thomas S. 1977. *The essential tension: Selected studies in scientific tradition and change.* Chicago: University of Chicago Press.

Kuriyama, Shigehisa. 1994. The imagination of winds and the development of the Chinese conception of the body. In *Body, subject and power in China,* ed. Angela Zito and Tani E. Barlow, 23–41. Chicago: University of Chicago Press.

———. 1995. Interpreting the history of bloodletting. *JHM* 50:11–35.

———. 1999. *The expressiveness of the body and the divergence of Greek and Chinese medicine.* New York: Zone Books.

L., C. A. 1839. Review of *Flora medica: A statistical account of all the more important plants used in medicine, in different parts of the world. NYJMS* 1:151–155.

La Beaume, Michael. 1820. *Remarks on the history and philosophy but particularly on the medical efficacy of electricity in the cure of nervous and chronic disorders,* 2nd ed. London: F. Warr.

———. 1826. *On galvinism: With observations on its chymical properties and medical efficacy in chronic diseases.* London: Highley.

Lach, Donald F. [1965]1997. *Asia in the making of Europe: II(2). The Literary Arts.* Chicago: University of Chicago Press.

————. 1977. *Asia in the making of Europe: II(3). The scholarly disciplines.* Chicago: University of Chicago Press.

Lafitau, Joseph François. [1716] 1858. *Memoire concernant la plante du ginseng de Tartarie, découverte en Amerique.* Montreal.

Lafosse, Pierre-Edouard de. 1817. A case of paralysis, illustrative of the curative effects of the application of moxa. *LMR* 7 (Jan.–June):332–333.

Lai, H. Mark, and Philip Choy. 1971. *Outlines: History of the Chinese in America.* San Francisco: Chinese-American Studies Planning Group.

Lai, Walton Look. 1999. Developments in the world at large. In *Encyclopedia of the Chinese overseas,* ed. Lynn Pan, 52–54. Cambridge, MA: Harvard University Press.

Lallemand, François. 1843. Acupuncture in neuralgia. *MT* 8 (198):231.

————. [1847] 1848. *A practical treatise on the causes, symptoms, and treatment of spermatorrhoea,* trans. Henry J. McDougall. Philadelphia: Lea and Blanchard.

Lambert, M. l'Abbé. 1750. *Histoire générale, civile, naturelle, politique et religieuse de tous les peuples du monde,* vols. 10–11. Paris: Prault Fils.

Laner, A. 1830. *De acupunctura.* Pestini.

Langridge, D. W. 1992. *Classification: Its kinds, systems, elements and applications.* London: Bowker-Saur.

Langworthy, Charles Cunningham. 1798. *A view of the Perkinean electricity; or, An enquiry into the influence of metallic tractors,* 2nd ed. Bath: Printed for the author by R. Cruttwell.

Larrey, Dominique Jean. 1819. Moxa. In *Dictionnaire des sciences médicales* 34:459–474. Paris: Panckoucke.

————. 1822. *On the use of the moxa, as a therapeutical agent,* trans. Robley Dunglison. London: Thomas and George Underwood.

Laurent, A. 1826. *Acupunctura.* Leoden.

Lawrence, Mr. 1830. Mr. Lawrence: Lecture LXXXIX. (Conclusion of the course.) *Lancet* 1 (Sept. 18):958–962.

Lay, G. Tradescant. 1838. Means of doing good in China. *CR* 7 (4):193–204.

————. 1839. Human anatomy and physiology, as understood by the Chinese. *LMG,* n.s. 2:378–383.

————. 1840a. Chinese surgery. *Lancet* 2 (Sept. 5):877–878.

————. 1840b. Diseases among the Chinese: Tumours. *Lancet* 2 (Sept. 5):851–853.

————. 1840c. Hospitals at Canton and Macao. *BosMSJ* 23 (9):437–439.

————. 1840d. Tumors among the Chinese. *BosMSJ* 23 (13):214.

————. 1841a. *The Chinese as they are: Their moral, social, and literary character; A new analysis of the language; with succint views of their principal arts and sciences.* London: William Ball.

————. 1841b. Chinese surgery: Diseases of the eye. *Lancet,* May 29, pp. 326–328.

————. 1841c. An outline of Chinese anatomy. *Lancet*, Feb. 20, pp. 751–754.

Lazich, Michael C. 1998. E. C. Bridgman and the coming of the millennium: America's first missionary to China. Paper presented at the Third Annual Conference of the Center for Millennial Studies, Boston University. www.mille.org/confprodec98/lazich (downloaded 11/09/2004).

Lecointe, L.-M. 1812. *Dissertation médico-chirurgicale sur l'emploi du moxa.* Strasbourg.

le Comte, Louis. 1696. *Nouveaux mémoires sur l'état present de la Chine.* Paris: Jean Anisson.

————. 1698. *Memoirs and observations topographical, physical, mathematical, mechanical, natural, civil, and ecclesiastical made in a late journey through the empire of China.* London: Benjamin Tooke.

Lee, William Markley. 1836a. Acupuncture as a remedy for rheumatism. *SMSJ* 1(3):129–133.

————. 1836b. Acupuncture as a remedy for rheumatism. *BosMSJ* 15(6):85–87.

————. 1837a. Acupuncture, as a remedy for rheumatism. *DJMS* 11:157–160.

————. 1837b. De l'acupuncture comme remède contre le rheumatism. *GMP* 5(19):298.

Leney, John. 1842. Use of moxa in rheumatism. *WJMS* 6:309–311.

Lepage, François-Albin. 1813. *Recherches historiques sur la médecine des Chinois.* Paris: Didot Jeune.

Leung, Angela Ki Che. 1987. Organized medicine in Ming-Qing China: State and private medical institutions in the lower Yangzi region. In *Late Imperial China* 8(1):134–166.

————. 1993. Diseases of the premodern period in China. In *The Cambridge world history of human disease,* 354–361. Cambridge: Cambridge University Press.

————. 2003. Transmission of medical knowledge from the Sung to the Ming. In *The Song-Yuan-Ming transition in Chinese history,* ed. Paul Jakov Smith and Richard von Glahn, 374–398, 461–467. Cambridge, MA: Harvard University Asia Center.

Lewis, D. 1836. New method of treating hydrocele (Letter to the editor). *Lancet* 2(May 7):206.

————. 1837a. Mr. Lewis's method of treating hydrocele (Letter to the editor). *Lancet,* Jan. 14, pp. 559–560.

————. 1837b. Mr. Lewis's cure of hydrocele by one acupuncture (Letter to the editor). *Lancet,* Feb. 18, p. 750.

————. 1837c. New(?) method of treating hydrocele. In reply to Mr. Travers. *LMG,* Feb. 18, p. 788.

————. 1838a. Acupuncture in hydrocele and in ascites. *LMG,* n.s. 1:55–56.

———. 1838b. On the treatment of hydrocele by acupuncture. *SMSJ* 2:537–538.

Lewis, M. G. 1839. Black and white. *LMG*, n.s. 2:735.

Liautaud, M. 1844a. On anatomy among the Chinese. *MT* 9(227):284.

———. 1844b. Anatomy of the Chinese. *MCRJPM*, n.s. 40:505.

———. 1844c. Chinese anatomy. *DMP* 11:294.

Libertas. 1841. From our Washington correspondent. *CA*, n.s. 1(49).

Lim, Genny, ed. 1984. *The Chinese American experience: Papers from the second National Conference on Chinese American Studies (1980).* San Francisco: Chinese Historical Society of America and Chinese Culture Foundation of San Francisco.

Lindley, John. 1838. *Flora medica: A botanical account of all the more important plants used in medicine in different parts of the world.* London: Longman, Orme, Brown, Green, and Longmans.

Linnaeus. *See* von Linné, Carl.

Lisfranc, M. 1835. Lecture on the treatment of white swelling. *Lancet* 2:337–339.

Liu, Jiantang. 1996. Martino Martini in Confucian China. In *Martino Martini: A humanist and scientist in seventeenth century China*, ed. Franco Demarchi and Riccardo Scartezzini, 343–351. Trento: Università degli Studi di Trento.

Liutaud, M. 1768. *Précis de la matière médicale*, vol. 1. Paris: Mgr. Le Comte de Provence.

Livingstone, John. 1819a. Chinese botany. *ICG* 2(9):122–124.

———. 1819b. Dr. Livingstone's letter to the Horticultural Society of London. *ICG* 2(9):126–131.

———. 1821a. Treatment of certain diseases by Chinese doctors. *ICG* 3(15):5–8.

———. 1821b. An account of a monster, or lusus naturae. *ICG* 3(15):53–55.

Lockhart, William. 1841. Medical profession in China. *AMI* 4(20):305–311.

———, trans. 1842. A treatise on midwifery. *DJMS* 20:134–169.

———, trans. 1843. On the preservation of infants by inoculation. Translated from the Chinese. *MCRJPM* 38:560–561.

London Medical Society. 1837. Treatment of hydrocele by acupuncture. *Lancet*, Jan. 7, p. 539.

Longhi, M. 1839. Bons effets de l'acupuncture dans un cas de convulsions douloureuses dans un moignon de cuisse amputée. *GMP*, 2nd ser., 7:123.

Lopez, Donald S., Jr. 1996. *Religions of China in practice.* Princeton: Princeton University Press.

Lottes, Günther. 1991. *China and Europe: Images and influences in sixteenth to eighteenth centuries.* Hong Kong: Chinese University Press.

Loudon, Irvine. 2000. Why are (male) surgeons still addressed as Mr.? *BMJ* 321:1589–1591.

Louis, Pierre. 1838. Louis on the application of statistics to medicine. *AJMS* 21:525–528.

Lu, Gwei-Djen, and Joseph Needham. 1980. *Celestial lancets: A history and rationale of acupuncture and moxa.* Cambridge: Cambridge University Press.

Lukes, Steven. 1971. The meanings of individualism. *JHI* 32(1):47–66.

Lundbaek, Knud. 1995. Notes on Abel Rémusat and the beginning of academic sinology in Europe. In *Échanges culturels et religieux entre la Chine et l'Occident. Variétés sinologiques,* n.s. No. 83, ed. Edward J. Malatesta, Yves Raguin, and Adrianus C. Dudink, 207–221. Paris: Institut Ricci-Centre d'Études Chinoises.

M. 1838a. Review: The Fanqui in China. *CR* 7(6):328–334.

———. 1838b. Memorial recommending that tea, rhubarb, and silk, be sold to foreigners at fixed prices. *CR* 7(6):311–314.

M., A. 1814. Case of ascites and general anasarca, cured after tapping. *LMSPR* 1(Jan.–June):102–105.

Ma, Kan-wen. 2000. Hare-lip surgery in the history of traditional Chinese medicine. *Medical History* 44:489–512.

Maciet, M. 1839. *Catalogue des livres imprimés, des manuscrits et des ouvrages chinois, tartares, japonais, etc., de feu M. Klaproth.* Paris: R. Merlin.

Mackerras, Colin. 1989. *Western images of China.* New York: Oxford University Press.

Madden, Mr. 1829. Opium eaters: From Mr. Madden's travels in Turkey. *BosMSJ* 2(32):503–504.

Maffei, Giovanni Pietro. 1589. *Historiarum indicarum libri XVI.* Venice: D. Zenarium.

Magalhães [Magaillans], Gabriel de. 1688. *A new history of China, containing a description of the most considerable particulars of that vast empire.* London: Thomas Newborough.

Magalotti, Lorenzo. 1676. *China and France; or, Two treatises.* London: Samuel Lowndes.

Mahoney, James W. 1846. *The Cherokee physician or Indian guide to health, as given by Richard Foreman, a Cherokee doctor.* Chattanooga, TN: Gazette Office.

de Mailla, Fr. Joseph-François-Marie-Anne de Moyriac. 1777–1785. *Histoire générale de la Chine,* ed. M. l'Abbé Grosier. Paris: Ph. D. Pierres . . . Clousier.

Malmsheimer, Richard. 1988. *"Doctors only": The evolving image of the American physician.* New York: Greenwood.

de Malon, M. 1766. *Le conservateur du sang humain.* Paris: Antoine Boudet.

de Malpière, D. B. 1825. *La Chine: Moeurs, usages, costumes, arts et métiers, peines civiles et militaires, cerémonies religieuses, monuments et paysages,* vols. 1–2. Paris: L'Éditeur.

Marat, Jean-Paul. 1784. *Mémoire sur l'électricité médicale*. Paris: L. Jorry.

Mareschal, M. 1825. Faits relatifs à l'emploi de l'acupuncture. *JSMSADL* 1:183–188.

Margotta, Roberto. 1967. *The story of medicine*. New York: Golden.

Martin, R. Montgomery. 1847. *China: Political, commercial, and social*, vols. 1–2. London: James Madden.

Martius, Theodore. 1847. On Kien; or, Native Chinese carbonate of soda. *PJT* 6:182–183.

Mason, George Henry. 1801. *The punishments of China*. London: W. Miller.

Maundeville, Sir John. 1887. *The voiage and travayle of Sir John Maundeville Knight*, ed. John Ashton. London: Pickering and Chatto.

Maw, S. 1839. *A catalogue of surgical instruments, pharmaceutical implements, dispensary utensils and vessels . . . Manufactured and sold by S. Maw*. London: J. Masters.

McCarthy, D. 1847. Treatment of varicose veins by galvano-puncture. *MT* 16(413):553.

McGlinchee, Claire. 1940. *The first decade of the Boston Museum*. Boston: Bruce Humphries.

McLeod, John, M.D. [1817]1820. *Voyage of H.M.S. Alceste, to China, Corea, and the island of Lewchew*, 3rd ed. London: John Murray.

McNeill, William H. 1976. *Plagues and peoples*. Garden City, NY: Anchor.

McPherson, Duncan. 1842. *Two years in China*. London: Saunders and Otley.

McVaugh, Michael R. 1997. Medicine in the Latin Middle Ages. In *Western medicine: An illustrated history*, ed. Irvine Loudon, 54–65. New York: Oxford University Press.

Meares, John. 1791. *Voyages made in the years 1788–1789, from China to the northwest coast of America*. London: Sold by J. Walter.

Medhurst, W. H. 1838. *China: Its state and prospects*. London: John Snow.

Medicus. 1802. On domestic quackery. *MPJ* 7(39):396.

Mencius. 1970. *Mencius*, trans. D. C. Lau. Harmondsworth, UK: Penguin Books.

Mendoza, Juan Gonzalez de. [1585]1586. *Historia de las cosas más notables*. Madrid: Pedro Madrigal.

———. 1588. *The historie of the great and mightie kingdome of China*, vols. 1–2, trans. R. Parke. London: Edward White.

Mentelii, D. Christiani. 1686. De radice Chinensium gîn-sen. In *Miscellanea curiosa sive ephemederidum medico-physicarum Germanicarum Academiae Naturae Curiosorum, decuriae ii annus quintus*, 73–78. Norimbergae: Wolfangi Mauritii Endteri.

Mérat, F. V., and A. J. de Lens. 1831. *Dictionnaire universel de matière médicale, et de thérapeutique générale*, vol. 3. Paris: J.-B. Baillière, Méquignon-Marvis.

Meyranx, Dr. 1825a. Observations sur l'acupuncture, faites à l'hôpital de la Pitié, sous les yeux de M. Bally [Bailly], et quelques reflexions sur sa manière d'agir. *AGM* 7:231–249.

———. 1825b. Réflexions sur la manière d'agir de l'acupuncture. *AGM* 7:387–396.

Michael, Emily. 2000. Renaissance theories of body, soul, and mind. In Wright and Potter, eds., 2000, 147–172.

Middleton, William Shainline. 1925. John Bartram, botanist. *SM* 2:191–216.

Midelfort, H. C. Erik. 1999. *A history of madness in sixteenth-century Germany.* Stanford: Stanford University Press.

Milani, Dr. 1846. Closure of several varices of the left leg, by means of the electro-puncture. *MJMS,* n.s. 71(5):377.

Miller, Amy Bess. 1998. *Shaker medicinal herbs: A compendium of history, lore, and uses,* ed. Deborah E. Burns. Pownal, VT: Storey Books.

Miller, Stuart Creighton. 1969. *The unwelcome immigrant: The American image of the Chinese, 1785–1882.* Berkeley: University of California Press.

Missionaries of Beijing (Missionaires de Pekin). 1784. *MCHSAMUC,* vol. 10. Paris: Nyon, Libraire.

Mitchell, Dr. 1832. Electro-puncturation. *WMG* 1:84–85.

Mitchell, John K. 1821. An account of a monster. *PJMPS* 3:78–86.

Monardes, Nicolás Bautista. 1565. *Dos libros. El uno trata de todas las cosas que traen de nuestras Indias Occidentales; . . . El otro libro, trata de dos medicines maravillosas.* Seville: Sebastian Trugillo.

Monchet, M. 1847. Lettre sur l'emploi de la galvano-puncture dans le traitement des anévrismes. *GMP,* 3rd ser, 2:11–12.

Mongiardini, Anthony. 1807. On the application of galvanism in the cure of diseases. *EMSJ* 3:29–34.

Morand, J. 1825a. *Dissertation sur l'acupuncture, et ses effets thérapeutiques.* Paris.

———. 1825b. *Memoir on acupuncturation, embracing a series of cases drawn up under the inspection of M. Julius Cloquet, Paris, 1825,* trans. Franklin Bache. Philadelphia: Robert Desilver.

Morantz, Regina Markell. 1977. Nineteenth century health reform and women: A program of self-help. In *Medicine without doctors: Home health care in American history,* ed. Guenter B. Risse, Ronald L. Numbers, and Judith Walzer Leavitt, 73–94. New York: Science History Publications.

Moreau, Jacques L. 1805. Oeuvres de Vicq-d'Azyr, recueillies et publiées, avec des notes et un discours sur sa vie et ses ourvrages; II.ᵉ partie.—II.ᵉ extrait. *JGMCP* 23:81–92.

Morel, Jean. 1813. *Mémoires et observations sur l'application du feu au traitement des maladies; guerison d'une maladie du foie operée par le moxa.* Paris: Le Normant.

Morelot, Simon. 1797–1798 [6th year of the Republic]. Mémoire sur la racine de rhubarbe et sur sa culture en France. *RPSMP* 13:301–313.

Morison, Samuel Eliot. 1921. *The maritime history of Massachusetts, 1783–1860.* Boston: Houghton Mifflin.

Morrison, Robert. 1817. *A view of China for philological purposes.* Macao: P. P. Thoms.

———. 1819a. Chinese metaphysics. *ICG* 2(9):144–153.

———. 1819b. Letter to John Livingstone, Esq. *ICG* 2(9):124–126.

———. 1820. *A memoir of the principal occurrences during an embassy from the British government: To the court of China in the year 1816.* London: Printed for the editor.

———. 1823. Chinese literature: To the editor of the *Asiatic Journal. AJMR* 15(Jan.–June):459–460.

———. 1835. Some account of charms, talismans, and felicitous appendages worn about the person, or hung up in houses, &c., used by the Chinese. *TRASGBI* 3:285–290.

———. 1839. *Memoirs of the life and labours of Robert Morrison, compiled by his widow,* vols. 1–2. London: Longman, Orme, Brown, Green, and Longmans.

Morus, Iwan Rhys. 1998. *Frankenstein's children: Electricity, exhibition, and experiment in early-nineteenth-century London.* Princeton: Princeton University Press.

Most, Dr. 1829. Acupuncturation in rheumatic paralysis. *ME* (8):126.

Mote, Frederick W. 1977. Yüan and Ming. In *Food in Chinese culture: Anthropological and historical perspectives,* ed. K. C. Chang, 193–258. New Haven: Yale University Press.

Mundy, Peter. [1634–1637]1919. *The travels of Peter Mundy, in Europe and Asia, 1608–1667,* vol. 3, ed. Sir Richard Carnac Temple. London: Hakluyt Society.

Myers, Norma. 1996. *Reconstructing the black past: Blacks in Britain, c. 1780–1830.* London: F. Cass.

Nacquart, M. 1812. Dictionnaire des sciences médicales, par une Société de médecins et de chirurgiens. *JGMCP* 64:162–171.

Namias, Giacinto. 1840. Di una nevralgia, o tic doloroso, combattuta utilmente coll'agopuntura, dell'efficacia di questo mezzo, e della natura di quel malore. *GSPPT* 4:135–150.

———. 1846. On the efficacy of acupuncture in causing obliteration of the arteries. *MJMS,* n.s. 71(5):378.

———. 1847. On the efficacy of acupuncture in causing obliteration of the arteries. *AJMS,* n.s. 13:191–192.

Naquin, Susan. 1985. The transmission of White Lotus sectarianism in late imperial China. In *Popular culture in late imperial China*, ed. David Johnson, Andrew J. Nathan, and Evelyn S. Rawski, 255–291. Berkeley: University of California Press.

Nash, George V. 1898. *American ginseng: Its commercial history, protection and cultivation*. Washington: Government Printing Office.

National Medical Convention. 1831. *The pharmacopoeia of the United States*. Philadelphia: John Grigg.

———. 1842. *The pharmacopoeia of the United States*. Philadelphia: John Grigg.

Navarrete, Domingo de. 1676. *Tratados historicos, políticos, éticos y religiosos de la monarchía de China*. Madrid: Juan García Infançon.

Needham, Joseph. 1954. Science and civilisation in China, vol. 1: *Introductory orientations*. Cambridge: Cambridge University Press.

———. 1970. *Clerks and craftsmen in China and the West*. Cambridge: Cambridge University Press.

———. 1981. *Science in traditional China: A comparative perspective*. Cambridge, MA: Harvard University Press.

Needham, Joseph, with Ho Ping-Yü and Lu Gwei-Djen. 1980. Science and civilisation in China, vol. 5: *Chemistry and chemical technology*, pt. 4: Spagyrical discovery and invention: Apparatus, theories and gifts. Cambridge: Cambridge University Press.

Neligan, John Moore. 1844. *Medicines, their uses and mode of administration*. New York: Harper.

Neuhausen, Dr. 1845. Clonic spasm of the muscles of the face, and of the orbicularis palpebrarum cured by galvano-puncture. *MT* 12(299):202.

Newman, John B. 1846. Vitalism. *NYMSR* 1(3):44–46.

Newton, Sir Isaac. 1718. *Opticks; or, A treatise of the reflexions, refractions, inflexions and colours of light*, 2nd ed. London: W. and J. Innys.

Nieuhof, Johannes. [1665]1669. *An embassy from the East-India Company of the United Provinces, to the Grand Tartar Cham, emperour of China*, trans. Jacob van Meurs. London: John Macock.

Nihell, James. 1741. *New and extraordinary observations concerning the predictions of various crises by the pulse . . . made first by Dr. Don Francisco Solano de Luque . . . and subsequently by several other physicians*. London: James Crokatt.

———. 1748. *Observations nouvelles & extraordinaires sur la perfection des crises, &c., par D. Francisco Solano de Luques, enrichies de plusieurs cas nouveaux*, trans. M. Lavirotte. Paris: Debure l'aîné.

Nitchie, John. 1818. A letter, relative to a Chinese in America. *ICG* 1(3):78–83.

Nutton, Vivian. 1995. Medicine in medieval western Europe. In Conrad et al., eds., 1995, 139–205.

Ogier, Thomas L. 1846. A case of hydrocele cured by electro-magnetism. *MERMS*, n.s. 2:368.

Olschki, Leonardo. 1960. *Marco Polo's Asia: An introduction to his "Description of the world" called "Il milione,"* trans. John A. Scott. Berkeley: University of California Press.

O'Neill, Robert K. 1986. The role of private libraries in the dissemination of knowledge about Asia in sixteenth century Europe. In *Asia and the West: Encounters and exchanges from the age of explorations—Essays in honor of Donald F. Lach*, ed. Cyriac K. Pullapilly and Edwin J. Van Kley, 277–308. Notre Dame: Cross Cultural Publications.

O'Reiley, E. 1845. On camphor. *AJP*, n.s. 10:56–58.

Origo, Iris. 1955. The domestic enemy: Eastern slaves in Tuscany in the fourteenth and fifteenth centuries. *Speculum* 30(3):321–366.

Orta, Garcia d'. 1563. *Coloquios dos simples, e drogas he cousas medicinales da India.* Goa: Ioannes de Endem.

Overmyer, Daniel L. 1986. *Religions of China: The world as a living system.* Prospect Heights, IL: Waveland.

Packard, Francis R. 1932. How London and Edinburgh influenced medicine in Philadelphia in the eighteenth century. *AMH* n.s. 4:210–244.

Page, M. 1815. State of medicine in China. *MPJ* 33(193):247–248.

Pallas, M. 1847. Effects of electricity on the human organism. *AJMS*, n.s. 14:468–469.

Pan, Lynn. 1990. *Sons of the yellow emperor: The story of the overseas Chinese.* London: Secker and Warburg.

Pantoja, Diego de. 1606. *Relación de la entrada de algunos padres de la Compañia de Iesus en la China.* Valencia: Iuan Chrysostomo Garris.

Paper, Jordan. 1995. *The spirits are drunk: Comparative approaches to Chinese religion.* Albany, NY: SUNY Press.

Paravey, M. 1837. Rhubarb. *AJP*, n.s. 2:263.

Paris, Dr. 1843. Ingredients of stamped and patent medicines. *MT* 8(186):44.

Paris, M. 1766. *Dissertation physico-medicale sur l'usage de l'electricité dans la médecine.* Paris.

Parker, Peter. 1836. Excision of a tumor in the Ophthalmic Hospital, under the charge of Rev. Dr. Parker. *BrMSJ* 15(2):29–30.

———. 1839. Sarcomatous tumor. *BosMSJ* 19(26):410–412.

Pascalis, Felix. 1818. Desultory remarks on the cause and nature of the black colour in the human species; Occasioned by the case of a white woman suddenly turned black. *MROEI*, n.s. 4(4):366–371.

Passamaquaddy. 1807. On the objects of the association. *MAR* 1(21):327.

Patton, Kimberley C., and Benjamin C. Ray, eds. 2000. *A magic still dwells:*

Comparative religion in the postmodern age. Berkeley: University of California Press.

Pauthier, M. G. 1831. Mémoires sur l'origine et la propagation de la doctrine du Tao, fondée par Lao-tseu. *NJA*, 2nd ser., 7:465–493.

de Pauw, Cornelius. 1795. *Philosophical dissertations on the Egyptians and Chinese,* trans. Capt. J. Thomson, vol. 1. London: T. Chapman.

Payen, M. 1843. Importation of Bengal opium into China. *MT* 9(215):62.

Pearson, A. 1826a. Abstract of the contents of a work on Chinese medicine, compiled by the order of the Emperor Kien Lung, intended to be used, and resorted to as a standard work on the subject. *TMPSC* 2:122–136.

———. 1826b. Some notices illustrative of Chinese medical opinion and practice in paralysis. *TMPSC* 2:137–150.

Pecchioli, Zanobi. 1841. Hydrocèle double de la tunique vaginale guérie au moyen de l'électro-puncture. *GMP,* 2nd ser., 9:805–806.

Pechlin, Johann Nicolas. 1691. *Observationum physico-medicarum libri tres.* Hamburg: Ex Officina Libraria Schultziana.

Pegolotti, Francesco Balducci. [1340]1936. *La pratica della mercatura,* ed. Allan Evans. Cambridge, MA: Mediaeval Academy of America.

Pelletan, Pierre, fils. 1825a. Notice sur l'acupuncture, contenant son historique, ses effets et sa théorie, d'après les expériences faites à l'hôpital Saint Louis. *RMCP* 1(Jan.):74–103.

———. 1825b. On acupuncture. *MCR,* n.s. 3:257–264.

———. 1825c. *Traité élémentaire de physique générale et médicale.* Paris: Gabon.

———. 1826. On acupuncture. *OMR* 1(6):23–24.

Pelletier, B. 1828a. Cas d'hystérie avec paralysie et contracture des membres, guérie par l'acupuncture. *RMFEJC* 4:328–331.

———. 1828b. Observations de paralysie qui durait depuis sept ans, guérie par l'acupuncture. *RMFEJC* 4:331–332.

———. 1828c. Observations recueillies à la clinique de M. Trouvé, médecin en chef des hôpitaux de Caen, par B. Pelletier, élève interne. *AGM* 7:196–204.

Pelliot, Paul. 1934. Michel Boym (a critique of Chabrié). *T'oung Tao: Archives concernant l'histoire, les langues, la geographie, l'ethnographie, et les arts de l'Asie Orientale* (Leiden) 31:95–151.

———. 1995. *Inventaire sommaire des manuscrits et imprimés chinois de la Bibliothèque Vaticane,* ed. Takata Tokio. Kyoto: Istituto Italiano di Cultura.

Pendleton, James M. 1827. Observations on monstrosities, part I. *PJMPS,* Nov., 289–297.

Percival, Edward. 1818. On the deleterious and medicinal effects of green tea. *MCJR* 5(Jan.–June):481–483.

Percy, Pierre-François. 1792. *Pyrotechnie chirurgicale-pratique, ou l'art d'appliquer le feu en chirurgie.* Paris.

———. 1819. Moxa. In *Dictionnaire des sciences médicales,* 459–492. Paris: Panckoucke.

———. 1826. Moxibustion. In *Dictionnaire des sciences médicales.* Paris: Panckoucke.

Pereira, Jonathan. 1843a. *The elements of materia medica and therapeutics,* 2nd ed., vols. 1–2. London: Longman, Brown, Green, and Longmans.

———. 1843b. Notice of a Chinese article of the materia medica, called "summer-plant-winter-worm." *PJT* 2:591–593.

———. 1844. Observations on the Chinese gall, called "woo-pei-tsze," and on the gall of Bokhara, termed "gool-i-pista." *PJT* 3:384–387.

———. 1845. Further notices respecting Siberian and Bucharian rhubarbs, with some remarks on Taschkent rhubarb. *PJT* 4:500–502.

———. 1847. Note on Banbury rhubarb. *PJT* 6:76–78.

Perez de la Flor. 1847a. L'acupuncture appliquée au traitement des taches de la cornée. *GMP,* 3rd ser., 2:423.

———. 1847b. L'acupuncture appliquée au traitement des taches de la cornée. *JMCP* (Aug.): 636–637.

———. 1848. Application de l'acupuncture au taches de la cornée. *GMP,* 3rd ser., 3:521–522.

Person, M. 1844. Traitement galvano-punctural des amauroses. *GMP,* 2nd ser., 2(Mar. 23):188.

Peters, John R. [1845]1846. *Miscellaneous remarks upon the government, history, religions, literature, agriculture, arts, trades, manners, and customs of the Chinese.* Boston: Eastburn's Press.

Peterson, Arthur G. 1930. Commerce of Virginia, 1789–1791. *WMCQHM,* 2nd ser., 10(4):302–309.

Pétrequin, M. 1845a. Nouvelle méthode pour guérir certains anéurismes sans opération a l'aide de la galvano-puncture. *GMP,* 2nd ser., 13:704–705.

———. 1845b. Aneurism treated by electro-galvanic action. *MT* 13(320):147–148.

———. 1845c. On the treatment of certain aneurisms by galvano-puncture. *DMP* 14:343–344.

———. 1846a. Aneurism treated by electro-galvanic action. *SMSJ,* n.s. 2:185.

———. 1846b. *Nouvelle méthode pour guérir certains anévrysmes sans opération, á l'aide de la galvano-puncture artérielle. 2. Memoire.* Lyon: Marie.

———. 1847a. Cure of aneurism by electro-puncturation. *WL* 5:305–306.

———. 1847b. Treatment of certain aneurisms by galvano-puncture. *AJMS,* n.s. 13:188–190.

Peyrefitte, Alain. 1993. *The collision of two civilisations: The British expedition to China in 1792–94.* London: Harvill.

Peyron, M. 1826. D'un rhumatisme du coeur, traité par l'acupuncture. *RMFEJC* 2:275–281.

Pfister, Louis. 1976. *Notices biographiques et bibliographiques sur les jesuites de l'ancienne mission de Chine, 1552–1773.* San Francisco: Chinese Materials Center.

Philibert, M., and Mme. Celliez. 1823. Historique de l'instruction du Chinois qui a été présenté au roi. *JA* 2:45–52.

Phillips, B. 1845. Treatment of aneurism by electro-puncture. *MT* 13(327):253.

Phillips, J. R. 1988. *The medieval expansion of Europe.* New York: Oxford University Press.

Phillips, Seymour. 1994. The outer world of the European Middle Ages. In *Implicit understandings: Observing, reporting, and reflecting on the encounters between Europeans and other peoples in the early modern era,* ed. Stuart B. Schwartz, 23–63. New York: Cambridge University Press.

Phillips, William D., Jr. 1985. *Slavery from the Roman times to the early transatlantic trade.* Minneapolis: University of Minnesota Press.

Pigou, F. 1836. Memoir on tea. *AJP,* n.s. 1:151–157.

Pipelet, Dr. 1823. Observation de maladie convulsive, avantageusement modifiée par l'acupuncture. *JCDSM* 5:186–187.

Pitcher, Edward W. R., and D. Sean Hartigan, eds. 2000. *Sensationalist literature and popular culture in the early American republic.* Lewiston, NY: Edwin Mellen Press.

Plumb, J. H. 1961. *The Horizon book of the Renaissance,* ed. Richard M. Ketchum. New York: American Heritage.

Polhman, Mr. 1846. The opium trade in China. *DAPMFN* 2(46):731.

Polo, Marco. 1579. *The most noble and famous trauels of Marcus Paulus.* London: Ralph Nevvbery.

Porter, Roy. 1995. The eighteenth century. In Conrad et al. 1995, 371–476.

Pouchelle, Marie-Christine. 1990. *The body and surgery in the Middle Ages,* trans. Rosemary Morris. New Brunswick, NJ: Rutgers University Press.

Pouillet, M. 1825a. Note sur les phénomènes électromagnétiques qui se manifestent dans l'acupuncture. *JPEP* 5(Apr.):1–16.

———. 1825b. On the electro-magnetic phenomena observed in acupuncture. *Lancet* 8(5):152–153.

———. 1825c. On the electro-magnetic phenomena observed in acupuncture. *BMI* 3(25):98.

———. 1825d. Upon the electro-magnetic phenomena which are manifested in acupuncturation. *LMRR* 24(141):273–275.

Pouteau, Claude. 1783. *Ouevres posthumes,* vol. 1. Paris.

Prichard, James Cowles. 1844. *Researches into the physical history of mankind,* 3rd ed., vol. 4. London: Sherwood, Gilbert, and Piper.

Princept, James. 1836. Library. *JASB* 5:246–247.

Pritchard, Earl H. 1936. The crucial years of early Anglo-Chinese relations, 1750–1800. *RSSCW* 4(3–4):1–311.

Procter, William. 1839. Observations on some of the camphorous essential oils. *AJP,* n.s. 4:17–24.

Provincial Surgeon. 1848. The apothecaries' physic garden at Chelsea. *MT* 19(472):14.

P'u, Sung-ling. [1740]1925. *Strange stories from a Chinese studio,* trans. Herbert A. Giles. New York: Boni and Liveright.

de Puisaye, Charles. 1846. On the therapeutic application of electricity. *SMSJ,* n.s. 2:51.

Purchas, Samuel. 1625. *Purchas his pilgrimes in five books.* London: Henrie Fetherstone.

————. [1625]1905–1906. *Hakluytus postumus; or, Purchas his pilgrimes: Contayning a history of the world in sea voyages and lande travells by English-men and others,* vols. 11–12. Glasgow: James MacLehose and Sons.

Purefoy, T. 1848. Cases of hydrocele and ascites, treated by acupuncture. *DQJMS* 5:264–265.

Purmann, Matthias Gottfried. 1706. *Chirurgia curiosa; or, The newest and most curious observations and operations in the whole art of chirurgery.* London: D. Browne.

Purvis, Robert. 1842. Letter to Henry Clarke Wright, Aug. 22, 1842. Anti-Slavery Collection, Boston Public Library.

Quen, Jacques. 1975. Acupuncture and Western medicine. *BHM* 49:196–205.

Quincey, Thomas De. 1948. *The confessions of an English opium-eater.* London: Folio Society.

Quincy, John. 1749. *Pharmacopoeia officinalis & extemporanea; or, A compleat English dispensatory,* 12th ed. London: T. Longman.

R., S. 1840. Notices of China. *CR* 9(8):617–620.

Raciborski, M. 1846a. On the use of galvanism in lumbago, sprains, and some other painful affections of the muscles and joints. *BMS* 4(6):199.

————. 1846b. On the use of galvanism in lumbago, sprains, and some other painful affections of the muscles and joints. *MCRJPM* 48:553–554.

Read, Bernard E. 1977. *Chinese materia medica: Insect drugs, dragon and snake drugs, fish drugs.* Taipei: Southern Materials Center.

Reeves, John. 1828. An account of some of the articles of the materia medica employed by the Chinese. *Transactions of the Royal Medico-Botanical Society of London,* pp. 24–27.

Rehmann, Dr. 1838. A few remarks on the state of medicine amongst the Chinese. *Lancet,* Jan. 27, p. 645.

Reinders, Eric. 2004. *Borrowed gods and foreign bodies: Christian missionaries imagine Chinese religion.* Berkeley: University of California.

Renton, John. 1830. Observations on acupuncture. *EMSJ* 34:100–107.

Restelli, M. 1847a. Cas d'anévrisme du pli du coude, guéri par l'électro-puncture; considérations propres à assurer la réussite de ce moyen. *GMP,* 3rd ser., 2:586

———. 1847b. Cure of aneurism by galvano-puncture. *MT* 16(407):436.

Revue Médicale. 1826–1827. Case of rheumatism of the heart cured by acupuncture. *PJMPS* (Nov. 1826–Feb. 1827): 177–178.

Ricci, Matteo. [1615]1942. *China in the sixteenth century: The journals of Matthew Ricci: 1583–1610.* Trans. Louis J. Gallagher, SJ. New York: Random House.

Ricci, Matteo, and Nicolas Trigault. 1616. *Histoire de l'expedition chrestienne au royaume de la Chine entreprise par les PP. de la compagnie de Jesus,* trans. D. F. de Riquebourg-Trigault. Lyon: Horace Cardon.

Richardsone, C. P. 1839. A case of aneurism, successfully treated by the needle. *SMSJ* 3(10):577–581.

Ricketson, Shadrach. 1806. *Means of preserving health and preventing disease.* New York: Collins, Perkins.

Ripa, Father. 1846. Medicine in China. *MNL* 4(42):59.

———. 1855. *Memoirs of Father Ripa during thirteen years' residence at the court of Peking in the service of the emperor of China,* ed. Fortunato Prandi. London: John Murray.

Roberts, William C. 1848. The encouragement given to quackery by ministers of the gospel. *Annalist* 2:190–194.

Rochat de la Vallée, Elisabeth. 1980. La transmission de l'herbier chinois en Europe au XVIIIe siècle. In *Actes du IIIe Colloque International de Sinologie,* 177–193. Paris: Les Belles Lettres.

Rochemonteix, Camille de. 1915. *Joseph Amiot et les derniers survivants de la mission française à Pekin (1750–1795).* Paris: A. Picard and Son.

Rolfe, W. D. Ian. 1985. William and John Hunter: Breaking the great chain of being. In *William Hunter and the eighteenth-century medical world,* ed. W. F. Bynum and Roy Porter, 297–319. Cambridge: Cambridge University Press.

Roper, Thomas W. 1817. The history of a remarkable tumour, arising from the left side of a woman's head. *MROEI,* n.s. 3(1):71–75.

Rosas, Dr. 1836. Amaurosis cured by electro-puncture. *AJMS* 20:239–240.

Rosen, George. 1970. Sir William Temple and the therapeutic use of moxa for gout in England. *BHM* 44:31–39.

Rosenberg, Charles E. 1987. *The care of strangers: The rise of America's hospital system.* New York: Basic Books.

Rothstein, William G. 1972. *American physicians in the nineteenth century: From sects to science.* Baltimore: Johns Hopkins University Press.

Rouleau, Francis A., S.J. 1959. The first Chinese priest in the Society of Jesus. *AHSI* 28:5–50.

Roy, David Tod, trans. 1993. *The plum in the golden vase; or, Chin P'ing Mei.* 2 vols. Princeton: Princeton University Press.

Royal Asiatic Society. 1835. Appendix. *TRASGBI* 3:xlii–xciv.

Royal College of Physicians of London. 1655. *Pharmacopoeia Londinensis Collegarum.* London: Peter Cole.

Rubinstein, Murray A. 1996. *The origins of the Anglo-American missionary enterprise in China, 1807–1840.* Lanham, MD: Scarecrow.

Rule, Paul Louis. 1995. Fan Shou-I: A missing link in the Chinese rites controversy. In *Échanges culturels et religieux entre la Chine et l'Occident,* ed. Edward J. Malatesta, Yves Raguin, and Adrianus C. Dudink, 277–294. Taipei: Ricci Institute.

Ruschenberger, William Samuel. 1838. *Narrative of a voyage round the world, during years 1835, 36, and 37,* vol. 2. London: R. Bentley.

Rush, Benjamin. 1948. *The autobiography of Benjamin Rush: His "Travels through life" together with his "Commonplace book" for 1789–1813,* ed. George W. Corner. Princeton: Princeton University Press.

Russel, R. C. 1832. Case of chronic hydrocephalus treated by puncture. *AJMS* 11:209–210.

Rutten, A. M. G. 2000. *Dutch transatlantic medicine trade in the eighteenth century under the cover of the West India Company.* Rotterdam: Erasmus.

S., E. 1837. Proposal of the London Missionary Association to introduce Christianity into China by the agency of English surgeons. *Lancet* 2(July 1):520–521.

Sackville-West, Vita. 1991. *Knole and the Sackvilles.* London: National Trust.

Said, Edward. 1979. *Orientalism.* New York: Vintage.

Sarlandière, Jean Baptiste. 1822. Mémoire sur la circulation du sang, éclairée par la physiologie et la pathologie. *AMP* 1(Jan.):135–192.

———. 1825. *Mémoires sur l'électro-puncture . . . Suivi d'un traité de l'acupuncture et du moxa, principaux moyens curatifs chez les peuples de la Chine, de la Corée et du Japon.* Paris: Chez l'auteur, Rue de Richelieu, no. 60; et chez Mlle Delaunay, Libraire.

Scheider, C. A. L. 1825. *De acupunctura.* Berolini.

Schlossberger, Dr. I., and Dr. O. Doepping. 1845. Chemical examination of rhubarb root. *PJT* 4(7):136–138, 232–236, 318–322.

Schott, M. 1843. On the natural-historical writings of the Chinese. *ENPJ* 34:153–155.

Schuster [Shuster], Dr. 1843. Researches on electro-puncture. *MT* 7(180):355.

————. 1844. Electro-puncture as a therapeutic agent. *LEMJMS* (June): 510–511.

Schutz, Charles. 1989. The sociability of ethnic jokes. *Humor* 2(2):165–177.

Sczesniak, Boleslaw. 1954. John Floyer and Chinese medicine. *Osiris* 11:127–156.

Secor, Robert. 1993. Ethnic humor in early American jest books. In *A mixed race: Ethnicity in early America,* ed. Frank Shuffelton, 163–193. New York: Oxford University Press.

Seeger, C. L. 1833. Letter to the editor: Opium eating. *BosMSJ* 9(8):117–120.

Semedo, Alvaro. 1643. *Relatione della grande monarchia della Cina.* Rome: Sumptibus H. Scheus.

————. 1655. *The history of that great and renowned monarchy of China.* London: John Crook.

Shapiro, Hugh. n.d. Interpreting the idea of nerves in nineteenth-century China. Manuscript. www.ihp.sinica.edu.tw/~medicine/ashm/lectures/Shapiro-ft.pdf (downloaded 11/27/04).

Sharp, Samuel. 1761. *A critical enquiry into the present state of surgery,* 4th ed. London: J. and R. Tonson.

Shaw, Samuel. 1847. *Journals of Major Samuel Shaw: The first American consul at Canton,* ed. Josiah Quincy. Boston: Wm. Crosby and H. P. Nichols.

Shuck, Henrietta. 1847. China. *DAPMFN* 3(14):218–219.

————. 1849. *A memoir of Mrs. Henrietta Shuck, the first female missionary to China,* ed. J. B. Jeter. Boston: Gould, Kendall, and Lincoln.

Siame, E. 1831. *Essai sur l'acupuncture.* Paris.

Sigmond, G. G. 1837a. Opium. *BosMSJ* 16(2):21–25.

————. 1837b. Opium. *BosMSJ* 16(4):55–58.

————. 1837c. Opium. *BosMSJ* 16(7):101–105.

————. 1839. On the properties and therapeutic powers of camphor. *AJMS* 24:198–201.

Silvestre de Sacy, Jacques. 1970. *Henri Bertin dans le sillage de la Chine (1720–1792).* Paris: Éditions Cathasia.

Simpson, Dr. 1845. Description of the bones of a Chinese woman's foot. *LL* 2:528.

Siraisi, Nancy G. 1990. *Medieval and early Renaissance medicine: An introduction to knowledge and practice.* Chicago: University of Chicago Press.

Sivin, Nathan. 1988. Science and medicine in imperial China—A state of the field. *JAS* 47(1):41–90.

————. 1998. The history of Chinese medicine: Now and anon. *Positions* 6(3):731–762.

Slack, D. B. 1844. An essay on the human color. *BosMSJ* 30(24):475–479; 30(25):495–499; 30(26):518–522.

Slade, John. 1843. Regulations of the medical missionary society. *CReg* 16(19):85.

Slotkin, James Sydney, ed. 1965. *Readings in early anthropology.* New York: Wenner-Gren Foundation for Anthropological Research.

Smedley, Audrey. 1993. *Race in North America: Origin and evolution of a worldview.* Boulder, CO: Westview.

Smith, Elias. 1824. The gastric juice of dead bodies, used by physicians as a remedy for diseases of the living. *MNP* 1(24):95.

Smith, George H. 1842. On opium-smoking among the Chinese. *Lancet* 1(Feb. 19):707–710.

———. 1847a. Violations of physiological laws in China. *BMSJ* 37(19):385–386.

———. 1847b. *A narrative of an exploratory visit to each of the consular cities of China, and to the islands of Hong Kong and Chusan.* London: Seeley, Burnside and Seeley.

Smith, Lyndon A. 1839. Acupuncturation for hydrocele. *BosMSJ* 20(25):398.

Smith, Richard J. 1992. *Fortune tellers and philosophers: Divination in traditional Chinese society.* Boulder, CO: Westview.

Smith, Samuel Stanhope. 1814. An essay on the varieties of complexion and figure in the human species. *AMPR* 2:70–90.

Solano de Luque, Francisco. 1741. *New and extraordinary observations concerning the prediction of various crises by the pulse,* trans. James Nihell. London: James Crokatt.

Sollers, Werner. 1997. How Americans became white: Three examples. In *MultiAmerica: Essays on cultural wars and cultural peace,* ed. Ishmael Reed, 3–5. New York: Viking.

Son of Han. 1820. Man a microcosm. *ICG* 2(11):371–373.

Spear, J. S. 1845. The Chinese. *BGHJAS* 1:189–190.

Spence, Jonathan D. 1974. *Emperor of China: Self-portrait of K'ang-hsi.* New York: Knopf.

———. 1975. Opium smoking in Ch'ing China. In *Conflict and control in late imperial China,* ed. Frederick Wakeman and Carolyn Grant, 143–173. Berkeley: University of California Press.

———. 1988. *The question of Hu.* New York: Vintage.

———. 1998. *The Chan's great continent: China in Western minds.* New York: Norton.

Sprengel, Kurt Polycarp Joachim. 1815. *Histoire de la médecine, depuis son origine jusqu'au dix-neuvième siècle,* vol. 1, trans. A. J. Jourdan. Paris: Deterville.

Standaert, Nicolas. 2001. *Handbook of Christianity in China* 1:635–1800. Leiden: Brill.

Stannard, Jerry. 1999. *Herbs and herbalism in the Middle Ages and Renaissance*, ed. Katherine E. Stannard and Richard Kay. Brookfield, VT: Ashgate Variorum.

Starr, Paul. 1982. *The social transformation of American medicine.* New York: Basic Books.

Staunton, Sir George Leonard. 1797. *An authentic account of an embassy from the king of Great Britain to the emperor of China*, vols. 1–2. London: G. Nicol.

Staunton, Sir George Thomas. 1822. *Miscellaneous notices relating to China, and our commercial intercourse with that country, including a few translations from the Chinese language.* London: J. Murray.

Stearns, Samuel. 1801. *The American herbal; or, Materia medica.* Walpole, NH: Thomas and Thomas.

Steiner, Stan. 1979. *Fusang: The Chinese Who Built America.* New York: Harper and Row.

Stephenson, John, and James Morss Churchill. 1834. *Medical botany; or, Illustrations and descriptions of the medicinal plants of the London, Edinburgh, and Dublin pharmacopoeias*, 2nd ed., vols. 1–3, ed. Gilbert T. Burnett. London: Printed for J. Churchill.

Stevens, Alexander H. 1843. A case of spina bifida successfully treated by repeated punctures; with practical remarks. *NYJM* 1(Sept.):149–151.

———. 1844. A case of spina bifida successfully treated by repeated punctures; with practical remarks. *MCRJPM*, n.s. 41:260.

Stewart, F. Campbell. 1843. On electro-puncture in hydrocele, with cases. *NYJMCS* 1:60–64.

———. 1844. On electro-puncture in hydrocele. *MCRJPM*, n.s. 41:260–261.

———. 1846. Hydrocele cured by electricity. *SMSJ*, n.s. 2:125.

St. John de Crevecoeur, J. Hector. [1782]1957. *Letters from an American farmer.* New York: E. P. Dutton.

Stockwell, W. Hamilton. 1836. On moxa. *TJMAS* 8(2):151–169.

Stokes, Dr. 1834. Dr. Stokes, on electro-puncturation and magnetism in paralysis, rheumatism, &c. *MM* 3(8):237–244.

Strambio, Gaetano, A. Quaglino, A. Tizzoni, and A. Restelli. 1847. *Sperimenti di galvano-ago-puntura istituiti sulle arterie e sulle vene . . .* Milan: G. Chiusi.

Sue, Pierre. 1796–1797a [5th year of the Republic]. Mémoire sur l'état de la chirurgie à la Chine. *RPSMP* 9:16–58, 121–145.

———. 1796–1797b [5th year of the Republic]. Notice sur deux ouvrages sur la médecine chinoise. *RPSMP* 9:145–156.

Sung, Tz'u. 1981. *The washing away of wrongs: Forensic medicine in thirteenth-century China*, trans. Brian E. McKnight. Ann Arbor: Center for Chinese Studies, University of Michigan.

Sutleffe, Edward. 1820–1821. The history of medicine in China. *ICG* 2(14):424–430; 3(15):1–5; 3(16):57–59; 3(17):125–129; 3(18):185–186.

————. 1825. *Medical and surgical cases; Selected during a practice of thirty-eight years,* vol. 2. London: T. and G. Underwood.

———— [Published anonymously]. 1844. The history of medicine in China. *CPCOTT,* Oct. 3, pp. 178–179.

Sydenham, Thomas. 1850. A treatise on gout and dropsy. In *The works of Thomas Sydenham, M.D.,* vol. 2, trans. R. G. Latham, 121–184. London: Sydenham Society.

Szczesnik, Boleslaw. 1949–1955. The writings of Michael Boym. *MSer* 14:481–538.

T., P. P. 1820a. Divination in China. *ICG* 2(12):318–320.

————. 1820b. Superstitions and customs of the Chinese. *ICG* 2(13):359–360.

Tartre, Fr. de [1701]1762. Father de Tartre, to Mr. de Tartre. In *Travels of the Jesuits, into various parts of the world: Particularly China and the East-Indies,* 2nd ed., vol. 1, ed. and trans. John Lockman, 107–155. London: T. Piety.

Tatar, Maria. 1978. *Spellbound: Studies on mesmerism and literature.* Princeton: Princeton University Press.

Tavernier, Alphonse. 1829. *Elements of operative surgery,* trans. S. D. Gross. Philadelphia: John Grigg, James Crissy, Towar and Hogan, J. G. Auner.

Tchen, John Kuo Wei. 1999. *New York before Chinatown: Orientalism and the shaping of American culture, 1776–1882.* London: Johns Hopkins University Press.

Teiser, Stephen F. 1988. *The ghost festival in medieval China.* Princeton: Princeton University Press.

————. 1996. The spirits of Chinese religion. In *Religions of China in practice,* ed. Donald S. Lopez, 3–37. Princeton: Princeton University Press.

Temkin, Owsei. 1973. *Galenism: Rise and decline of a medical philosophy.* Ithaca: Cornell University Press.

Temple, Sir William. 1814. *The works of Sir William Temple, Bart.,* vol. 3. London: F. S. Hamilton, Weybridge.

Tennent, John. 1734. *Every man his own doctor,* 2nd ed. Williamsburg, VA: William Parks.

ten Rhijne, Willem. 1683. *Dissertatio de arthritide: Mantissa schematica; De acupunctura . . .* London: R. Chiswell.

Thilorier, M., and M. Lafontaine. 1843. Nervous fluid. *MNL* 2(20):67.

Thion, M. 1826. Observations sur l'acupuncture. *ASRS* 8:5–29.Thomaz de Bossierre, Yves de. 1982. *François Xavier Dentrecolles Yin Hong-siu Ki-Tsong et l'apport de la Chine à l'Europe du XVIIIe siècle.* Paris: Les Belles Lettres.

Thompson, Laurence G. 1975. *Chinese religion: An introduction,* 2nd ed. Encino, CA: Dickenson.

Thomson, Samuel. 1825. *New guide to health; or, Botanic family physician.* Boston: E. G. House.

Thonching. 1845. Thonching's letter. *DAPMFN* 1(45):718–719.

Thunberg, Carl Peter. 1795. *Travels in Europe, Africa, and Asia, made between the years 1770 and 1779,* vol. 4. London: W. Richardson.

Ticknor and Fields. 1844. *Catalogue of medical books.* Boston.

———. 1847. *Catalogue of medical books.* Boston.

Tindall, George Brown, with David E. Shi. 1992. *America: A narrative history,* 3rd ed. New York: Norton.

Travers, Benjamin. 1837. Account of a method of operating for hydrocele. *LMG,* Feb. 11, 737–738.

Travers, Lewis. 1837. Nouveau mode de traitement de l'hydrocèle testiculaire à l'aide de l'acupuncture. *GMP,* 2nd ser., 5:522–523.

Trouvé, Dr. 1828. Influence de l'acupuncture, dans un cas d'hystérie avec paralysie et contracture des membres. *AGM* 18:196–200.

Tu, Wei-ming. 1984. Pain and suffering in Confucian self-cultivation. *PEW* 34(4):379–387.

———. 1985. *Confucian thought: Selfhood as creative transformation.* Albany, NY: SUNY Press.

Tweedale, John. 1823. Case of anasarca successfully treated by acupuncture. *LMR* 20(118):313–314.

Twitchett, Denis. 1989. China's Manchu overlords. In *Powers of the crown: Timeframe A.D. 1600–1700,* ed. Tony Allan, 34–53. Alexandria, VA: Time-Life Books.

Unschuld, Paul U. 1985. *Medicine in China: A history of ideas.* Berkeley: University of California Press.

———. 1986a. *Medicine in China: A history of pharmaceutics.* Berkeley: University of California Press.

———. 1986b. *Nan-Ching: The classic of difficult issues.* Berkeley: University of California Press.

———. 1987. Traditional Chinese medicine: Some historical and epistemological reflections. *SSM* 24(12):1023–29.

———. 1990. *Forgotten traditions of ancient Chinese medicine.* Brookline, MA: Paradigm.

———. 2003. *Huang Di nei jing su wen: Nature, knowledge, imagery in an ancient Chinese medical text.* Berkeley: University of California Press.

Ure, Andrew. 1819. An account of some experiments made on the body of a criminal immediately after execution, with physiological and practical observations. *ERAR* 9:347–358.

Vaidy, J.-V.-F. 1820a. Faits constatant l'efficacité du moxa dans le traitement des phlegmasies chroniques des organes de la respiration. *JGMCPFE* 72:55–68.

———. 1820b. Observation sur les bons effets du moxa dans le traitement des inflammations chroniques des organes de la respiration. *JCDSM* 6:9–16.

Vaillant, Mr. 1717–1719. A new genus of plants, call'd araliastrum, of which the famous nin-zin or ginseng of the Chineses, is a species. *PT* 30:705–707.

Valmont de Bomare, M. 1775. *Dictionnaire raisonné universel d'histoire naturelle,* vols. 4 and 6. Paris: Brunet Libraire.

Van Braam Houckgeest, André Everard. 1797. *Voyage de l'ambassade de la compagnie des Indes Orientales Hollandaises, vers l'empereur de la Chine, dans les années 1794 & 1795,* trans. M. L. E. Moreau de Saint-Méry. Philadelphia: Imprimeur-Libraire.

Veith, Ilza. 1975. Sir William Osler—Acupuncturist. *BNYAM* 51(3):393–400.

Velpeau, M. 1831. On the acupuncturation of arteries in the treatment of aneurism. *AJMS* 8(16):510–512.

Verlinden, Charles. 1995. Colonial techniques from the Mediterranean to the Atlantic. In *The global opportunity,* vol. 2, ed. Felipe Fernández-Armesto, 226–254. Brookfield, VT: Variorum.

Vernant, J. P. 1984. Parole et signes muets. In *Divination et rationalité,* ed. J. P. Vernant, 9–25. Paris: Éditions du Seuil.

Versluis, Arthur. 1993. *American transcendentalism and Asian religions.* New York: Oxford University Press.

———. 2000. *The esoteric origins of the American Renaissance.* New York: Oxford University Press.

Vicq-d'Azyr, Felix. 1805. *Oeuvres de Vicq-d'Azyr, recueillies et publiées avec des notes,* vol. 5, ed. Jacques L. Moreau. Paris: L. Duprat-Duverger.

Viesseaux, M. 1824. Chinese college in Italy. *AJMR* 18:266–267.

Villeneuve, M. 1817. Review of *Mémoires sur les malades chroniques, les évacuations sanguines et l'acupuncture,* by L. V. J. Berlioz. *JMCP* 38(Jan.–Feb.):265–267.

Voltaire. 1878. *Oeuvres complètes de Voltaire,* vols. 11–13. Paris: Garnier Frères, Libraires Éditeurs.

von Klaproth, Julius. 1823. Sur les ambassades en Chine. *JA* 3:361–364.

———. 1824. Liste des noms des thés les plus célèbres de la Chine (Traduite d'un manuscrit chinois appartenant à M. le baron de Schilling). *JA* 4:120–22.

———. 1825. *Mémoires relatifs a l'Asie.* Paris: Dondey-Dupré.

von Linné, Carl [Linnaeus]. 1735. *Systema naturae.* Lugduni Batavorum: Theodorum Haak.

———. 1753. *Species plantarum.* Holmiae: Impensis Laurentii Salvii.

Voss, Stephen. 2000. Descartes: Heart and soul. In Wright and Potter 2000, 173–196.

Vossius, Isaac. 1685. *Isaaci Vossii variarum observationum liber.* London: Robert Scott.

Vowell, J. N. 1838. Acupuncture of Ganglions (Letter to the editor). *Lancet* 2(Aug.):769–770.

W—. 1824a. Voyages on wings: Singular female beauties. *AMM* 1:434–447.

———. 1824b. Voyages on wings: Chinese small feet and long nails. *AMM* 2:3–17.

Wagner, Roy. 1981. *The invention of culture,* rev. ed. Chicago: University of Chicago Press.

Wakefield, Priscilla. 1811. *Sketches of human manners.* Philadelphia: Johnson and Warner.

Wakley, Thomas. 1825. Analysis of foreign medical journals . . . Reflections on the nature of the action of acupuncture. *Lancet* 7(6):181–183.

———. 1826a. Chinese method of examining medical candidates. *Lancet* 10(158):794.

———. 1826b. Review of *Medical and surgical cases: Selected during a practice of thirty nine years,* by Edward Sutleffe. *Lancet* 10(138):102–109.

———. 1826c. Therapeutics: Acupuncturation. *Lancet* 10(157):719.

———. 1826d. Case of sciatica, cured by acupuncturation. *Lancet* (Nov. 25): 272.

———. 1827a. Paralysis nearly complete, of the lower extremities . . . . Cured by application of moxas. *Lancet* (Feb. 3): 590.

———. 1827b. Review of *A physiological enquiry respecting the action of moxa . . .* by William Wallace. *Lancet,* Mar. 24, pp. 795–799.

———. 1827c. The true moxa; or, The *Foy-cong* of the Chinese. *Lancet* 11(170):285.

———. 1828a. Case of paralysis, in which the moxa was successfully employed. *Lancet,* June 21, p. 359.

———. 1828b. Cases of rheumatism cured by acupuncturation (St. Thomas's Hospital). *Lancet* 2:409–410.

———. 1830. Mountains of muriate of ammonia in China. *LL* 2(Apr. 16):76.

———. 1831a. Acupuncturation. *Lancet* 20(pt. 2):129.

———. 1831b. Operation on Hoo Loo. *Lancet* 2(Apr. 16):83–84.

———. 1831c. Removal of a tumour fifty-six pounds in weight, extending from beneath the unvilicus to the anterior border of the anus. *Lancet* 2(Apr. 16):86–89.

———. 1831d. Edinburgh Medical and Surgical Journal. *Lancet* 2:836–837.

———. 1832. Practical considerations on the use of cauteries and moxae. *Lancet,* Feb. 16, pp. 643–644.

———. 1837a. Medical establishments in China and Siam. *Lancet,* Dec. 30, pp. 481–484.

————. 1837b. Efficacy of the moxa in wrist-drop. *Lancet,* July 8, p. 560.

————. 1839a. Blenheim Street free dispensary and infirmary: Ovarian dropsy—puncturation—recovery. *Lancet,* May 25, pp. 344–345.

————. 1839b. Epilepsy cured by acupuncture. *Lancet,* Aug. 17, p. 768.

————. 1840a. Report on Mr. Ley's [Lay's] paper on Chinese surgery. *Lancet,* Mar. 28, p. 104.

————. 1840b. Report on Mr. Ley's [Lay's] paper on medicine in China. *Lancet,* May 19, p. 209.

————. 1841. Review of *The Chinese as they are . . .* , by G. Tradescant Lay. *Lancet,* May 8, pp. 235–236.

Wallace, William. 1827. *A physiological enquiry respecting the action of moxa, and its utility in inveterate cases of sciatica, lumbago, paraplegia, epilepsy, and some other painful, paralytic, and spasmodic diseases of the nerves and muscles.* Dublin: Hodges and M'Arthur, and Curry.

Wallich, N. 1829. An account of the Nipal ginseng. *TMPSC* 4:115–120.

Wallis, Roy, and Peter Morley, eds. 1976. *Marginal medicine.* New York: Free Press.

Walravens, Hartmut. 1996. Medical knowledge of the Manchus and the Manchu anatomy. *Études Mongoles et Sibériennes* 27:359–374.

Walsh, Mary Roth. 1977. *"Doctors wanted: No women need apply": Sexual barriers in the medical profession, 1835–1975.* New Haven: Yale University Press.

Waltner, Ann. 1994. Demerits and deadly sins: Jesuit moral tracts in late Ming China. In *Implicit understandings: Observing, reporting, and reflecting on the encounters between Europeans and other peoples in the early modern era,* ed. Stuart B. Schwartz, 422–448. New York: Cambridge University Press.

Wansbrough, T. W. 1826. Acupuncturation. *Lancet* 10(161):846–848.

————. 1828. Case of rheumatism successfully treated by acupuncturation. *Lancet* 2:366–367.

Warner, John Harley. 1986. *The therapeutic perspective: Medical practice, knowledge, and identity in America, 1820–1885.* Cambridge, MA: Harvard University Press.

————. 1987. Medical sectarianism, therapeutic conflict, and the shaping of orthodox professional identity in antebellum American medicine. In *Medical fringe and medical orthodoxy, 1750–1850,* ed. W. F. Bynum and Roy Porter, 234–260. London: Croom Helm.

Warren, Jonathan Mason. 1978. *The Parisian education of an American surgeon: Letters of Jonathan Mason Warren, 1832–1835.* Philadelphia: American Philosophical Society.

Warrington, Mr. 1844a. Extensive adulteration of tea by the Chinese. *MNL* 2(19):58.

————. 1844b. Extensive adulteration of tea by the Chinese. *LL* 2:219.

Watson, John. 1839. A summary view of the progress of medicine in America. *NYJMS* 1(July–Oct.):1–22.

Watson, Walter. 1980. Interprétations de la Chine à l'époque des lumières: Montesquieu et Voltaire. In *Actes du IIIe Colloque International de Sinologie,* 15–37. Paris: Les Belles Lettres.

Wear, Andrew. 1995. Medicine in early modern Europe, 1500–1700. In Conrad et al., eds., 1995, 215–361.

Weber, Eugen. 1971. *A modern history of Europe.* New York: Norton.

Webster, J. 1825a. Case of a painful affection of the arm, following venesection, cured by acupuncturation. *LMPJ* 54(July–Dec.):31–33.

———. 1825b. Dr. Webster on acupuncturation. *MJM* 6(July–Dec.):293–295.

———. 1825c. Acupuncturation. *MCR,* n.s. 3:562–563.

Wesley, Charles H. 1935. *Richard Allen: Apostle of freedom.* Washington: Associated Publishers.

Wesley, John. 1747. *Primitive physick; or, An easy and natural way of curing most diseases.* London: Thomas Trye.

Whorton, James C. 1977. Tempest in a flesh-pot: The formulation of a physiological rationale for vegetarianism. *JHM,* Apr., 115–139.

———. 1989. The first holistic revolution: Alternative medicine in the nineteenth century. In *Examining holistic medicine,* ed. Douglas Stalker and Clark Glymour, 29–48. Buffalo, NY: Prometheus.

Wilkes, Richard. 1775. *An historical essay on the dropsy.* London.

Williams, Samuel Wells. 1838. Notices of natural history. *CR* 7(1):45–49; 7(2):90–92; 7(3):136–141; 7(4):212–217; 7(5):250–255; 7(6):321–327; 7(8):392–399; 7(9):485–490.

———. 1848. *The Middle Kingdom,* vols. 1–2. New York: Wiley and Putnam.

Williams, William H. 1976. *America's first hospital: The Pennsylvania Hospital, 1751–1841.* Wayne, PA: Haverford House.

Wilson, John. 1846a. Chinese ideas respecting the anatomy of the circulating system. *DMP* 16:415.

———. 1846b. On Chinese pharmacy. *PJT* 5(12):567–569.

———. 1846c. Mode of inoculation in China. *MJMS,* n.s. 68(2):160.

———. 1847a. Chinese ideas respecting the anatomy of the circulating system. *MERMS,* n.s. 3:201–202.

———. 1847b. Chinese ideas respecting the anatomy of the circulating system. *NYJMCS* 8:285–286.

———. 1847c. On Chinese pharmacy. *AJP,* n.s. 13:129–131.

Wines, E. C. 1840. A peep at China, in Mr. Dunn's Chinese collection. *CR* 8(Mar.):581–587.

Winkley, Francis, Israel Sanborn, and David Parker. 1835. The village of the United Society of Shakers. *AMUEK* 2:133–135.

Winterbotham, W. 1796. *An historical, geographical, and philosophical view of the Chinese empire . . . To which is added a copious account of Lord Macartney's embassy,* vols. 1–2. Philadelphia: Richard Lee.

Witek, John W. 1995. Reporting to Rome: Some major events in the Christian community in Peking, 1686–1687. In *Échanges culturels et religieux entre la Chine et l'Occident,* ed. Edward J. Malatesta, Yves Raguin, and Adrianus C. Dudink, 129–146. Taipei: Ricci Institute.

Withering, M. 1808. Botanical description of British plants. *MPJ* 19(110):353–361.

Wittie, Robert. 1680. *Some observations made upon the root called nean or ninsing imported from the East-Indies.* London: Printed for the author.

Wood, George B. 1865. *Biographical memoir of Franklin Bache, M.D.* Philadelphia: Lippincott.

Wood, George B., and Franklin Bache. 1834. *The dispensatory of the United States of America,* 2nd ed. Philadelphia: Grigg and Elliot.

———. 1847. *The dispensatory of the United States of America,* 7th ed. Philadelphia: Grigg, Elliot.

Wood, Kinder. 1818. Some observations on the cure of hydrocele of the tunica vaginalis testis. *MCT* 9:38–51.

Wood, William Wrightman. 1830. *Sketches of China.* Philadelphia: Carey and Lea.

Woost, Gustav Eduard. 1826. *Quaede acupunctura Orientalium ex oblivionis tenebris ab Europaeis medicis nuper revocata: Dissertatio inauguralis medico-chirurgica.* Leipzig: Richter.

Wotton, William. 1694. *Reflections upon ancient and modern learning.* London: J. Leake.

Wright, Arthur F. 1992. The study of Chinese civilization. In *Discovering China: European interpretations in the Enlightenment,* ed. Julia Ching and Willard G. Oxtoby, 189–211. Rochester, NY: University of Rochester Press.

Wright, John P., and Paul Potter, eds. 2000. *Psyche and soma: Physicians and metaphysicians on the mind-body problem from Antiquity to Enlightenment.* Oxford: Clarendon.

Wu, Lien-The. 1931. Early days of Western medicine in China. *JNCBRAS* 62:1–31.

Yamada, Keiji. 1979. The formation of the *Huang-ti Nei-ching. AA* 36:67–89.

———. 1991. Anatometrics in ancient China. *CS* 10:39–52.

Yang, C. K. 1961. *Religion in Chinese society.* Berkeley: University of California Press.

Yoon, Chong-kun. 1982. Sinophilism during the Age of Enlightenment: Jesuits, philosophes and physiocrats discover Columbus. In *Western views of China,* vols. 1–2, ed. Henry A. Myers, 149–182. Hong Kong: Asian Research Service.

Yule, Colonel Sir Henry, trans. and ed. 1914. *Cathay and the way thither: Being a collection of medieval notices of China,* vols. 1–2. New York: Paragon Book Gallery.

Yung, Judy. 1986. *Chinese women of America: A pictorial history.* Seattle: University of Washington Press.

Yuria, Mori. 2002. Identity and lineage: The *Taiyi jinhua zongzhi* and the spirit-writing cult to Patriarch Lü in Qing China. In *Daoist identity: History, lineage, and ritual,* ed. Livia Kohn and Harold D. Roth, 165–184. Honolulu: University of Hawai'i Press.

Xu, Mingde. 1996. The outstanding contribution of the Italian sinologist Martino Martini to cultural exchanges between China and the West. In *Martino Martini: A humanist and scientist in seventeenth century China,* ed. Franco Demarchi and Riccardo Scartezzini, 23–38. Trento: Università degli Studi di Trento.

Zboray, Ronald J., and Mary Saracino Zboray. 2004. Between "crockery-dom" and Barnum: Boston's Chinese Museum, 1845–47. *American Quarterly* 56(2): 271–307.

Zhang, Lanqing. 1996. Martino Martini and cultural exchanges between China and Italy. In *Martino Martini: A humanist and scientist in seventeenth century China,* ed. Franco Demarchi and Riccardo Scartezzini, 91–108. Trento: Università degli Studi di Trento.

Zhang, Qiong. 1999. Demystifying Qi: The politics of cultural translation and interpretation in the early Jesuit mission to China. In *Tokens of exchange: The problem of translation in global circulations,* ed. Lydia H. Liu, 74–106. Durham: Duke University Press.

Zhu, Xi, and Lu Ziqian, comps. 1967. *Reflection on things at hand: The neo-confucian anthology,* trans. Wing-tsit Chan. New York: Columbia University Press.

Zürcher, Erik. 1990. The Jesuit mission in Fujian in late Ming times: Levels of response. In *Development and decline of Fukien province in the 17th and 18th centuries,* ed. E. B. Vermeer, 417–458. New York: Brill.

Index